Statistical Methods for Dose-Finding Experiments

STATISTICS IN PRACTICE

Advisory Editor

Stephen Senn
University of Glasgow, UK

Founding Editor

Vic Barnett
Nottingham Trent University, UK

Statistics in Practice is an important international series of texts which provide detailed coverage of statistical concepts, methods and worked case studies in specific fields of investigation and study.

With sound motivation and many worked practical examples, the books show in down-to-earth terms how to select and use an appropriate range of statistical techniques in a particular practical field within each title's special topic area.

The books provide statistical support for professionals and research workers across a range of employment fields and research environments. Subject areas covered include medicine and pharmaceutics; industry, finance and commerce; public services; the earth and environmental sciences, and so on.

The books also provide support to students studying statistical courses applied to the above areas. The demand for graduates to be equipped for the work environment has led to such courses becoming increasingly prevalent at universities and colleges.

It is our aim to present judiciously chosen and well-written workbooks to meet everyday practical needs. Feedback of views from readers will be most valuable to monitor the success of this aim.

A complete list of titles in this series appears at the end of the volume.

Statistical Methods for Dose-Finding Experiments

Edited by

S. Chevret

*INSERM U717, Hôpital Saint-Louis
Paris, France*

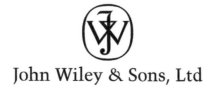

John Wiley & Sons, Ltd

Other Wiley Editorial Offices

John Wiley & Sons Inc., 111 River Street, Hoboken, NJ 07030, USA

Jossey-Bass, 989 Market Street, San Francisco, CA 94103-1741, USA

Wiley-VCH Verlag GmbH, Boschstr. 12, D-69469 Weinheim, Germany

John Wiley & Sons Australia Ltd, 42 McDougall Street, Milton, Queensland 4064, Australia

John Wiley & Sons (Asia) Pte Ltd, 2 Clementi Loop #02-01, Jin Xing Distripark, Singapore 129809

John Wiley & Sons Canada Ltd, 22 Worcester Road, Etobicoke, Ontario, Canada M9W 1L1

Wiley also publishes its books in a variety of electronic formats. Some content that appears
in print may not be available in electronic books.

Library of Congress Cataloging-in-Publication Data

British Library Cataloging in Publication Data

A catalogue record for this book is available from the British Library

ISBN-13   978-0-470-86123-3 (HB)
ISBN-10   0-470-86123-1 (HB)

Typeset in 10/12 pt Times by TechBooks, New Delhi, India

Contents

7   Using Bayesian decision theory in dose-escalation studies   149
John Whitehead

8   Dose-escalation with overdose control   173
Mourad Tighiouart and André Rogatko

Contributors

B. NEBIYOU BEKELE, M. D. Anderson Cancer Center, Department of Biostatistics and applied Mathematics, The University of Texas, Houston, Texas, USA

YING KUEN CHEUNG, Department of Biostatistics, Mailman School of Public Health, Columbia University, New York, USA

SYLVIE CHEVRET, Département de Biostatistique et Informatique Médicale, INSERM U717, Hôpital Saint-Louis, Paris, France

J.D. COOK, M.D. Anderson Cancer Center, Department of Biostatistics and Applied Mathematics, The University of Texas, Houston, Texas, USA

JANET DANCEY, Investigational Drug Branch, CTEP, DCTD, NCI, Bethesda, Maryland, USA

NANCY FLOURNOY, Department of Statistics, University of Missouri-Columbia, Columbia, MO 65211, USA

BORIS FREIDLIN, Biometric Research Branch, DCTD, NCI, Bethesda, Maryland, USA

ROBERT HEMMINGS, Medicines and Healthcare Products Regulatory Agency, Room 13-206, Market Towers, 1 Nine Elms Lane, London SW8 5NQ, UK

ANNA IVANOVA, Department of Biostatistics, The University of North Carolina at Chapel Hill, Chapel Hill, NC 27599-7420, USA

YONG LIN, Department of Biostatistics, School of Public Health, University of Medicine and Dentistry of New Jersey, Room 216, 683 Hoes Lane West, PO Box 9, Piscataway, NJ 08854, USA, and Division of Biometrics, The Cancer Institute of New Jersey, University of Medicine and Dentistry of New Jersey, 195 Little Albany Street, Room 5538, New Brunswick, NJ 08903, USA

ANDRE ROGATKO, Department of Biostatistics and Winship Cancer Institute, Emory University, 1518 Clifton Road NE, Atlanta, GA 30322, USA

LARRY RUBINSTEIN, Biometric Research Branch, DCTD, NCI, Bethesda, Maryland, USA

WEICHUNG JOE SHIH, Department of Biostatistics, School of Public Health, University of Medicine and Dentistry of New Jersey, Room 216, 683 Hoes Lane West, PO Box 9, Piscataway, NJ 08854, USA, and Division of Biometrics, The Cancer Institute of New Jersey, University of Medicine and Dentistry of New Jersey, 195 Little Albany Street, Room 5538, New Brunswick, NJ 08903, USA

PETER F. THALL, M.D. Anderson Cancer Center, Department of Biostatistics and Applied Mathematics, The University of Texas, Houston, Texas, USA

MOURAD TIGHIOUART, Department of Biostatistics and Winship Cancer Institute, Emory University, 1518 Clifton Road NE, Atlanta, GA 30322, USA

JOHN WHITEHEAD, Medical and Pharmaceutical Statistics Research Unit, The University of Reading, UK

Y. ZHOU, Medical and Pharmaceutical Statistics Research Unit, The University of Reading, UK

SARAH ZOHAR, Département de Biostatistique et Informatique Médicale, INSERM U717, Hôpital Saint-Louis, Paris, France

Preface

After examining the dose-finding studies for the first time, I was surprised by the usual concepts that commonly surround their standard design, such as the choice of dose levels according to the Fibonacci scheme. Another example dealt with the first safe starting dose level that is commonly derived from the LD10 in mice, i.e., the dose that is lethal to 10% of the animals. This seemed somewhat magical to me, and certainly lacked a sound statistical basis!

Moreover, the ethical requirement of minimizing sample size, which is particularly limiting in these early phase trials, has deeply governed the design of the studies and even their analysis – to the extent that no analysis is usually made, with the justification that the number of observations was too small.

A further examination of the literature shows that many researchers in biostatistics have been interested in this field for the last decade. Innovative designs with ad hoc inference have been proposed throughout the world. However, although some of these new methods have been known for several years, few dose-finding trials have made use of them.

The goal of this book is to present and disseminate many of the innovative statistical approaches for dose-finding studies, in a way that can be comprehensible to any scientist involved in such trials. As a statistician who has worked on the design, conduct and analysis of many dose-finding trials based on new methods, I am convinced of the practicability of these methods.

It is my hope that a large number of medical statisticians, including those studying medical statistics or embarking on a career in drug development, as well as interested clinicians planning early phase trials, will find this book useful.

This publication would have been impossible without the collaboration of many statisticians and scientists who detailed their own methods clearly, demonstrating methods by presenting extensive examples and applications. I am very grateful to all those who participated in the preparation of this manuscript.

Finally, I wish to thank Rob Calver, Jane Shepherd, and Wendy Hunter at Wiley for being so patient with the repeated excuses for delay. Many thanks also to Pooja Naithani.

Sylvie Chevret

Introduction

Sylvie Chevret

Département de Biostatistique et Informatique Médicale, U717 Inserm, Hôpital Saint-Louis, Paris, France

The purpose of this book is to review the main innovative statistical approaches for dose-finding in phase I/II clinical trials, with emphasis on general concepts and practical considerations. Since formal statistical methods for dose-finding experiments have been mostly proposed for cancer drugs, a large place of this book is devoted to this particular setting. Nevertheless, these methods could be seen as an illustration of what can be achieved in other settings, as depicted further in the book, notably when dealing with healthy volunteers.

From a statistical point of view, we choose to deal with the common setting where the patient's outcome is characterized by a binary variable that indicates whether he(she) experienced any event of interest, though other settings will be discussed specifically in some chapters. In the setting of phase I dose-finding trials, the event of interest is usually the dose-limiting toxicities, whereas in phase II dose-finding trials, it is rather some measure of treatment response or failure.

Finally, most of these statistical approaches are still poorly used in practice. The final aim of this book is to promote their further use and appropriate implementation. Moreover, to address medical readers, we have attempted to exemplify through illustrations the methods developed in the book.

The book is organized as follows.

- Firstly, Part I aims at summarizing the main concepts in dose-findings, mostly from a statistical or a philosophical point of view.

- Part II focuses on the main algorithm-based approaches, namely the traditional "3 + 3" design, as well as designs including dose de-escalation (so-called up-and-down designs) and those with intrapatient dose-escalation.

Statistical Methods for Dose-Finding Experiments   Edited by S. Chevret
© 2006 John Wiley & Sons, Ltd

- Part III refers to model-based approaches such as the continual reassessment method (CRM) and some related methods, namely the dose-escalation with overdose control (EWOC) design and the Bayesian decision theory approaches, with special attention to dose-findings in healthy volunteers.

- Part IV highlights main issues in dose-findings such as how to stop such trials early, how to cope with delayed or ordinal outcomes, with two cytotoxic drugs or with both efficacy and toxicity.

- Finally, Part V reports some of the main websites and softwares to implement published methods.

Part I

General Principles and Controversial Issues in Dose-Findings

1

Basic concepts in dose-finding

Sylvie Chevret

Département de Biostatistique et Informatique Médicale, U717 Inserm, Hôpital Saint-Louis, Paris, France

1.1 Main concepts

Dose-finding trials aim at coming up with a safe and efficient drug administration in humans [1]. They are defined as early phase clinical experiments in which different doses of a new drug are evaluated to determine the optimal dose that elicits a certain response to be recommended for the treatment of patients with a given medical condition. They are to be distinguished from preclinical quantal bioassays, though statistical analysis of both experiments may be closely related [2–5], as detailed below. They should also be distinguished from dose-ranging experiments, though there is a frequent confusion in literature between dose-ranging and dose-finding [6]. Actually, we will consider dose-ranging as the (often random) comparison of two or more doses of a drug in terms of response, which is not within the scope of this book.

Besides this controversy, the definition of dose-finding studies always uses several distinct concepts of *dose*, *response* and *optimal dose*, which should be clearly defined. The *dose* is the amount of active substance given in a single administration or repeated over a given period, according to a certain administration schedule of equal or unequal single doses at equal or unequal intervals. Of note, it is sometimes important to include the patient's body weight (notably in children) in the expression of doses. The *response* is the patient's outcome of interest, defined either in terms of toxicity/tolerability or therapeutic points of view. The tolerability is commonly measured

Statistical Methods for Dose-Finding Experiments   Edited by S. Chevret
© 2006 John Wiley & Sons, Ltd

by the appearance of unwanted signs and symptoms and changes in some clinical and laboratory findings, denoting some adverse reactions following drug administration. By contrast, the therapeutic response is measured by the change observed in one or more variables taken as indications of the intensity of the patient's condition, i.e. depending on the disease under study. According to the measured outcome, either toxicity or therapeutic response, two *optimal doses* are defined in dose-finding, namely the maximal tolerated dose (MTD) and the minimal effective dose (MED). The maximal tolerated dose is often defined as the dose that produces an 'acceptable' level of toxicity [7] or which, if exceeded, would put patients at 'unacceptable' risk for toxicity, or the dose producing a certain frequency of (medically unacceptable) reversible, dose-limiting toxicity (DLT) within the treated patient population. DLT includes host effects up to the point that is acceptable to the patient, based on several severity grading scales of adverse events, such as the common toxicity criteria developed by the National Cancer Institute of the United States. For instance, in oncology, DLT is usually defined as any nonhaematological grade III or grade IV toxicity (except alopecia, nausea, vomiting or fever, which can be rapidly controlled with appropriate measures), or an absolute neutrophil count <500/ml for at least 7 days, or febrile neutropenia (absolute neutrophil count <500/ml for at least 3 days and fever above 38.5 °C for 24 hours), or thrombocytopenia grade IV. The minimal effective dose (MED) is the dose that elicits a prescribed lowest therapeutic response. Such definitions are particularly important by conditionning the definition of the endpoint in dose-finding experiments; they will be discussed in Section 1.3.3.2. The difference between these two doses defines the therapeutic area (window) of interest.

Dose-finding experiments are common for evaluating tolerability, while dose-finding studies of efficacy are unusual. Dose-finding experiments that focus on the evaluation of MTD are referred to as phase I clinical trials, whereas those focusing on the evaluation of MED are referred to as (early) phase II clinical trials. Most of the time, dose-finding experiments are restricted to phase I trials.

Traditionally, phase I trials are considered 'first in human' studies, following extensive preclinical testing. However, it is important to recognize that phase I studies are not limited to 'first in human' studies. Subsequent phase I trials often evaluate new schedules or combinations with established drugs. In addition, these secondary phase I studies may focus on a particular population that was excluded in prior studies, such as children.

The primary goal of phase I trials is to determine the appropriate dose for phase II evaluation, i.e. attempting to define a standardized treatment schedule to be safely applied to humans and worth being further investigated for efficiency. Phase I clinical trials are performed in many medical areas, but are particularly important in cancer, where they are the essential gateways to the development of new therapies. Otherwise, for most drugs, as long as the expected toxicity is mild and can be controlled without harm, dose-finding phase I trials involve the administration of usually subtherapeutic doses of a new agent to healthy adult volunteers, in specially dedicated clinical pharmacology units, to investigate the initial safety and tolerability, and also the pharmacokinetic drug profile and the pharmacodynamics [8]. By contrast, in life-threatening diseases, such as cancer and AIDS, because of the toxicity that generally is observed in preclinical studies, phase I trials of new agents cannot be conducted in healthy volunteers. In these settings, participants in phase I trials are almost always patients with refractory disease or for whom there is no standard therapy, often at a very high risk of death, who consent to participate in the trial only as a last resort in seeking a cure.

Actually, most attention has been devoted to the design, conduct and analysis of phase I dose-finding experiments in cancer patients. Besides the main difference described above in enrolled subjects, there are many other differences in the design, the endpoints and the analysis of dose-finding phase I experiments conducted in healthy volunteers and those conducted in cancer patients. Therefore, dose-finding methods for phase I healthy volunteer studies will be treated separately (in Chapter 9).

By contrast, there are fewer differences in statistical methods between dose-finding experiments for cancer phase I studies and those for phase II studies than between dose-finding phase I studies in cancer and in healthy volunteers. Most of the methods presented below focus on dose-finding in phase I cancer studies, but would be extended easily to dose-finding phase II studies in noncancer populations.

1.2 Main issues from a pharmaceutical point of view

Drug development is a continuous process through which the knowledge of efficacy and safety of an experimental drug is gradually accumulated. For designing confirmatory (phase III) trials, it is essential to have sufficient knowledge of one or two doses of the drug that can be considered as optimal for safety and efficacy. A well-designed dose-finding study should provide valuable information for this purpose. Actually, it constitutes one of the most important steps in the drug's development [9].

Notably, it should be kept in mind that failure to identify an appropriate dose can cause delays throughout the drug development process, increase cost and, at last not at least, compromise the commercial success of the marketed drug, and even cause widespread harm to patients. This underlines the need for understanding the scientific and regulatory aspects of dose selection, as well as effective statistical methods for identifying dosing regimens with maximized likelihood of efficacy and minimized risk of toxicity. This will be detailed in Chapter 2.

1.3 Statistical issues of dose-finding phase I trials

As stated above, the dose-finding phase I trials usually represent the first application of a proposed drug to humans. Despite the centrality of these early-phase trials to the process of drug evaluation, they are not well understood, are subject to many popular misconceptions [10] and are still unfamiliar to most physicians. Moreover, besides some guidelines established for phase I trial execution during the 1970s, statistical considerations have been mostly absent from the design, analysis and reporting of these studies until the 1990s. Nevertheless, phase I trials pose challenging problems for the ethical conduct, for efficient design and for inference (with increased confidence that our estimate is accurate) of these studies, all of which have important statistical content [11].

1.3.1   Ethical concerns

Dose-finding studies involve humans, either healthy volunteers or patients. Therefore, investigators conducting dose-finding trials must adhere to the ethical norms of clinical research. Moreover, as first-in-man studies, the safety of the participating subjects is of primary concern. Phase I trials are studies of, for and (increasingly) with patients. However, the research goals may differ from the patients' goals, and there is no consensus on how to achieve the researcher's goals in the most efficient and ethically appropriate way. Actually, ethical issues have markedly influenced the sample size and the design of these studies.

Firstly, typical sample sizes of dose-finding studies are small, commonly about 20 subjects. As mentioned by Gatsonis and Greenhouse [12], perhaps the limited sample size and the ethical concerns, closely related, are the two most serious problems currently facing phase I study designs.

Secondly, some rather special designs are used in dose-finding. Indeed, the design has long been governed by the ethical constraint of minimizing subjects treated at toxic doses. Therefore, randomly assigning patients between several dose levels appeared unacceptable. Doing so, some subjects will be assigned to low doses that are known to be suboptimal in terms of efficacy while other subjects will be exposed to high doses that are very toxic. Initial standard phase I designs were rule-based (or algorithm-based) dose-escalation schemes in which the dose is gradually increased throughout the experiment from the lowest dose level until some desired response or unwarranted toxicity is observed (see Chapter 3). Intrapatient dose-escalation is frequently not permitted because of concerns about cumulative toxicity obscuring effects at a subsequent dose level. However, accelerated titration designs have been developed using such an within-patient dose escalation [13], notably in healthy volunteers. Such designs will be developed in Chapter 4.

In traditional between-patient group escalation designs, because of fears for safety, an escalation of doses by group takes place. Thus, the first dose will be examined in one group of patients before proceeding to study the next dose and so forth. The starting dose and the escalation scheme, which both determine the distribution of patients at potentially toxic dose levels, deal with the issue of safety. Issues raised in determining the starting dose and escalation scheme will be discussed below (Section 1.3.2).

Nevertheless, when conducted in AIDS or cancer patients, phase I trials also have a therapeutic aim. Thus, another ethical obligation, more recently reported, is to maximize the chance that the dose which an individual receives has the potential for therapeutic value or, in other words, that the number of patients treated at ineffective doses should also be minimized [14]. Therefore, the process of dose escalation is governed by a fundamental conflict. On the one hand, there is a need to go slowly in order to avoid a sudden jump from no observable toxicity to a lethal dose; on the other hand, there is a need to go rapidly, so that large numbers of patients are not treated at ineffective doses. In this setting, there is a need to balance the concern for patient safety when being treated with an unknown agent, as reflected in careful dose escalation and the desire to treat at doses that will be close to the recommended phase II dose, thus increasing the likelihood of benefit. Thus, one should design cancer phase I trials to minimize both the number of patients treated at low, nontherapeutic doses, as well as the number given severely toxic overdoses. Attention has been directed towards the objective of treating as many phase I patients as possible close to the MTD (see Chapter 6). Alternate designs were developed to treat as few patients as possible at a biologically inactive dose level. This will be discussed in Chapter 8.

Finally, two fundamental ethical challenges are often raised about phase I cancer trials, namely the risk–benefit ratio and informed consent, but available data do not support these objections [15].

1.3.2 Design

During the past decade, the importance of properly designed early (phase I) trials has led to dramatic changes in their traditional $3 + 3$ design (see Chapter 3), including selection of starting dose and rapidity of dose-escalation.

1.3.2.1 Starting dose

To begin human testing, a safe starting dose is needed. This is an important step in dose-findings for anticancer drugs [16]. Guidelines for determining phase I starting doses for chemotherapeutic agents were developed following retrospective reviews that compared specific toxic dose levels in animals and in humans [17]. Actually, the current preclinical toxicology does provide the basis for a safe starting dose, tailored to potency in rodents. As safety was the primary concern, the starting dose has been long calculated as the highest fraction of a specific toxic dose level, in a particular animal species. Early in the history of the development process for phase I trials, preclinical toxicology studies were used to define the toxic dose low (TDL), or first toxic dose, in dogs and monkeys for safety considerations in clinical trials; one-third of the TDL in the more sensitive species was chosen as a safe starting dose for phase I trials of antitumor agents [18]. However, later studies suggested that the LD10 in mice, i.e. the dose that was lethal to 10 % of animals, would be a safe starting dose and would decrease the number of dose-escalation steps required to reach the MTD as compared with one-third of the TDL in dogs and monkeys [19]. One-tenth of the mouse LD10, expressed in milligrams per meters squared, has historically been found to be a safe starting dose in humans, as long as that dose is not lethal or life-threatening to a second species (e.g. rat, dog). This provides the commonly used basis for initial doses in phase I studies [20]. The question of whether higher starting doses can be safely used was recently pointed out [21], notably through the use of interspecies scaling [16]. This could help to save time and avoid unecessary steps in attaining MTD in dose-finding experiments.

1.3.2.2 Dose-escalation

Standard phase I design is a rule-based dose-escalation scheme, in which the dose is gradually increased throughout the experiment until some desired response or unwarranted toxicity is observed. Until recently, it was expected that dose-escalation for all anticancer drugs would continue until limited by toxicity.

The traditional phase I design is algorithm-based. For escalating doses above the starting dose, the modified Fibonacci search scheme [22] with escalations in decreasing increments was initially applied to phase I studies on nitrosourea [23]. Once the starting dose has been evaluated, the rate of escalation is empirically defined by a modified Fibonacci series. The initial dose escalation is thus rapid (100 %, or doubling of the dose) and narrows down with successive increases until the 30–35 % range is reached (actually, dose increases of 100 %, 65 %, 50 %, 40 % and 30–35 % thereafter). In theory, this approach would decrease the risk of overshooting the MTD as it is approached, but scientific justification for it is lacking.

The widely used standard phase I design (so called 3 + 3 design) is very simple. It uses three patients at each dose level until one of three patients have DLT; then three more patients are added. If none of the three additional patients have DLT, escalation continues; if one or more of the additional patients have DLT and only three patients were evaluated at the next lower dose, additional patients are added to the lower dose level. Otherwise, the trial is stopped.

This standard approach treats the MTD as being identifiable from the data [24], and thus is a statistic rather than a parameter. Actually, no estimation is involved. Of note, the derivation of exact formulae for statistical quantities of interest has recently been proposed [25, 26].

By design, the MTD estimate relies heavily on the actual cohort of patients treated and the order in which they enter the study. A review of phase I studies undergone during the period 1977–89 has documented that the usual methods for choosing starting doses and dose-escalation schemes for phase I studies are overly conservative and delay opportunities for therapeutic benefit in phase I and subsequent phase II trials [27]. Because of the small number of patients who actually receive the recommended phase II dose, there is a large uncertainty in the toxicity rate associated with that dose. For instance, if all three patients of a hypothetical cohort experience dose-limiting toxicity, most investigators would agree that the recommended phase II dose has been exceeded. However, even in that setting, one must acknowledge that the 95 % exact confidence interval for the incidence of dose-limiting toxicity is 37–100 %. Many investigators would not accept a 33% rate of dose-limiting toxicity (two out of six patients) at the recommended phase II dose; however, the 95 % exact confidence interval for this dose-limiting toxicity rate is quite broad (6–73 %). Otherwise, statisticians feel that conventional methods in widespread use for dose-finding in phase I clinical trials are unrealiable, pointing out the need for alternative methods [28]. As an illustration, all participants in a workshop on phase I trial designs in cancer drug development stated that they no longer would routinely use standard dose escalation when designing a phase I trial [21].

Therefore, other rules for escalating and de-escalating dose levels have been proposed. For more rapid and efficient dose-escalation schemes, pharmacologically based designs have been proposed in recent years. Like the traditional modified Fibonacci-based design, these methods use toxicity, and specifically DLT, as the endpoint of the trial, using toxicologic projections that are based on pharmacological information from preclinical models. Such pharmacokinetically guided determination of the MTD has been suggested in cancer [11, 14, 29], using preclinical and pharmacokinetical information in the choice of starting dose, rate of escalation and design. They will be discussed in Chapter 4.

Finally, statistical-based designs, which treat the MTD as a population parameter, are driven by accumulating patient observations that refine a model predictive of the optimal dose. They will be developed below. Whatever the inference, iterative fitting of the dose–effect model, as data accumulate, allows model-guided dosing. A new data-driven dose-escalation method, adaptative dose-finding (ADF), has been proposed, which combines the standard rule-based method with a model-guided method [30].

Most of these new proposals will be discussed in Parts III, IV and V.

1.3.3 Inference

The primary purpose of a phase I clinical trial is efficiently and accurately to determine the dose of a new drug or therapeutic agent being studied for future applications (in phase II and then in phase III trials). Thus, phase I trials address an estimation problem rather than the testing of a hypothesis. The fact that phase I clinical trials are not hypothesis-driven has been considered as potentially the reason why statistical considerations have largely been ignored in these trials [24]. Moreover, as exposed above, for a long time phase I studies were often done in small numbers of patients, with the optimal dose usually administered to only a minority of the patients treated in the trial. As a result, neither efficacy nor safety data were considered to be reliable.

In the traditional algorithm-based designs, it is common to define the MTD as the previous lower dose level reached in the trial. Nonetheless, designs for phase I clinical trials should be concerned with efficiency of estimation of the MTD. Actually, it has been argued that efficiency is a more relevant consideration than convergence in such very small trials [31]. Notably, any statistical discussion of issues in dose–finding trials should begin with a proposal for a formal inferential framework for analysis. Within this framework, one would specify a form for the dose–response relationship, define the quantities of interest and proceed to quantify the degree of uncertainty about these quantities.

1.3.3.1 Specify a form for the dose–response relationship

The basic and cental assumption in cancer dose-finding is that the therapeutic and toxic effects of a treatment are related to the concentration of the treatment in blood,

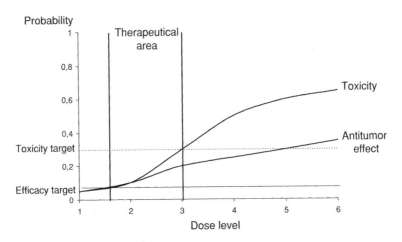

Figure 1.1   Dose–response relationships.

which are dose-dependent (Figure 1.1). In the case of cytotoxic agents, this concept of dose response has greatly influenced the thought process of oncologists, assuming that the higher the dose, the greater the likelihood of efficacy ('more seems better' [32]). A monotonic relationship is commonly stated, although some authors have developed methodology for the design and analysis of nonmonotonic relationships.

The mathematical function describes the hypothetized relationship between the incidence of DLT and dose in the target population. This parametric quantal response model is reasonably predicted to assume a sigmoid shape that can be generically described by a probit or logit function, and for which the MTD must be estimated first [6, 12, 33, 34]. This is more in line with the statistical development in bioassay with a binary response, which dates back from more than five decades [35]. Usually, maximum likelihood or least-squares techniques are used to estimate the model parameters [6, 13, 26], though Bayesian approaches have also been proposed since 1972 [5], such as the original continual reassessment method (CRM) [34] (see Chapter 6), the decision–theoretic approach of Whitehead and Brunier [36] (see Chapter 7), escalation with overdose control (EWOC) [33] (see Chapter 8) and Bayesian optimal designs for phase I trials of Haines, Perevozskaya and Rosenberger [31].

Of note, completely nonparametric approaches have been proposed more recently [33, 37–41].

1.3.3.2   Define the quantities of interest

Because most of these agents exhibit a monotonic dose-toxicity relationship, dose–related toxicity is regarded, in general, as a surrogate for efficacy. In this setting, the achievement of significant, but reversible, toxicity becomes desirable, so that most statistical methods for dose-finding in cancer phase I clinical trials determine a maximum tolerabled dose (MTD) based on toxicity alone, while ignoring therapeutic response [34, 42–46]. Virtually, all designs for dose-finding in phase I characterize patient response by a binary [45, 47] or possibly ordinal [48] toxicity variable.

In the traditional algorithm-based designs (either the 3 + 3 design, see Chapter 3, or the up-and-down designs, see Chapter 5), the MTD was first defined as the dose level at which at least one-third (conventionally in no more than two of six patients) of the patients experience DLT. Many use the term MTD for the next lower dose, which is frequently the recommended phase II dose. It is important to note, however, that the MTD will depend upon the criteria set for DLT. These sometimes vary because investigators may be more conservative or more agressive in their definition of acceptable and unacceptable toxicity. In all cases, the MTD is treated as being observable from the data. Such a definition of MTD appeared vague from a statistician's point of view. As stated by Storer [45], a strict quantitative definition of the MTD is seldom acknowledged, although it is often taken as a specific percentile of the tolerance distribution of the treatment, i.e. the dose that would be expected to produce a toxic response in a specified proportion of patients. The percentile of interest could vary according to the nature and seriousness of the toxicities produced by the drug under investigation. The 33rd percentile has been proposed for cancer chemotherapy drugs [45], but other percentiles may be reasonable choices. In this setting, the MTD is an unknown population parameter that can be estimated from the data. Such an interpretation of the MTD is more in line with historical statistical developments in bioassay with quantal response curves for a binary response.

Phase I trials are designed to determine the recommended phase II dose for a population, not an individual patient. Since there is usually substantial interpatient variability in toxic effects, the recommended phase II dose will always be an imprecise estimate of the optimal dose for the individual patient. An alternative target dose, the patient-specific MTD, has been proposed explicitly to take into account a patient's history via an augmented dose–response model [49]. Recently, other researchers have defined the MTD as the highest dose with toxicity risk not exceeding the tolerable toxicity [33, 50]. Otherwise, some authors have developed methods to account for differences among toxicities, using ordinal-valued toxicities according to severity (or grade). This will be developed in Chapter 12. Strategies for dose-finding where both toxicity and efficacy are considered have been developed. They will be discussed in Chapter 14.

Finally, toxicity may no longer be an appropriate endpoint in some phase I studies [51], so it is no longer expected that determination of the MTD will be the universal endpoint of a phase I investigation. These include studies of drugs characterized by a dose–response curve that reaches a plateau at nontoxic doses, or that have the desired effect at doses without significant toxicity. Probable examples include angiogenesis inhibitors and colony stimulating factors. Toxicity would also not be an appropriate endpoint for phase I studies of agents with a bell-shaped dose–response curve and a dose–toxicity curve that rises after the maximal therapeutic dose. There are already several classes of molecules undergoing clinical evaluation for which the MTD was not determined and/or relevant to the drug's use. Probable examples include interferons, some interleukins and negative regulators of hematopoiesis. Thus, with the development of novel biologic agents such as these, the use of toxicity as an endpoint would result in unnecessary toxicity and wasted resources. The need for new endpoints is also apparent for new modalities including monoclonal antibodies and gene therapy, which may produce nonspecific and sporadic toxicities that are not clearly dose-related. In many cases, plasma concentration has served as the alternative endpoint. Pharmacokinetics assessment and correlation of drug levels with target effects, in addition to pharmacodynamic measures, will be necessary. At last, it is critical to validate that the proposed target endpoints are correlated with activity [52].

Of note, a recent survey of completed phase I trials for targeted, noncytotoxic agents showed that nontraditional endpoints (such as measures of molecular drug effects in tumor or surrogate tissue) were not routinely incorporated in the study design and rarely formed the basis for dose selection, which is still based on toxicity traditional endpoints [53].

1.3.3.3 Proceed to quantify the degree of uncertainty about these quantities

Finally, it is important to include measures of variability in such studies. They are usually nonreported from traditional algorithm-based designs, in contrast to statistical-based designs.

The main approach is to quote confidence limits. Confidence limits, due to Neyman, are the limits of usually the 95 % confidence interval, which represents all the parameter values compatible with the data accumulated in the trial. In a Bayesian framework, credible intervals for the model parameter can be computed. This gives an interval such that (say) the model parameter lay between these limits with 95 % probability. Of note, the numerical integration procedures are often ignored in reporting these Bayesian studies, though of prime interest in evaluating its reliability [24].

1.4   Conclusion

Dose-finding experiments refer to a broad class of early development trial designs whose purpose is to find a dose of treatment that is optimal with respect to simple criteria, namely toxicity, efficacy and a low risk of side effects. The tendency has been to focus on a dose–safety association. Therefore, dose-finding studies are typically phase I clinical trials, based on very small, uncontrolled, sequential studies of subjects to determine the maximum tolerated dose (MTD) of an experimental drug that will be used in further phase II or III trials. While performed in many areas of medicine, they are mostly devoted to cancer studies due to the severe toxicity of cytotoxic drugs, assumed to be related to the dose and, expectedly, to the efficacy of the drug. Such phase I trials are mostly concerned with protecting patients from being assigned to highly toxic doses and with efficiency of estimation.

A number of philosophical and statistical issues emerge from the design and analysis of dose-finding studies, with two main divergent schools. While algorithm-based designs define the MTD as a statistic computed from data, statistical (or model)-based designs consider the MTD as a parameter of a monotonic dose–response curve to be estimated from data. However, whatever the statistical grounds of the proposed techniques, there is still an obvious gap between the statistical approaches developed in this setting and the common use of standard methods that have been shown to be inefficient for several decades. Indeed, despite proposed new methodologies for phase I trials, very few are being used in practice and many of the methods currently used in phase I trial design date back to the 1970s [52]. This was notably observed through a review of 46 phase I trials of single cytotoxic agents in adult solid tumors published between 1993 and 1995 [54].

The purpose of this book is to review the main innovative statistical approaches for dose-finding in phase I/II clinical trials, from both algorithm- and model-based designs, with emphasis on general concepts and practical considerations.

References

1. J. Kotz, Z. Knapik, W. Lubczynska-Kowalska, M. Houszka, J. Lapinska and M. Rybak (1988) Effect of a single dosis of 96 % ethanol on rat gastric mucosa. Part I. Morphological studies. *Mater. Med. Policy*, **20**(2), 67–9.
2. P.R. Freeman (1970) Optimal Bayesian sequential estimation of the median effective dose. *Biometrika*, **57**, 79–89.
3. M. Mendoza (1990) A Bayesian analysis of the slope ratio bioassay. *Biometrics*, **46** (4), 1059–69.
4. F.L. Ramsey (1972) A Bayesian approach to bioassay. *Biometrics*, **28** (3), 841–58.
5. R. K. Tsutakawa (1972) Design of experiment for bioassay. *J. Am. Statist. Assoc.* **67**, 584–90.
6. J.R. Murphy and D.L. Hall (1997) A logistic dose-ranging method for phase I clinical investigations trials. *J. Biopharm. Statistics*, **7**(4), 635–47.
7. B.E. Storer (2001) Phase I trials, in *Biostatistics in Clinical Trials* (eds C. Redmond and T. Colton), John Wiley & Sons, Ltd, Chichester, pp. 337–42.
8. G. Emilien, W. van Meurs and J.M. Maloteaux (2000) The dose-response relationship in phase I clinical trial design and beyond: use, meaning and assessment. *Pharmacology and Therapeutics*, **88**, 33–58.
9. D.D. Von Hoff, J. Kuhn and G.M. Clark (1984) Design and conduct of phase I trials, in *Cancer Clinical Trials: Methods and Practice* (eds M.E. Buyse, M.J. Staquet and R.J. Sylvester), Oxford University Press, Oxford, pp. 210–20.
10. ASCO (1997) Clinical practice guidelines for the treatment of unresectable non-small-cell lung cancer. Adopted on May 16, 1997 by the American Society of Clinical Oncology, *J. Clin. Oncology*, **15** (8), 2996–3018.
11. M.J. Ratain, R. Mick, R.L. Schilsky and M. Siegler (1993) Statistical and ethical issues in the design and conduct of phase I and II clinical trials of new anticancer agents. *J. Natl Cancer Inst.*, **85**(20), 1637–43.

12. C. Gatsonis and J.B. Greenhouse (1992) Bayesian methods for phase I clinical trials. *Statistics in Medicine*, **11**(10), 1377–89.

13. R. Simon, B. Freidlin, L. Rubinstein, S.G. Arbuck, J. Collins and M.C. Christian (1997) Accelerated titration designs for phase I clinical trials in oncology. *J. Natl Cancer Inst.*, **89**(15), 1138–47.

14. J.M. Collins, D.S. Zaharko, R.L. Dedrick and B.A. Chabner (1986) Potential roles for preclinical pharmacology in phase I clinical trials. *Cancer Treatment Rep.*, **70**(1), 73–80.

15. M. Agrawal and E.J. Emanuel (2003) Ethics of phase 1 oncology studies. *JAMA*, **290**(8), 1075–82.

16. I. Mahmood (2001) Interspecies scaling of maximum tolerated dose of anticancer drugs: relevance to starting dose for phase I trials. *Am. J. Therapeutics*, **8**(2), 109–16.

17. E.J. Freireich, E.A. Gehan, D.P. Rall, L.H. Schmidt and H.E. Skipper (1966) Quantitative comparison of toxicity of anticancer agents in mouse, rat, hamster, dog, monkey, and man. *Cancer Chemotherapy Rep.*, **50**(4), 219–44.

18. D.J. Prieur, D.M. Young, R.D. Davis, D.A. Cooney, E.R. Homan, R.L. Dixon and A.M. Guarino (1973) Procedures for preclinical toxicologic evaluation of cancer chemotherapeutic agents: protocols of the laboratory of toxicology. *Cancer Chemotherapy Rep. 3*, **4**(1), 1–39.

19. J.S. Penta, M. Rozencweig, A.M. Guarino and F.M. Muggia (1979) Mouse and large-animal toxicology studies of twelve antitumor agents: relevance to starting dose for phase I clinical trials. *Cancer Chemotherapy and Pharmacology*, **3**(2), 97–101.

20. M. Rozencweig, D.D. Von Hoff, M.J. Staquet, P.S. Schein, J.S. Penta, A. Goldin, F.M. Muggia, E.J. Freireich and V.T. DeVita Jr (1981) Animal toxicology for early clinical trials with anticancer agents. *Cancer Clin. Trials,* **4**(1), 21–8.

21. E.A. Eisenhauer, P.J. O'Dwyer, M. Christian and J.S. Humphrey (2000) Phase I clinical trial design in cancer drug development. *J. Clin. Oncology*, **18**(3), 684–92.

22. M.A. Goldsmith, M. Slavik and S.K. Carter (1975) Quantitative prediction of drug toxicity in humans from toxicology in small and large animals. *Cancer Res.*, **35**(5), 1354–64.

23. H.H. Hansen, O.S. Selawry, F.M. Muggia and M.D. Walker (1970) Clinical studies with 1-(2-chloroethyl)-3-cyclohexyl-1-nitrosourea (nsc 79037). *Cancer Res.*, **31**(3), 223–7.

24. W.F. Rosenberger and L.M. Haines (2002) Competing designs for phase I clinical trials: a review. *Statistics in Medicine*, **21**(18), 2757–70.

25. Y. Lin and W.J. Shih (2001) Statistical properties of the traditional algorithm-based designs for phase I cancer clinical trials. *Biostatistics*, **2**(2), 203–15.

26. M. Stylianou and N. Flournoy (2002) Dose finding using the biased coin up-and-down design and isotonic regression. *Biometrics*, **58**(1), 171–7.

27. J.S. Penta, G.L. Rosner and D.L. Trump (1992) Choice of starting dose and escalation for phase I studies of antitumor agents. *Cancer Chemotherapy and Pharmacology*, **31**(3), 247–50.

28. T.L. Smith, J.J. Lee, H.M. Kantarjian, S.S. Legha and M.N. Raber (1996) Design and results of phase I cancer clinical trials: three-year experience at M.D. Anderson Cancer Center. *J. Clin. Oncology*, **14**(1), 287–95.

29. J.M. Collins, C.K. Grieshaber and B.A. Chabner (1990) Pharmacologically guided phase I clinical trials based upon preclinical drug development. *J. Natl Cancer Inst.*, **82**(16), 1321–26.

30. D.M. Potter (2002) Adaptive dose finding for phase I clinical trials of drugs used for chemotherapy of cancer. *Statistics in Medicine*, **21** (13), 1805–23.
31. L.M. Haines, I. Perevozskaya and W.F. Rosenberger (2003) Bayesian optimal designs for phase I clinical trials. *Biometrics*, **59**(3), 591–600.
32. W.M. Hryniuk (1988) More is better. *J. Clin. Oncology*, **6**(9), 1365–7.
33. J. Babb, A. Rogatko and S. Zacks (1998) Cancer phase I clinical trials: efficient dose escalation with overdose control. *Statistics in Medicine*, **17**(10), 1103–20.
34. J. O'Quigley, M. Pepe and L. Fisher (1990) Continual reassessment method: a practical design for phase I clinical trials in cancer. *Biometrics*, **46**(1), 33–48.
35. J. Berkson (1944) Applications of the logistic function to bio-assay. *J. Am. Statist. Assoc.*, **39**, 357–65.
36. J. Whitehead and H. Brunier (1995) Bayesian decision procedures for dose determining experiments. *Statistics in Medicine*, **14**(9), 885–93.
37. Y.K. Cheung and R. Chappell (2002) A simple technique to evaluate model sensitivity in the continual reassessment method. *Biometrics*, **58**(3), 671–4.
38. S.D. Durham, and N. Flournoy (1994) Random walks for quantile estimation, in *Statistical Decision Theory and Related Topics V* (eds S.S. Gupta and J.O. Berger), Springer, New York, pp. 467–76.
39. M. Gasparini and J. Eisele (2000) A curve-free method for phase I clinical trials. *Biometrics*, **56**(2), 609–15.
40. J. O'Quigley (2002) Curve-free and model-based continual reassessment method designs. *Biometrics*, **58**(1), 245–9.
41. J. O'Quigley, X. Paoletti and J. Maccario (2002) Non-parametric optimal design in dose finding studies. *Biostatistics*, **3**(1), 51–6.
42. S.N. Goodman, M.L. Zahurak and S. Piantadosi (1995) Some practical improvements in the continual reassessment method for phase I studies. *Statistics in Medicine*, **14**(11), 1149–61.
43. E.L. Korn, D. Midthune, T.T. Chen, L.V. Rubinstein, M.C. Christian and R.M. Simon (1994) A comparison of two phase I trial designs. *Statistics in Medicine*, **13**(18), 1799–806.
44. S. Moller (1995) An extension of the continual reassessment methods using a preliminary up-and-down design in a dose finding study in cancer patients, in order to investigate a greater range of doses. *Statistics in Medicine*, **14**(9–10), 911–22.
45. B.E. Storer (1989) Design and analysis of phase I clinical trial. *Biometrics*, **45**(3), 925–37.
46. P.F. Thall, J.J. Lee, C.H. Tseng and E.H. Estey (1999) Accrual strategies for phase I trials with delayed patient outcome. *Statistics in Medicine*, **18**(10), 1155–69.
47. N.L. Geller (1984) Design of phase I and II clinical trials in cancer: a statistician's view. *Cancer Invest.*, **2**(6), 483–91.
48. B.N. Bekele and Y. Shen (2004) A Bayesian approach to jointly modeling toxicity and biomarker expression in a phase I/II dose-finding trial. Technical report, M. D. Anderson Cancer Center, The University of Texas.
49. A.T.R. Legedza and J.G. Ibrahim (2001) Heterogeneity in phase I clinical trials: prior elicitation and computation using the continual reassessment method. *Statistics in Medicine*, **20**(6), 867–82.
50. D.H. Leung and Y.G. Wang (2002) An extension of the continual reassessment method using decision theory. *Statistics in Medicine*, **21**(1), 51–63.

51. E.L. Korn, S.G. Arbuck, J.M. Pluda, R. Simon, R.S. Kaplan and M.C. Christian (2001) Clinical trial designs for cytostatic agents: are new approaches needed? *J. Clin. Oncology*, **19**(1), 265–72.

52. S.G. Arbuck (1996) Workshop on phase I study design. Ninth NCI/EORTC New Drug Development Symposium, Amsterdam, March 12, 1996. *Ann. Oncology*, **7**(6), 567–73.

53. W.R. Parulekar and E.A. Eisenhauer (2004) Phase I trial design for solid tumor studies of targeted, non-cytotoxic agents: theory and practice. *J. Natl Cancer Inst.*, **96**(13), 990–7.

54. S.F. Dent and E.A. Eisenhauer (1996) Phase I trial design: are new methodologies being put into practice? *Ann. Oncology*, **7**(6), 561–6.

2

Philosophy and methodology of dose-finding – a regulatory perspective

Robert Hemmings

Medicines and Healthcare Products Regulatory Agency, London, UK

2.1 Introduction

It is well known that pharmaceutical interventions are associated with both risks and benefits. For any given formulation, the precise nature of these risks and benefits will differ from individual to individual based on a complicated (and usually unknown) algorithm accounting for disease characteristics and demographic characteristics, including, but not limited to, gender, weight, age, renal and hepatic functions and, perhaps, genetic make-up. The risks and benefits might also differ between treatment episodes within the same patient. In addition to these characteristics, it is intuitive that the balance of risks and benefits will also be affected by the dose of intervention received. Indeed, for the individual, the dose of treatment would appear to be of paramount importance [1–3], with different doses providing different combinations of risks and benefits and no one dose, or dose regimen, being optimal for all patients.

In order to identify the 'optimal dose' for an individual, it is necessary to address a realm of questions too broad in scope for a standard clinical development programme. These include not only the identification of the most appropriate dose of treatment, conditional on the relevant disease and demographic characteristics of that 'type'

Statistical Methods for Dose-Finding Experiments   Edited by S. Chevret
© 2006 John Wiley & Sons, Ltd

of patient, but the optimal dosing frequency, the duration of treatment and whether dose modifications are useful in the event of inadequate efficacy or unacceptable toxicity. This chapter considers the extent to which answers to these questions are firstly feasible and secondly necessary during prelicensure drug development. It will also highlight the difficulties faced by drug regulators in giving generic advice on dose-finding. It is highlighted a number of times through the chapter, and is worth stating up-front that requirements for data supporting the choice of dose and dose regimen at the time of regulatory review will depend not only on clinical expectation in the particular therapeutic indication, precedent and on the precise wording of the proposed posology, but also on the strength of the evidence for a favourable risk–benefit for the product in question. It is clear that the precise posology and the overall evidence on risks and benefits are unlikely to be known at the time at which regulatory advice is sought.

Scientific aspects of dose-finding are the focus of this chapter. Nevertheless, the resource constraints of drug development cannot be ignored. Any company with a commitment to research and development runs the risk of not recuperating their costs in terms of eventual sales. In particular the costs associated with potential medicines 'failing' in or after phases II and III of development are well documented [4–10]. It is unsurprising therefore that there are pressures to limit both costs (in terms of both time and money) of prelicensure drug development [4–10]. It will be argued that these pressures can compromise those aspects of the trial programme concerned with providing the information necessary to establish optimal dosing. It is further argued that additional information on dose response, which may in some circumstances be desirable in order to refine the posology, will not be investigated at all. In particular, 'dose-finding' is commonly the objective for phase II (sometimes called phase IIb) of drug development. However, there has been reported [4–10] an upward pressure on the costs of developing a new chemical entity, which some authors argue is unsustainable [4–10]. Given the extensive guidance from drug regulators, including the Food and Drug administration (FDA) and the European Medicines agency (EMEA), on drug development in preclinical, phase I (e.g. pharmacokinetic requirements) and phase III, perhaps phase II is the first target for reducing development costs and decreasing time to market. The relationship between risk–benefit and requirements for data on dose-response is highlighted by the closing statement of ICH E4 [1], the global guidance document on 'Dose response information to support drug registration', which states: 'Thus, informative dose-response data is expected, but might, in the face of a major therapeutic benefit or urgent need, or very low levels of observed toxicity, become a deferred requirement'. Does this open the door for the sponsor, in certain circumstances, to pay only lip service to data on dose-response? Does this encourage, even permit, development programmes that identify only the dose, or doses, with the greatest chance of success in phase III, which may or may not be the optimal dosing regimen for even a majority of patients?

There is clearly a trade-off between spending time and money on a full and complete investigation of dose-response and providing only those data that are nec-essary to achieve licensure and are beneficial in promoting sales. A full and complete investigation may expend considerable resources. However, the benefits of a thorough investigation of dose-response are not only limited to an increased probability of success in phase III, but also to achieving the desired product licence, and hence promotional material, and to the continued success of the product postlicensure. Reliable data in the early phase of drug development can also assist in directing resources across a portfolio of potential medicines and, importantly, can contribute to the overall evidence for efficacy and safety, potentially reducing the amount of work necessary in phase III.

In light of the financial constraints, the chapter introduces the questions that might be posed and answered in the investigation of dose-response and the clinical trial designs likely to be favoured by regulators in providing these answers. The relevant questions include determining the dose and duration of treatment and the circumstances under which either single or multiple doses should be proposed for licensure. Demonstrating the benefits and risks of dose modifications in the event of inadequate response or unacceptable toxicity is also discussed. The chapter will focus on the information to provide in support of the choice of dose and the preferred trial designs from which to provide this information. The chapter does not describe or express preferences for particular statistical techniques. It is not usually the role of the regulator to pronounce on preferred statistical methodology.

The chapter considers also how the role of the drug regulators affects the dose-finding phase of clinical development. Particular attention is paid to the role of the regulators in the EU. The FDA have greater (mandatory) involvement with pharmaceutical companies in the earlier phases of drug development than do EU regulators and, therefore, a greater opportunity to influence the investigation of dose-response and the ultimate selection of dose. The regulations governing drug regulation in the UK set out requirements on the quality, safety and efficacy of medicines, not specifically on dose, though dose is, of course, inextricably linked to both efficacy and safety. This does, however, mean that the choice of dose is usually 'the sponsor's risk' rather than a decision taken in partnership. The risk of choosing a dose that is too low is that the product is likely to be viewed as having inadequate efficacy, thus precluding marketing authorisation. The risk of choosing a dose too high is that the product is likely to be associated with unacceptable toxicity (noted either pre- or postmarketing) which might also preclude authorisation, lead to marketing withdrawal or lead to a product that cannot be readily marketed. This is particularly true for applications where the majority of data on safety and efficacy are at a single dose. For applications in which multiple doses have been investigated, the regulator has the opportunity for greater influence as the different risk–benefit profiles of each different dose can be considered.

The chapter concludes with an introduction to novel methods investigating dose-response. A large amount of work has been done in the area of dose-response for cytotoxic compounds. However, similar methods are now being used in other indications. These methods include, in particular, Bayesian approaches and the use of adaptive designs. Brief comment will be made on the circumstances in which these approaches are acceptable from a regulatory perspective, firstly with regards to evidence of dose-response and secondly with regards to providing supportive or confirmatory evidence of efficacy and safety relative to a more traditional design.

2.2 In search of the optimal dose

2.2.1 What is an optimal dose?

Prior to discussing 'how', it is important to be clear on 'what' is being sought during the dose-finding phase of clinical development – that which I have referred to above as the 'optimal dose'. Arguably, the definition of this concept differs between the different stakeholders. Certainly, patients and treating physicians will want a medicine that is effective and tolerably safe for the individual. This will be equally desirable to the ethical pharmaceutical company, as a product liked by the patients and physicians is likely to satisfy two of the primary objectives of all pharmaceutical companies: successfully treating patients and making a profit from licensed medicines.

These objectives, however, are perhaps not fully aligned with the primary objectives of phases II and III drug development. It may be argued that, here, the primary objective for the sponsor is to provide sufficient data to the regulator and to the marketing department such that the product can be licensed and then successfully sold, all in a cost-efficient manner. As introduced above, this means that questions on dose for any given individual, even a given 'type' of individual, are unlikely to be fully answered. Instead, the sponsor-led development concentrates on mean response, assessing subgroups by demography or disease characteristics, usually only when there is a biological plausibility that response to treatment will differ or when sufficient benefit cannot be demonstrated in the whole population of patients assessed. The regulator is also complicit in this and for a good reason. There is clearly a trade-off between ensuring adequate provision of data on dose (and, indeed, on efficacy and safety) and stifling development. The good of public health is unlikely to be served by requiring data that establish optimal dosing for every type of individual. However, as discussed in Section 2.3, where to draw the line is a point of debate and contention and will differ for each development programme. How important are regulatory concerns relating to a failure to precisely define the optimal dose, and other aspects relating to the posology, when a favourable risk–benefit profile has been demonstrated for the majority?

What then is the optimal dose? As stated above, this may differ from individual to individual, and for a development programme that aims to define a single dose, an answer will usually be reached only at the population level. From a regulatory perspective, the optimal dose can only be estimated as the dose from those tested which appears to have the most favourable risk–benefit balance. For indications where there is a need (and indeed an expectation) for more than one dose, the identification of an optimal dosing strategy is more complicated. Dosing strategies are required, for example, for treatments requiring dose titration (defined here as the progression through a number of subtherapeutic doses in order to reach a therapeutic dose that, usually because of adverse experiences, could not reasonably be the first dose a patient receives) or for treatments where dose increases might be explored in the event of inadequate efficacy at a recommended starting dose. In these cases, the optimal dose is the range of doses and the strategy for using these doses that is established as providing the most favourable risk–benefit balance. These doses will form the basis of the licensed posology (the dosing instructions), along with further information on the duration of dosing and advice on how to amend dosing in the event of adequate or inadequate efficacy and unacceptable toxicity. As a minimal requirement it will usually be necessary to establish that licensing more than one dose will increase the usefulness of the product (see Section 2.2.5).

2.2.2   When to determine the dose and duration of treatment?

To some extent, aspects of the posology for a potential medicine will be determined, at least hypothesised, prior to the availability of any information on dose. There will be clinical expectations for medicines to treat certain indications. For example, Actilyse, a recombinant tissue plasmin activator (rt-PA), indicated for fibrinolytic treatment of acute ischaemic stroke, requires a one-off treatment without the possibility for dose adjustment. On the other hand, medicines for chronic conditions, e.g. hyperlipidaemia, might seek a dose regimen that benefited from the availability of multiple doses over the course of the treatment period such that patients might be titrated according to response (enabling at least some individualisation of the risk–benefit balance). Similarly, there will be steer from inside the pharmaceutical company as to the posology that is likely to be both suitable for licensure and, perhaps more importantly, readily marketed. These preconceptions lead to dose-finding programmes that will not necessarily attempt to answer all of the questions that might be of interest. For example, a treatment for pain might be proposed for once-daily dosing based on a combination of clinical expectations, preclinical data and sponsor desire rather than on data examining once-daily versus twice-daily dosing, which might have indicated that twice-daily dosing would have provided improved efficacy for the patient. It is important that a sponsor company clearly delineates those conclusions on dose that are supported by data from those that are supported only by clinical hypothesis and expectation. From a regulatory perspective, conclusions drawn in the absence of data will be examined just as rigorously as those derived from the clinical trial database.

Historically, phase II has served more than one purpose: in particular, to provide preliminary evidence of efficacy, often by way of hypothesis generation, and to provide evidence on dose-response, even to identify a single dose to examine in phase III. However, it can be reasonable for dose-finding to continue to the end of the phase III confirmatory studies and perhaps beyond. To my mind this commonly happens for two reasons. Firstly, even when a comprehensive phase II programme has been completed, there might well be questions on dose-response outstanding, which require greater number of patients and/or a more appropriate clinical setting to answer. Obvious examples include phase II data being based on a surrogate endpoint but with dose-response on an outcome variable being desirable and eliminating extreme low or high doses in phase II but needing greater numbers of patients to differentiate between the doses likely to have the most favourable risk–benefit.

Phase IV trials will rarely address the subject of dose if conducted in patients already covered under the terms of the present licence. Such trials could in fact explore the issue of dose in greater detail, albeit without a placebo if rendered unethical, and without the pressures of time associated with trials prelicensure. This may lead to finding a dose or dosing regimen with an improved risk–benefit compared with the licensed posology. Nevertheless, it is readily understood that further studies would not appeal to the sponsor who is, at this stage, looking to recuperate rather than increase costs and to focus resources elsewhere in their development programme. Phase IV dose-finding will be limited therefore to licence extensions (where information on dose-response cannot simply be extrapolated) and for rare cases where further information on how dose relates to efficacy and safety will help defend a favourable risk–benefit balance in the event that this is questioned based on findings postlicensing.

The important aspect from a regulatory point of view is that the phase of development in which data on 'dose' are generated is unimportant. What matters is the design and the quality of the trials used to provide evidence in support of the proposed posology. In particular, information on dose would, ideally, be viewed as being of sufficient importance to address in adequately powered clinical trials utilising all available design features to minimise bias. This is discussed further in Section 2.5.

2.2.3   Limitations of clinical trials

As introduced above, it is understandable that a pharmaceutical company will not wish to spend time and money generating data that are not pivotal for registration or marketing. Nevertheless, to achieve the desired product information and to smooth the regulatory process, a robust evidence base on dose-response is desirable. In the vast majority of cases, this means data from phase II and phase III clinical trials. It is therefore important to consider the limitations of clinical studies, in particular phase II studies, where, for many indications, the initial explorations into dose-response are conducted.

2.2.3.1   Patient population, sample size, choice of endpoint and trial duration

It is well known that clinical trials utilise inclusion and exclusion criteria which limit their applicability to 'the real world'. Further, it is known that these criteria are likely to be more restrictive in phase II than in phase III. The issue of extrapolation is therefore important when considering the data generated on dose-response. Likewise it may be that the population in which the product is hypothesised as effective, and therefore tested in the early stages of development, will differ to that in which it ultimately proves to be effective. It is therefore reasonable to assume that the population of patients treated postlicensure will differ, to at least some extent, to those included in these clinical trials. However, although the limitations of extrapolation are clear, the impact of the inclusion/exclusion criteria is never reliably estimated and neither the regulator nor the sponsor knows therefore whether the dose(s) identified as optimal in phases II and III will remain optimal postlicensure. The pharmaceutical company should address the patient population studied, and this extrapolation, in their submission. The regulator will aim to minimise this problem by ensuring that the patient population described in the indication matches as closely as is reasonable the population treated in the clinical studies (expanded to include only those additional patients where extrapolation is clearly warranted), i.e. the population in whom a favourable risk–benefit has been demonstrated.

Another limitation of phase II studies is that they are traditionally constrained in terms of size and duration. Limitations to the number of patients recruited means limitations to the precision with which questions of efficacy relative to placebo and relative efficacy between doses can be answered. In addition, the exploration of important subgroups will be difficult. Furthermore, for some indications, the estimation of dose-response will be based on surrogate endpoints, or on treatment durations shorter than those employed in phase III or in clinical use. It is clear that decisions on dose and posology will frequently be complicated by a lack of full and complete information. The situation improves in applications where the investigation of dose has continued into phase III, though some extrapolation is almost always necessary. Nevertheless, if important questions on dose are imprecisely answered, the regulator may feel the need to take a conservative position with regards to the doses that can be licensed. This will usually entail licensing the lowest dose and the shortest duration for which there is a clearly favourable risk–benefit.

2.2.3.2 Replication of evidence

There are other limitations to dose-finding programmes that have parallels to other phases of clinical development. One is that clinical trial results are more readily interpreted if there is replication of the evidence. Data on efficacy will usually be replicated in at least two studies, thus limiting the 'regulator's risk', i.e. the probability of licensing a nonefficacious treatment. As a rule, such replication is neither sought nor required on dose-response data. Given that replication of evidence on 'dose' is not usually a regulatory requirement it will rarely be produced. Of course, replication of evidence is not only of benefit to the regulator and the patient, but potentially to the sponsor as an aid to resolving unexpected and inconsistent results. For example, prior expectation might lead one to believe that a particular treatment will have a linear (at least monotonically increasing) dose-response curve. If a single dose-response trial is presented that does not confirm this pattern, one is left wondering whether the original hypothesis was incorrect, requiring a biologically plausible explanation of the results observed, or whether the original hypothesis was correct and the observed data were due to chance. This may be due to a statistical artefact caused by, for example, patient withdrawals or measurement error. Clearly the conduct of a second trial not only increases the totality of the data available, but, if independent, provides

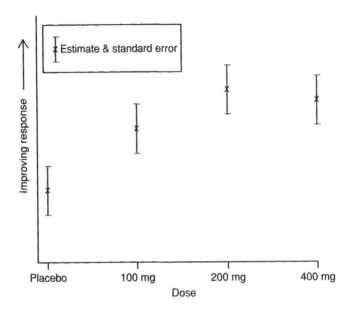

Figure 2.1   Example data on the dose-response.

a data source that may not be affected by the same observed or unobserved biases. It is important to note that replicating the dose-response study is likely not only to support better decisions regarding dose but also to provide additional evidence of efficacy, potentially reducing the amount of confirmatory evidence of efficacy required from future studies.

Figure 2.1 represents phase II dose-response data (in relation to an efficacy variable) presented to the regulator at a meeting to discuss the continued development of this product. The sponsor proposed that the highest dose was continued to phase III in light of their desire to market only one dose and their opinions that the dose-response was monotonically increasing and that there was no apparent dose-response in terms of adverse effects.

Setting aside the issue of whether one or two doses would ultimately be desirable for the licensed product, the advice from the regulator for this particular product was to continue with both 200 mg and 400 mg in phase III. The rationale was that the phase II data did not offer convincing evidence that the efficacy at 400 mg would be superior to that at 200 mg. Given this, and the mantra that all pharmaceutical interventions should be given at the lowest possible dose for the shortest possible time for a desired effect to be achieved, it was considered that a favourable risk–benefit might ultimately be more readily argued for the 200 mg dose. Let us consider three scenarios from the above example, each of which involves continuing the development of the higher dose. Firstly, the sponsor elects to continue with either 400 mg only and the drug proves in phase III to have a favourable risk–benefit. This is likely to be perfectly acceptable to the regulator, whose concern that the 200 mg dose might also have a favourable risk–benefit will be outweighed by the benefits to public health of licensing a medicine with a proven favourable risk–benefit. Secondly, the sponsor elects to continue with the 400 mg only and the phase III programme fails to establish a favourable risk–benefit. This will clearly be unacceptable to the regulator, who cannot then license the higher dose and will wish to know why the 200 mg dose was not progressed. Thirdly, the sponsor elects to continue with both doses into phase III. This would be welcomed by the regulator as the information forming the basis for dose selection is greatly increased. Importantly, decisions taken on posology, in particular which dose offers the most favourable risk–benefit, can then be made at the time of a regulatory review based on an increased clinical trial database rather than earlier in the development programme when the decision would be based predominately on clinical hypotheses.

2.2.3.3   When to obtain regulatory advice on dose

This simplistic example illustrates a further point relating to interactions with regulatory authorities on the subject of dose-response; the opinion of the regulators on dose will depend on when that opinion is sought. If opinion is sought during development, the regulator will advise that the clinical trial programme pays close attention to quantifying the optimal dose accurately. If the time of the regulatory review is the first opportunity a regulator has to consider the dose-response data, he/she will not be considering whether the trial data are adequate to identify the optimal dose or a dose-response. The regulator's concern will be whether the proposed posology is supported. If overall evidence on the risk–benefit is favourable, then the quantity and quality of the data provided in support of the posology are unlikely to be crucial. If, on the other hand, the risk–benefit is not clear-cut, the selection of dose is likely to receive greater attention as the regulator and the sponsor try to identify areas in which the risk–benefit might be improved.

2.2.3.4   Summary

Am I then arguing that dose-response should never be limited to phase II trials? Am I also taking the extreme position that information on dose should always be derived from at least two clinical studies that are adequately powered to answer all questions of interest, do not have excessive inclusion and exclusion criteria and are of adequate duration to reflect clinical practice, assessing 'dose' based on outcome rather than surrogate variables? The simple answer is, of course, 'no'. However, this question highlights not only the trade-off between providing sufficient information on dose while limiting the time and cost of development, but also the difficulties in providing generic advice on regulatory requirements with regards to dose. This is because both the precise questions on dose that a trial programme should aim to answer and the quality and quantity of evidence that should be provided by way of answers will differ not only from indication to indication but also from product to product, depending on the strength of evidence for a favourable risk–benefit ratio. The crucial point is that the decisions made on dose are based on incomplete and imperfect evidence. Such deficiencies are expected, even necessary, but the limitations and extrapolations should be appreciated and addressed by pharmaceutical companies and regulators during the course of development and at the regulatory review.

2.2.4   Identification of the therapeutic window

The therapeutic window is defined as the range of doses between the minimum effective dose (MED) and the maximum tolerated dose (MTD) (both obtained on the population level). For a new medicinal product, data on a minimally effective dose is useful from a regulatory point of view as it gives a lower bound to the range of doses that might be licensed. It is of particular use when a dose proposed by a sponsor has a risk–benefit that is adjudged unfavourable because of the incidence and/or severity of certain adverse effects. In these situations, it is of interest to consider other, usually lower, doses that might have improved safety without a clinically important reduction in efficacy. The absence of a clearly defined minimally effective dose complicates these considerations as it is unclear to what extent a dose might be reduced while maintaining efficacy. This highlights the benefits of exploring the attributes of more than one dose. While it is clearly cheaper and quicker to explore only one dose in any detail, it may prove to be a false economy. In the event that a favourable risk–benefit cannot be clearly established for this dose, a negative opinion is likely to ensue and the cost of repeating the development programme to identify a more appropriate dose will be large, perhaps prohibitive.

The clearest way to demonstrate the lowest dose that is effective is, obviously, to identify a marginally lower dose that is not effective. However, proof of an absence of benefit for a particular dose, say to placebo, is difficult to obtain. A nonsignificant P-value is clearly not proof on its own (the absence of evidence is not evidence of absence) because of concerns over type II error. Much more convincing is an appropriate upper confidence limit that excludes differences of clinical relevance. In practice, given the limitations of these studies described above and the consequent problems with obtaining precise estimates of effect for each dose level explored, assessment of the point estimate against a minimally clinical relevant difference is more usual. This can be acceptable from a regulatory point of view, though the former is clearly desirable.

The term 'maximum tolerated dose' is used frequently in trials of cytotoxics in oncology. There are some interesting dose-finding issues specific to this area, which will be discussed briefly in Section 2.5. However, the term is also used, more generally, to define the upper end of the therapeutic window. The precise identification of this upper limit is, understandably, not the usual focus of either the regulator or the sponsor once it has been established that doses included in phases II and III are below this value. However, there are exceptions to this rule. The cytotoxics are a good example where it is frequently necessary to give the highest tolerable dose to any given patient. Here it is necessary to define 'tolerable' for each indication separately; naturally the incidence and severity of an adverse event considered acceptable in certain indications will be greater and/or more severe than would be considered acceptable in other indications. Indeed, ICH E4 states that: 'For example, the lack of appropriate salvage therapy for life-threatening or serious conditions with irreversible outcomes may ethically preclude conduct of studies at doses below the maximal tolerated dose.' Nevertheless, even in these indications some information on dose-response is required – if only preclinical and phase I data aimed at identifying and accurately quantifying the maximum tolerated dose.

For medicinal products already licensed, licence variations may warrant further investigations on dose, though these will not generally be at the extremes of the therapeutic window. Whether further dose-finding studies are likely to be required will depend on the extension to the indication sought, whether the patient populations are sufficiently similar and whether the expected levels of risks and benefits have altered. In general, extensions of patient population to include, for example, the elderly or paediatrics are more likely to require additional data on dose-response, though clinical arguments may be sufficient.

2.2.5 How many dose levels should be licensed?

Whether a single dose or multiple doses are to be proposed will generally be determined prior to the conduct of any clinical trials based on clinical expectations and sponsor desire, including considerations relating to the ease with which the product might be marketed and manufactured. There are some indications e.g. the use of 'statins' in reducing LDL-C (bad cholesterol), where it will be expected that a range of doses will be available. This contrasts with some acute treatments where the identification of a single dose would be desirable.

From a patient's point of view, it is intuitive that the availability of more than one dose would be welcome in many indications, as the probability of an individual finding a dose with a favourable risk–benefit is increased. It is perhaps unfortunate then that sponsors frequently appear unwilling to provide the clinical trial data that might permit multiple doses of drug to be licensed, thus allowing some individual dose modifications in the case of inadequate efficacy or unacceptable adverse events. It is presumed that this is borne from the ease of marketing and manufacturing a single dose whenever possible and the desire to avoid the additional development costs associated with establishing a favourable risk–benefit for multiple dose levels. This is an example of where the sponsor's desire to minimise costs is, from the perspective of the patient, detrimental to the product ultimately made available as the patient is unable to identify which dose is 'right for them'.

2.2.5.1 Proposing a single dose

When a single dose is intended, determination of the dose-response and description of the posology can be relatively straightforward, though differences in interpretation of dose-response data can still lead to extensive discussions between sponsor companies and drug regulators, as highlighted in Figure 2.1 above. These differences in interpretation will frequently occur as the trials investigating the relative efficacy of the different dose levels will often not be powered to demonstrate differences between them or may not include a sufficient number of dose levels to adequately characterise the dose-response. Differences between dose levels may, of course, be relatively small, certainly compared with differences to placebo, and the trial results will more usually be presented in terms of trends towards differences rather than differences that reach statistical significance.

Of course, the discussion of which single dose is optimal will frequently not occur until the time of a regulatory review. If the sponsor has selected a single dose for their pivotal studies of efficacy and safety, thus putting all their eggs in one basket, the issue of dose will rarely be important; the product, at the dose selected, will either have demonstrated a favourable risk–benefit or will not. Where the sponsor has included more than one dose in phase III with a view to selecting only one dose, the issue of which to choose will, obviously, remain of great regulatory interest and the different risk–benefit profiles of each different dose can be considered. This latter strategy clearly increases development costs but, it is argued, with the benefits of increasing the chance of success. Whether the trade-off is worthwhile is usually a judgement for the sponsor. As stated previously, the regulator will generally recommend that multiple doses be tested in phase III if any doubt over the optimal dose remains following phase II.

2.2.5.2 Proposing multiple doses

For some applications, agreement to license more than one dose is desirable and sometimes necessary. A readily understood example is a product for which titration to an effective dose is required in order to avoid, early, undesirable effects. Another scenario would be a product for which differing pharmacokinetics by age indicated that different single doses were appropriate for different subgroups. Again, if the need for different doses can be justified, these can be relatively straightforward.

There are more interesting issues, however, in applications where a patient would eventually be treated with one of multiple doses. If multiple doses merit being licensed it can be presumed that each dose will offer a different efficacy and safety profile for each individual patient. In these cases the complicated question arises of how to optimise the regimen for using these multiple doses and which recommendations should be made in the product licence. The aim is to provide information on which patients should use which doses at which point in the treatment. In these applications it is necessary to define how a target dose might be identified (e.g. the highest tolerable dose for a particular patient or the lowest dose that provides satisfactory efficacy) and also how a patient is treated in the event of an adverse experience or nonresponse. The former of these is relatively straightforward; an adverse experience will lead either to down-titration of the dose received, to a temporary cessation of treatment, or to complete withdrawal of treatment. The latter is, perhaps, more complicated, particularly when the target dose is to be defined in terms of efficacy. The regulator is trying to avoid the situation where a patient receives a dose increase that does not result in improved efficacy for the patient. The remainder of the section is devoted to establishing evidence in support of such dose modifications. In applications where more than one dose of treatment is proposed, a sponsor will often propose posology along the following lines in the summary of product characteristics: 'Patients with inadequate response to DOSE X should receive a dose increase to DOSE Y'.

This is a good example of an aspect of the posology that generally requires support from clinical trial data (see Sections 2.4 and 2.5). Considering for the moment only the aspects of this problem relating to efficacy, this statement is intuitively reasonable. However, this intuition is based not only on the assumption that efficacy is monotonically increasing with dose received, but also that this increase might be clinically observable and useful. The question of greatest interest for statisticians and others involved in compiling a regulatory submission relates to the evidence that would ideally be provided in support of such a statement.

Clearly some evidence on the relative risk–benefit relationship for each dose is necessary along with a biologically plausible hypothesis for why beneficial responses should increase with increased doses. In fact, it is important to quantify the relationship between each of the proposed doses in relation to both efficacy and safety. As stated in the introduction, quantifying the relationship between doses with regards to safety will be difficult within a programme of clinical trials, unless a particular adverse event or set of adverse events is sufficiently common to allow for adequate statistical power. This will less commonly be problematic with regards to efficacy. It should be possible to demonstrate that increasing the dose leads, on average, to superior efficacy, either in terms of a mean response or the proportion of responders. This population-level dose-response is often the evidence provided in support of the claim that dose increases are beneficial in initial nonresponders. The list below details some ways in which evidence supporting a monotonically increasing dose-response within a proposed range of doses might be derived. It is assumed, for simplicity, that the dose-response is being examined within a randomised, parallel-group trial including all doses of interest plus placebo and that the response is being observed on clinically relevant endpoints after a sufficient duration of treatment. Note that the objective is to provide evidence in support of the statement above, not only to establish 'dose-response'.

1. Statistically significant evidence of a superior effect, on average, at a higher dose level (Y) compared to the starting or current dose level (X).

2. A statistically significant trend within the therapeutic window.

3. A statistically significant trend across all doses examined (including those outside the therapeutic window, possibly including zero, i.e. placebo).

4. A nonsignificant indication of a superior effect, on average, at a higher dose level (Y) compared to the starting or current dose level (X).

Which approach is pursued by the sponsor depends on the clinical setting, the strengths of prior beliefs and clinical expectations, and on the sponsor resource. Historically, evidence of the types described in 1 and 2 would be likely to be considered

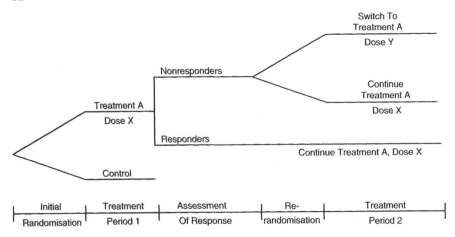

Figure 2.2   Schematics of trial designs to investigate dose increases in non-responders

sufficient in support of a posology that allowed dose increases in patients with an adequate initial response.

Evidence of this strength might be difficult to obtain. Furthermore, in patients with an inadequate initial response, these sources of evidence are not entirely relevant. This is because they are based on the mean response, the response across the entire patient population. The question of increasing the response in initial nonresponders actually bears on the specific subgroup of patients with an inadequate initial response and it is not clear that the answer can be reliably inferred from the whole trial population. Therefore, preferable to all of the above strategies is a design that investigates the dose-response in the relevant subgroup of patients, i.e. those with an inadequate initial response. One approach to this, indeed the preferred approach, is to re-randomise the subgroup of nonresponding patients, either to remain on their initial dose or to undergo a dose increase (Figure 2.2). This additional randomisation step avoids the complication of confounding by time on treatment that is problematic in the alternative design in which all patients with an inadequate response receive a dose increase (Figure 2.3). The interpretation of this latter design is complicated by the absence of a concurrent control group against which to compare the subsequent responses.

The inclusion of a re-randomisation phase in a phase II (or phase III) trial might be a substantial addition in terms of resource, in particular if it were required by regulators to demonstrate statistically significant advantages for the subgroup experiencing a dose increase over the subgroup who do not. Whether the additional resource is greater than might be required to substantiate options 1) or 2) could only be determined on a case-by-case basis. The number of patients included in the trial may need to be substantially increased to ensure an adequate level of statistical power within the re-randomised subgroup. However, while there is no written policy or guidance in

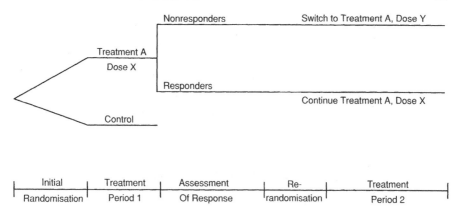

Figure 2.3 Schematics of trial designs to investigate dose increases in nonresponders.

this area, I would not necessarily look here for statistical significance between the groups, though this would obviously be preferable. Any credible separation of effects, indicative of potential clinical benefit for patients who otherwise would receive an inadequate response, is of great value. While this might appear to be a very woolly requirement, such data not only increase the totality of information available but also provide some evidence in the most relevant patient group – the group of patients with an inadequate response at a lower dose. This is an example of a balance being struck between the data that would be ideal to support an aspect of the posology (i.e. a re-randomised phase that could provide statistically significant evidence of superiority for the dose increase) and the cost and time it would take to derive these data.

The situation described above represents a good example of two of the arguments set out in the introduction. This is a situation where additional data, potentially of great use to both the sponsor and regulator (and hence, it is hoped, the wider users of medicines), could be readily obtained, albeit at the obvious costs in terms of both time and money. However, it is also a situation where the information could not be classed as being demanded by regulators or as being necessary for regulatory approval. This illustrates the difficult trade-off between restricting development costs while attempting to optimise the time to market and maximise the chances that the treatment is ultimately successful and therefore profitable, by increasing the data available on its use. An obvious question from a sponsor to a regulator would be to identify the types of application for which this particular information would be of benefit. In response to this it is important to indicate that no current regulatory guidance (in particular, in the EU or the USA) requires such re-randomisation in non-responders. One also has to appreciate that different products and different indications will require different levels of evidence on this point. Therefore, a general answer to this question is not possible. Nevertheless, there are avenues for discussion with regulators about specific development programmes where this point could be raised.

The sponsor must decide how important they consider the licensure of multiple doses and the opportunities to increase the dose in nonresponders, who would otherwise, presumably, seek alternative treatments. It is repeated that this aspect of the posology should be supported by clinical trial data and that the re-randomisation is the preferred approach. The increased likelihood of being able to support the desired posology leading, potentially, to additional market share might warrant the extra expense in providing higher-quality data on dose-response in patients with an initially inadequate response.

2.2.6   Determining the duration of treatment

There are other aspects to the posology than the dose of intervention. Aspects of dose-response rarely addressed relate to the optimal duration of treatment and frequency of dosing. Of course, for many acute conditions this is a moot point, e.g. the duration of treatment for migraine (usually a single dose of medication) will be contained by the episode of the condition. Chronic conditions will require long-term, effectively indefinite, treatment as without such treatment (or other curative intervention) the disease reverts to its natural course. In these indications the pivotal questions relating to the duration of treatment are around whether or not long-term safety and efficacy have been established.

2.2.6.1   Providing evidence of long-term efficacy and safety

Establishing long-term safety is complicated, because of both the difficulties in establishing the absence of an effect and the limitations of clinical trials, in particular limits to patient numbers and to durations of trials. This is nicely illustrated by the findings surrounding the class of medicines known as the Cox-2 inhibitors. These were licensed (among other things) for chronic, arthritic conditions based on data up to 1 year from active-controlled safety and efficacy studies. In nonlicensed indications, where long-term trials could be placebo-controlled and required longer durations of study (3 years or more) cardiovascular safety concerns have been highlighted relative to placebo. Whether these concerns are relevant in the licensed conditions and whether these medicines offer an increased risk compared with other medicines in these indications is still unclear [11] and outwith the scope of this chapter. Nevertheless, long-term safety, once thought acceptable, had to be questioned once more. These experiences may ultimately change the requirements for data on long-term safety, either in this class of medicines or for all pharmaceutical interventions. For now, the requirements in this area are set out in ICH E1A and other regulatory guidance documents and, despite the above limitations, are viewed as both necessary and, providing the data appear to be acceptable, sufficient.

It is clear that a patient with a chronic condition is likely to cease taking a particular licensed treatment when it ceases to be effective (or becomes intolerable). This would, presumably, override any advice on the duration of treatment given in the product literature. However, in order to avoid large numbers of patients receiving unnecessary exposure, more detailed specifications of treatment duration are desirable in a product's summary of product characteristics (SPC). Where possible, these should be based on clinical trial data. Three populations of patients are considered:

1. Those patients experiencing a serious adverse event on treatment. This is straightforward as such patients will require either a treatment holiday or withdrawal of treatment.

2. Those patients not responding to the treatment regimen which may or may not include dose increases. These patients will also be withdrawn from treatment but the question is 'when'? For how long should a patient be treated in the hope of observing a satisfactory response? This will usually be determined by clinical judgement on an indication by indication basis.

3. Relating to the long-term evidence of efficacy, and of greatest relevance here, are the patients who respond well to initial treatment. For how long should treatment continue in these patients? Again, evidence in support of treatment duration can be derived in more than one way.

Again it is assumed that a randomised placebo-controlled trial has been conducted to establish evidence of efficacy in the short or medium term:

- uncontrolled extension data following the controlled trial;

- continued controlled data;

- re-randomisation of responders to continue treatment or switch to placebo (often termed 'randomised withdrawal').

Data from uncontrolled extension phases are generally unhelpful unless the progression of the condition under study is well characterised in the absence of treatment. If clinical experience is sufficient to conclude that the response observed in the uncontrolled extension is certain to be superior to the response that would have been observed without treatment, then it may be concluded that long-term efficacy has been established. Clearly defined, relevant and comprehensive (i.e. free from selection bias) literature searches can assist in defining the average response without treatment, but such searches often give rise to highly variable results, and therefore a demonstration of superiority to the 'average' effect is rarely compelling. The interpretation of uncontrolled extension phases is also frequently complicated by patient withdrawals.

Much preferred are controlled extension phases, either to placebo, if ethical as in the scenario above, or against an active control. Although the issue of patient withdrawals can still be problematic, the addition of a concurrent control arm clearly eases interpretation. The primary shortfall with this method is that it does not establish the optimal duration of treatment; instead it merely establishes that long-term treatment with the test agent is superior to long-term treatment with placebo (or, perhaps, non-inferior to long-term treatment with a reference agent).

2.2.6.2 Establishing the optimal duration of treatment

Let us consider an example. A chronic treatment for psoriasis is proposed based on 30 week data from a placebo-controlled trial. The primary timepoint for the comparison to placebo is 18 weeks. Dosing in the trial was at weeks 0, 6 and 12. A similar treatment regimen is proposed for the SmPC, with dosing continuing indefinitely on a 6 weekly basis in patients responding well to treatment. It is known that, if left untreated, the psoriasis will again become problematic for many patients. At weeks 18 and 30, separation to placebo is large and can be seen to decrease between time-points, congruent with the absence of treatment (Figure 2.4). Regulatory advice on how to determine the duration of treatment is sought. Should treatment be indefinite, and does the trial substantiate the benefits of this? Should treatment be limited to the 12 week dosing period for which benefit was demonstrated in the trial?

As described above, although the trial demonstrates some benefit for three doses (12 weeks) of treatment compared with placebo, it cannot provide a reliable basis for determining the optimal duration of treatment. Perhaps the optimal duration for treatment is indefinite; perhaps it is 12 weeks; perhaps 16 weeks? What further data would be desirable?

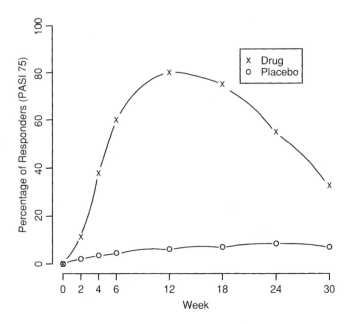

Figure 2.4 PASI 75 response to week 30 in patients with psoriasis.

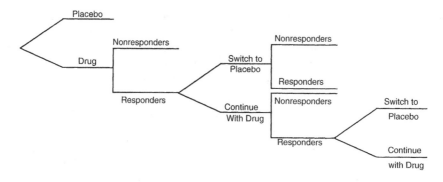

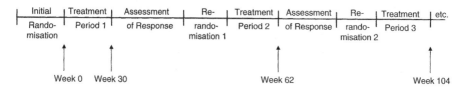

Figure 2.5   Schematic of a trial design to include randomised withdrawals.

Measurements of the efficacy endpoint, the psoriasis area severity index (PASI), could, in theory, be taken at even later timepoints in a continuation of the controlled phase of the trial. Such data would be welcomed, but fail to answer the question of whether continued dosing is beneficial and, as with any data from long-term extension studies, might eventually become so confused by patient withdrawals as to be rendered uninterpretable. Furthermore, one interpretation of the above data is that the effect of initial treatment has 'worn-off'. The ideal comparison would require a trial comparing groups of patients experiencing different durations of active treatment. If, at week 30, a benefit could be observed for treating patients every 6 weeks, compared with the week 30 response of patients treated only to week 12, for example, then the benefits of longer-term treatment would be clear. Note that the benefits of indefinite treatment would still require some extrapolation. In general, the preferred way in which to construct such data is to include a randomised withdrawal phase at the end of the treatment period. Separation in effects between those patients continuing on treatment from those patients switching to placebo is compelling evidence of the benefits of continued treatment. Naturally this can be repeated ad nauseam, with randomised withdrawals from treatment in our example at, for example, 30 weeks and 52 weeks (Figure 2.5).

A randomised withdrawal at 52 weeks, which demonstrated separation of those on treatment to those withdrawn from treatment, would confirm that at least 52 weeks of treatment was beneficial. Of course, analogous to the argument relating to providing evidence of efficacy from dose increases in nonresponders, it is clear that statistical power will eventually diminish to the stage where even large differences resulting from withdrawal of an effective treatment are not statistically significant. Nevertheless, any clear and biologically plausible separation of the re-randomised groups can be compelling for these data. This approach is preferred to having a separate treatment group who are treated for a shorter duration. In particular, the randomised withdrawal is a more efficient use of the patients in the trial; it assesses the question in the relevant subgroup of patients (i.e. those patients continuing with treatment) and, as illustrated, can be used to answer the question at more than one timepoint. This regulator has seen three re-randomisations in a single trial. The evidence for long-term efficacy, and for continued treatment, in that application was particularly compelling, even though an extrapolation from the final randomised withdrawal to indefinite treatment was still required.

Again, the sponsor will question whether the costs of providing these additional data are worthwhile. The consequences of not providing such information were, historically, negligible providing that the clinical rationale for long-term use was sensible and that there were no concerns over long-term safety. This may well remain the case for products clearly without long-term safety concerns (e.g. some topical products). However, with regards to the long-term safety of other medicines, considerations over how duration of treatment is specified in the posology will, in my opinion, increasingly rely on the safety and efficacy data generated in the clinical trial programme [12, 13]. It is hoped that this will lead to more reliable data on long-term safety and efficacy being provided in regulatory submissions, leading to more reliable decisions. For example, a reduction in the number of uncontrolled extension phases with controlled extension phases or randomised withdrawals are preferred. In applications where the necessity for long-term treatment is unclear, the duration of treatment might be limited to the length of time over which benefit has been demonstrated in the clinical trial programme; frequently this will be the duration of the randomised phase of the pivotal clinical trials.

It is worth noting that, in some indications, there exists the possibility of re-treatment following successful treatment of an initial disease episode and a period without treatment. Similar arguments over the necessity of providing data and the quality of data that might be provided to demonstrate that re-treatment is beneficial would apply. Of particular note is the regulatory desire to see controlled data.

2.2.6.3 Summary

While it is undoubtedly useful to the regulator for an application to include evidence on dosing frequency and duration, the necessity of providing such information will depend on the particular product and therapeutic indication under study. Again, it is the sponsor's risk as to whether time and money is spent addressing in detail the question of treatment duration. For some indications, clinical expectation will be so strong that using resources is unnecessary. In other indications the lack of quality data might limit the duration of treatment proposed in the SPC, with obvious consequences for clinical use. Again, there are sources of regulatory advice for questions on requirements in specific development programmes.

2.3   Regulatory requirements for drug licensure

2.3.1   Introduction

The sections above give some clues as to why giving general advice to the pharmaceutical industry on requirements surrounding determination of dose and duration of treatment is particularly complicated. Requirements, both in terms of what data should be provided and the strength of the evidence in support of each particular conclusion relating to the posology, will differ by product, by indication and by strength of evidence available across each of quality, safety and efficacy. Indeed, the law relating to the licensing of medicines [14–18] states that decisions on approvability should be based on quality, safety and efficacy. Dose is not specifically mentioned, but obviously bears on both efficacy and safety. The upshot of this is that a product that has demonstrated a favourable risk–benefit should be licensed regardless of the quality and quantity of data on dose-response. Indeed, in relation to the quantity of data on dose response that is *necessary*, ICH E4 states that: 'Informative dose-response data is expected, but might, in the face of a major therapeutic benefit or urgent need, or very low levels of observed toxicity, become a deferred requirement'. This is not to say that data on dose-response is of no use during regulatory assessment. Although the assessment of the risk–benefit is often described as a ratio, there is no scale on which it can be readily quantified, even when the numerator and denominator are well estimated.

Regulatory decision making is not, therefore, an exact science. Issues that constitute a problem for one regulator will not worry another. Where data on dose-response can help is to better quantify both risk and benefit. For example, if data on doses above that (those) proposed are available, one can often look at the risks at these doses in the knowledge that the risk at higher doses is likely to be increased compared to the proposed dose. If the risk remains sufficiently small, even at higher doses, a positive risk–benefit can be determined with greater confidence. Analogously, if efficacy can be established at doses lower than that proposed, it might be reasonable to be more confident on efficacy at the proposed dose, assuming that a monotonically increasing dose-response is plausible.

At the other extreme, when data on efficacy and safety are insufficient to conclude a favourable risk–benefit, the selected dose can, naturally, be the focus of much regulatory attention with a view towards finding out how further studies should be designed and the specific questions they should attempt to address. In the event that the evidence base for the choice of dose(s) is unclear, question marks over whether another dose might have a more favourable risk–benefit will usually lead to a request for further clinical trials. This highlights again the risk run by the sponsor in terms of up-front expenditure on determination of the dose. Spending less up-front when the risk–benefit balance is ultimately unclear may well turn out to be a false economy.

Certainly there are a number of examples where products have ultimately been withdrawn from the market due to an adverse risk–benefit. In a subset of these the choice of dose is certainly an issue [1, 2] and the absence of efficacy and safety data at other doses renders withdrawal from the market the only sensible regulatory decision.

Looking at the regulatory requirements at the time of licensing only might also be considered somewhat short-sighted. A license from a regulatory agency is not the final hurdle for a medicinal product. There may be cost-effectiveness or reimbursement considerations (e.g. NICE (National Institute for Clinical Excellence) in the UK). There are pharmacovigilance considerations and the need to review and renew licences on a regular basis. Perhaps most importantly of all, there is the question of whether those who prescribe and use the medicine find it acceptable. In order for a cogent argument to be made that the amount of information on dose provided to the regulator at the time of licensing should be more than that *necessary* for drug licensure, it must be shown that further information provided at this early stage in a product life-cycle might be of benefit further down the line. This benefit must be considered in relation not only to company returns but to whether or not patients have ultimately been exposed inappropriately and avoidably to a certain dose of a medicine (see Section 2.4).

2.3.2   The product licence

In the EU, the summary of product characteristics (SPC) represents the product licence. Section 4.2 of the SPC is devoted to the 'posology' of the treatment, i.e. recommendations for the doses and dosing frequencies at which the product is administered. The wording of this section is agreed between the sponsor and regulator at the time of licensing and is based on a combination of the clinical trial data provided and clinical judgement. Two contrasting examples of this SPC section are presented below. The first is straightforward, indicating only the dose to be administered and the dose frequency. This excerpt is taken from the SPC of a product called Zoladex (correct as of 1999). The latter is more complicated; it is taken from a 1999 centralised approval for Remicade, indicated, among other things, for fistulating, active Crohn's disease.

> 'Adult males (including the elderly): One depot of Zoladex LA injected subcutaneously into the anterior abdominal wall every 12 weeks'.

> 'Fistulating, active Crohn's disease: An initial 5 mg/kg infusion given over a 2-hour period is to be followed with additional 5 mg/kg infusion doses at 2 and 6 weeks after the first infusion. If a patient does not respond after these 3 doses, no additional treatment with infliximab should be given. In responding patients, the strategies for continued treatment are:
>
> • Additional infusions of 5 mg/kg every 8 weeks or
>
> • Readministration if signs and symptoms of the disease recur followed by infusions of 5 mg/kg every 8 weeks

In Crohn's disease, experience with readministration if signs and symptoms of disease recur is limited and comparative data on the benefit/risk of alternative strategies for continued treatment are lacking.

Clearly the latter posology is more detailed, indicating not only the dose and dosing frequency but what to do in the event of response or nonresponse, the duration of treatment and, to some extent, use in readministration (if required). For this type of posology, there are clearly many questions to answer: What is the optimal dose? What is the optimal dosing frequency? For how long should treatment continue in responders/nonresponders? Is readministration beneficial in the event of relapse? The requirements for data on questions surrounding dose-response are clearly greater for this type of product. Nevertheless, it is clear that this was a clinical programme that did not answer all of the above questions: 'Comparative data on the benefit/risk of alternative strategies for continued treatment are lacking'. Of course, the complexity of the posology will be driven to some extent by the indication (e.g. whether the indication is an acute or a chronic condition). However, it is also likely that Section 4.2 will continue to include a greater level of detail as regulatory interest in the wider questions on 'dose' increase. I expect that regulators will become more and more interested in having data-driven answers to questions similar to those posed in the above paragraph.

2.3.3   ICH E4

This guidance document sets out regulatory considerations on 'Dose response information to support drug registration'. Given the scope of the document, it is comprehensive. The reader of this chapter is urged to read ICH E4 as it contains regulatory considerations that are broader than those considered here and are a worldwide consensus on these topics. Some of the topics addressed in the guidance are covered elsewhere in this chapter. However, some statements warrant particular attention. The first section highlighted is actually written with reference to examining dose-response across the entire database. The section describes concisely many of the arguments presented in the section above. The paragraphs state that data on dose-response should be used to:

1. identify a reasonable starting dose, ideally with specific adjustments for the type of individual (or a firm basis for believing that none is needed);

2. identify reasonable, response-guided titration steps, and the interval at which they should be taken (for both desirable and undesirable effects);

3. identify a dose or a response (desirable or undesirable) beyond which titration should not ordinarily be attempted because of a lack of further benefit or an unacceptable increase in undesirable effects.

Another such statement deserving of attention is that: 'If development of dose-response information is built into the development process it can usually be accomplished with no loss of time and minimal extra effort compared to development plans that ignore dose-response'. This sentence is preceded by a sentence stating that assessment of dose-response is integral to drug development and its logic is unclear. I would argue that a sponsor and the regulator should expect costs in terms of time and effort in order to obtain good data on dose-response, but that these are prices worth paying in order to improve the likelihood of success in phase III, improve the probability of licensure and improve the likelihood that the treatment is of benefit to patients.

ICH E4 also indicates other obvious advantages to an extensive phase II programme, focusing, in particular, on dose. These are that (a) more extensive information is provided on whether continued development is sensible or whether continuing is likely to be a waste of resource; (b) the expensive phase III programme can focus on a specific dose or set of doses with greater confidence; (c) preliminary evidence of safety and, in particular, efficacy is provided that might reduce the scope or number of phase III trials needed; and (d) accumulation of data on dose groups higher than the dose ultimately proposed for licensing and therefore not directly applicable or useful to the regulatory assessment of risk is avoided. Point (c) is of particular interest. While regulatory guidance [19] indicates that conducting two pivotal studies is the preferred approach to confirming evidence of efficacy, it is known that some licences can be supported by a single, well-conducted pivotal study with levels of evidence more extreme than the usual $p = 0.05$. One of the usual prerequisites for accepting a single pivotal trial is that there is extensive evidence from elsewhere in the development programme in support of efficacy. This generally means either good evidence from closely related indications (relevant only to variations to existing product licenses) or to a good body of evidence from phase II.

It is conceivable, then, that two birds could be killed with one stone. A full and complete dose-finding programme, potentially randomising more patients than the phase III programme, cannot only support the desired posology and best define the phase III programme with the greatest probability of success but can also provide strong evidence of efficacy to be used in support of a marketing authorisation application. If clear and relevant evidence for efficacy were demonstrated across one or more phase II studies, it might be argued that the two pivotal studies requirement could be waived and that only a single confirmatory study would be required (albeit with the extreme level of evidence described). Because of this potential saving in phase III, it is argued that, for some products in some indications, increased spending in phase II would lead to a better trial programme, leading to more straightforward, evidence-based regulatory decision making.

A final advantage indicated in ICH E4 is that the provision of extensive data on dose-response may lead to an economical approach to drug development in that multiple regulatory agencies will reach their decisions from the same database. This is presumably because regulators will follow evidence-based decision making more easily than decisions than are made based on poor evidence or absence of evidence.

This, in turn, will lead to similar regulatory advice and decision making with regards to dose, presumably facilitating worldwide marketing.

2.4 Benefits to the sponsor and the patient of providing data on dose-response over and above those required for licensing

It has been stated above that the relevance of whether or not reliable data must be provided on the various aspects of dose-response depends on numerous factors including the indication and the strength of evidence for a favourable risk–benefit ratio. In addition, an absence of sufficient data on dose-response can be a handicap if the risk–benefit ratio is borderline. The benefits (to the sponsor, the regulator and the patient) of providing some data on dose-response are covered elsewhere in this chapter, but why might a sponsor attempt to provide more data on dose-response than is necessary for a favourable regulatory opinion? It is argued that providing additional data might benefit the sponsor (as well as the regulator and the patient) in a number of ways:

- reducing the number of phase III trials required to prove efficacy, thus decreasing the time to market;
- portfolio management;
- increasing the likelihood that the product is ultimately a success;
- achieving consistent product literature worldwide.

The first of these potential advantages has been discussed in the preceding sections. The second in the list is not directly a regulatory concern and is not discussed further here.

2.4.1 Increasing the likelihood that the product is a success

The third argument is not based on the fact that more data on dose-response is likely to increase the probability of achieving an initial product licence, but on decreasing the likelihood that unfavourable characteristics of the drug will be identified postlicensure. To explain this, it is necessary to consider again two limitations of clinical trials. Firstly, it is well known that a clinical trial is an artificial setting, with inclusion and exclusion criteria limiting the patient population included and meaning that, to be generally applicable, some faith must be put in extrapolation [20–24]. It is generally hypothesised that, compared to clinical trial populations, the expected effects of a medicine in a more general setting would lead to reduced efficacy and increased concerns over adverse events [20–24]. Secondly, clinical trials are of limited scope in terms of both duration and patient numbers. With regards to the former, it may be possible to demonstrate effectiveness in, for example, osteoarthritis with a trial of 6 months, and a further 6 months' worth of safety data might be considered adequate for initial regulatory approval. Under this framework adverse experiences that usually occur following durations of treatment greater than the 12 months over which the trials have been conducted are likely to be unknown at the time of approval. Likewise, even if a trial programme recruits 1000 patients, a particular event with an incidence (in the timeframe of the trial programme) of, say, 1 in 1000 is likely to be seen only 0–3 times. Set this against the likely background rate, and it is clear that even comprehensive clinical trial programmes leave many questions unanswered. Events with such low incidences may not appear important, but if hundreds of thousands of patients are likely to be exposed, the absolute increase in the particular event may well have a major impact on public health.

As argued above, this is necessary to avoid unacceptable delays to market for beneficial medicines, the majority of which, history tells us, are unlikely to be associated with adverse events so severe as to warrant the withdrawal of the product or a change to the product literature, in particular the dose.

Considering these two limitations and the conclusion drawn that much remains unanswered at the time of licensure, why might additional information on dose prelicensure be of benefit? In the event that postlicensure data indicates a problem once a product has been licensed, a number of regulatory options are available: withdrawal, suspension pending submission of further data, monitoring or amendment to the product literature. Which of these is chosen will depend on risk–benefit considerations and on the clinical trial data available in support of the original licence. For example, if unacceptable safety problems are highlighted, the availability of information on a minimally effective dose will assist in answering whether or not the licensed dose can be reduced while retaining a favourable risk–benefit. A risk–benefit evaluation may still be possible (and therefore additional clinical trial work rendered unnecessary) if dose-finding has been fully evaluated prelicensure. Similarly, clinical trial data may accurately quantify the dose-response relationship with regards to a particular efficacy or safety variable and might be considered more reliable than postmarketing data, usually observational data, claiming a contradictory effect. In such instances it might be concluded that the problems observed postmarketing might be more closely related to the patient population being administered the treatment or the conditions of use rather than, for example, the dose of treatment licensed. On the contrary, it is clear that in the absence of reliable clinical trial data, the regulator will be more prone to act (and indeed has a responsibility to act) on postlicensing reports of unfavourable risk–benefit.

A sponsor will rightly ask, however, whether this additional time and cost is worthwhile if only to guard against problems that might be found postmarketing. Of course, this is a similar argument to taking out house or car insurance. It is argued that a relatively small cost up-front (extending certain aspects of a dose-response programme that is already planned) will, on occasion, prevent a larger cost later on. On this point it is noted that the penalties for 'getting it wrong' with regards to dose can be severe. The penalties may relate not only to lost sales postmarketing, because of adverse publicity or marketing withdrawal, but also to additional costs arising from, for example, increased pharmacovigilence requirements, e.g.

constructing a patient registry or conducting a phase IV study. Even more important than the regulatory considerations are those of the patients to whom the products are administered.

2.4.2 Achieving consistent posology worldwide

Another reason for sponsors to conduct a full and complete dose-finding programme for a new medicinal product, also related to the eventual marketing of the product, relates to the eventual ease of product marketing. Clearly, if absolutely no work is done to compare safety and effectiveness across a range of doses then the single dose tested, if proven to be acceptably safe and efficacious, will receive a product licence. However, the probability of identifying the correct dose without information on dose-response is clearly limited. Once dose-finding work is commenced, those data are open to interpretation by the different regulatory authorities worldwide, which introduces personal prejudices and potentially different attitudes to risk, not just over choice of dose but also over the duration of treatment, etc. On completion and submission of a clinical development programme there exists the possibility that different regions will license different posologies based on the same dataset. This probability is surely increased where fewer data on dose-response are available or the dose-response relationship with regards to efficacy and safety are poorly defined. This may lead to different posologies in different parts of the world, which will not facilitate a worldwide marketing campaign.

2.5 Trial designs for determining dose-response

2.5.1 Introduction

As previously stated, it is outwith the scope of this chapter to provide guidance on regulatory requirements, or advice on preferences on trial designs or statistical analyses in all clinical trial programmes across all indications. Nevertheless, there are pros and cons to different trial designs and some specific issues will be addressed. Two aspects that are not addressed in detail are the merits of including a placebo and the quality of clinical trial design and conduct. Providing it is ethical, the inclusion of a placebo control would certainly be expected. Where unethical, inclusion of an additional active control would be highly beneficial. If neither placebo nor active control arm is included in addition to the different doses of test treatment, interpretation, for both regulator and sponsor, is complicated. In particular, while evidence of differences between the doses of test treatment could be sought, it would be difficult to gauge the absolute benefit of the new treatment. In order to establish preliminary evidence of efficacy it would be necessary to identify at least a 'no-effect dose' or a clear 'dose-response'. The second topic to bypass is that statistical considerations relating to trial quality, prespecification, blinding, randomisation, handling of missing data, multiplicity, etc., would ideally be adhered to with the same high level of diligence as for confirmatory studies [25–30].

2.5.2   Issues relating to the design of a dose-response programme

Certain limitations of clinical trials are outlined in Section 2.3. This section expands on those relating to sample size, trial objectives and use of surrogate endpoints.[1]

A tongue-in-cheek argument can be made that phase II offers the classic example of clinical trials being sized by the clinician rather than the statistician and the clinician combined. Once upon a time the clinician might have posed the question: 'What effect size should we write in the protocol to give us 80 % power and 40 patients?' Whether or not this is true, it is clear that there are cost implications that limit the scope of the dose-finding programme. This frequently leads to dose-finding trials that lack the statistical power to answer precisely the questions of interest. Too often in regulatory submissions, decisions are required to be made based on 'trends' in data, rather than on proven hypotheses. This clearly complicates the decision-making process for both the sponsor and the regulator.

The traditional phase II study might also be accused not only of answering the question of interest imprecisely but, in some cases, of not answering the most important question. For the sake of argument let us consider the 'traditional' objective of phase II as being the identification of a dose, or range of doses, with a potentially positive risk–benefit, to continue testing in phase III. This might have been achieved by randomising patients to fixed doses of treatment and comparing the response at each dose to placebo (or another control) to assess whether the benefits observed are likely to be clinically relevant. Perhaps a more appealing approach is not to answer the question 'what is the effect size on dose x?' but instead address the question 'which is the dose with effect size y?'. It is possible to model the dose-response curve with a particular effect size in mind. Under this framework, rather than generating estimates of effect on the response scale, the trial would aim to estimate a dose that gives the desired response and generates a confidence interval on the dose scale giving a range of doses to take forward for further study. This can be a more efficient use of patients (see Section 2.5.5 for an example). The desired effect size need not even be prospectively identified, as the purpose of the trial is to assist in the sponsor's decision-making process rather than to provide confirmatory evidence of efficacy.

The same cost implications described above may limit the duration of the study and hence, in some indications, the selection of the primary endpoint, in that a surrogate for clinical outcome may be used. Conditional on the surrogate being validated and appropriate, this is generally acceptable; nevertheless, the limitations of using a surrogate endpoint should be appreciated (and it should be noted that the same surrogate might not be acceptable for confirmatory evidence of efficacy – even if accepted for evidence of dose-response). Two limitations merit particular attention. One relates to the confidence with which the sponsor can predict the probability of success in phase III if no data on clinical outcome are available. A second limitation,

---

[1]For ease, the nomenclature used in this section is frequentist. This is no comment on the acceptability of alternative approaches.

more pertinent to this chapter, relates to whether or not the dose considered optimal for risk–benefit on the surrogate is also optimal for the outcome variable. Where data on outcome are required for submission, it is considered that the continuation of dose-finding into phase III would usually be highly beneficial, using phase II trials with a surrogate only to narrow the potential dose range rather than to select a single dose for the phase III study.

A similar argument relates to the provision of data on safety. Even at the end of the clinical trial programme it is clear that much remains unknown (or, at least, is imprecisely estimated) with regards to the side-effects of a medicinal product. It is likewise clear therefore that selection of only one dose from phase II is perhaps even more of a concern with regards the risk side of the equation than the benefit side of the equation (often preliminary evidence of efficacy will be available, although preliminary evidence of safety will rarely be as reliable). Where unforeseen adverse effects are detected in phase III it is clear that a different dose to that selected in phase II might ultimately be optimal for risk–benefit.

In all of these examples, the unsurprising conclusion is reached that more information on dose-response, for both safety and efficacy, will lead to better decisions – but is this additional information worthy of the additional costs? This is certainly an area in which statisticians can be of assistance, by using novel and efficient trial designs to answer the relevant questions of interest precisely, but using fewer resources than might traditionally be the case.

2.5.3 Designing a dose-finding trial for monotherapy

Either parallel-group or crossover trials might be appropriate. The choice of trial design merits no special considerations here. It is well known that there are certain considerations relating to when crossover trials are practical and, potentially, beneficial [31]. These arguments are not expanded here. Additional concerns might arise for crossover trials if a large number of doses require testing, as their duration might become unwieldy. However, there are examples in the literature of successfully designed and conducted crossover trials [32] that are still preferable in terms of patient numbers to parallel-group trials, which include many treatment arms.

Comparing the effect sizes of more than one fixed dose of treatment in the same study is the most common approach to the problems of dose selection and determining dose-response, though the use of fixed doses is dependent on the medicine and the therapeutic indication. When multiple fixed doses of test treatment are examined in the same study, the interesting questions surround the trial objectives and interpretation. The most common approach to addressing the choice of dose in a regulatory submission is based on pairwise comparisons between doses and, if included, to placebo, seeking statistically significant (and hopefully clinically relevant) differences, thus establishing that at least one dose is potentially useful. Frequently, this design will give insufficient information with regards to differences in the response between doses. Other methods, e,g., testing for a (linear) trend, might be preferred. Two points are made on these tests. Firstly, the evidence of dose-response from such tests is more convincing when they can be based on data that exclude doses outside the therapeutic window (including placebo). This is simply because the regulator will be interested in whether the dose-response exists within the therapeutic window rather than across the entire dose range. Secondly, a test including or excluding data on placebo does offer some preliminary evidence of activity/efficacy (separate to considerations of dose-response).

Difficulties with either approach arise when the conclusions drawn by the sponsor are based on differences that do not reach accepted levels of statistical significance rather than conclusions that are statistically robust (including linear trends that are established as being statistically different to zero). This is explained further by the examples given in Section 2.2. Whether nonsignificant differences are a sufficient basis for determination of dose-response or dose selection will depend on the need for precise determination of dose for a particular product in the particular therapeutic indication and the strength of the underlying biological plausibility of the conclusions drawn. As indicated by the paragraph above, arguably a more intuitive framework is to attempt to answer the relevant questions on the scale of 'dose' rather than on the scale of 'response'.

The interpretation of fixed-dose studies is relatively straightforward compared to flexible-dose studies. The term 'flexible dosing' is used here to denote a regimen allowing for dose increases or decreases over the course of treatment, but does not include the class of medicines that require titration in early use to minimise the likelihood of adverse effects. Dose increases or decreases would usually be according to 'investigator opinion' or in response to lack of efficacy or concerns over toxicity, but could, in theory, be based on other criteria. Almost without exception, such trials appear in regulatory submissions, in support of a flexible dosing posology, without adequate information (i.e. answers to the questions posed below) having been generated in phase II or other phase III studies. They are used effectively as a route of bypassing the investigation of dose-response. This is not valid.

Studies utilising 'flexible dosing' presume to test a real-life approach to dosing in some indications. However, from a regulatory point of view there are major methodological drawbacks to their use in establishing dose-response. Firstly, although a trial comparing a flexible dosing regimen with a control arm (say, concurrent placebo) might offer some evidence of efficacy, it will not provide information on optimal dose or, importantly, on how the regimen compares to a fixed dosing regimen. The regulator will generally be interested in whether the flexible dosing regimen offers any advantage to the lowest dose considered efficacious (often the starting dose). In particular, is the supposed benefit from exposure to higher doses worth any additional risk? For example, although a regimen allowing patients to find their optimal dose between 5 mg and 40 mg might be superior to placebo, it does not alone demonstrate superior efficacy to maintaining all patients at a dose of 5 mg. It is sometimes argued that the very fact that patients experienced dose increases in a randomised (double-blind) trial implies that such dose increases were necessary, and indeed beneficial, in some patients, 'x patients obviously benefited from a dose increase because they received one'. Such an argument is not reasonable as such conclusions are complicated by the will of investigators to explore the treatment, their confidence in the treatment and, perhaps more importantly, by time on the treatment. Just because a patient responds to a regimen of 5–40 mg over 6 months despite apparently not responding to 5 mg for 1 month does not mean that a longer duration of treatment with 5 mg would not have been effective – the data are confounded by time.

Of course, including a flexible dose arm in a study also testing fixed-dose regimens will provide precisely the information of interest and might be simpler than alternative strategies aimed at investigating the benefits of dose increases (see Section 2.2.5 for an explanation of the benefits of re-randomisation). In the absence of an appropriate fixed-dose control arm, selecting a recommended starting dose and titration scheme based only on data from a flexible dosing regimen is not only complicated but may well lead to a dose being licensed that is higher than necessary for some patients.

The complications with interpreting data from flexible dose studies are not limited to efficacy. The regulatory assessment of benefit–risk across doses of a particular medicine must also consider adverse experiences recorded. In studies employing a flexible dosing regimen, the time on treatment at lower doses will frequently be limited compared to higher doses. Furthermore, for many compounds, patients are likely to experience adverse events early in the treatment course. For these reasons it is clear that a comparison across doses of dose-response with regards to safety is likely to be biased in favour of demonstrating relatively fewer adverse events at higher doses. This will be particularly problematic if summaries by 'time on treatment' are used and if patients experiencing adverse events on lower doses are subsequently withdrawn from treatment. Of course, similar arguments apply to efficacy, in particular when patients are withdrawn due to lack of efficacy.

For all the reasons outlined above, a clinical trial programme based solely on studies examining flexible dosing is strongly discouraged.

2.5.4 Designing a dose-finding trial for a combination product

Fixed-dose combination products can offer clear benefits in terms of improvements in risk–benefit and in compliance compared with the administration of multiple single agents and therefore have a place in the therapeutic armoury [33].

Requirements for dose-response data will depend on the therapeutic rationale for the combination. If two products have completely different modes of action it is frequently desirable that the combination includes the therapeutic dose levels of each of the licensed components. In this case, further dose-finding work is unnecessary providing that the increase in risk is not of sufficient magnitude to offset any increased benefit. Alternatively, it may be that two subtherapeutic doses are combined in an attempt to achieve an acceptable level of efficacy, perhaps similar to that associated with either component administered individually, but with reduced risk. Here there is, clearly, a greater requirement for exploration of suitable combinations of doses. Again, pairwise comparisons traditionally form the basis of analysing such trials.

However, here the trade-off between sample size and statistical power is of even greater concern than for monotherapy, as the number of groups, and hence the number of potential comparisons, is potentially large. For example, two nonzero dose levels of each treatment give four possible combinations, leading to a trial of five treatment arms, potentially more, depending on the manner in which placebo is incorporated (i.e. whether doses of monotherapy are included). The study might soon become too large to power the relevant pairwise comparisons adequately and, as stated above, decision making based on nonsignificant differences is risky from the sponsor's point of view and highly undesirable from the point of view of the regulator. An alternative approach is to pool data on each dose of each component in turn and assess the dose-response for each component separately. This may decrease the number of subjects required in order to generate statistically persuasive results, but it is considerably more complicated to interpret as the results observed are conditional on the dose of the other component. For example, while it might appear that the dose-response for component A is linear, the interpretation is complicated by the possible interactions with each dose level of component B. A preferable alternative is a response-surface analysis [34]. Given sufficient precision to identify the most appropriate combination of doses, or to exclude differences of clinical importance between lower dose and higher dose combinations, this would usually be a welcome alternative.

2.5.5   Use of 'adaptive designs' in dose-response

2.5.5.1   What is an 'adaptive' design and why might it be useful?

The terms 'adaptive design' and 'flexible design' do not yet have one universally accepted definition. Included in these umbrella terms are group sequential trials and trials employing sample size reassessment in addition to trials that, for example, change an inclusion criteria or withdraw a dosage arm based on unblinded interim information.

It is not only the definition of these studies that is unclear; there are few precedents for their regulatory acceptability. An exception to this is the use of properly controlled and implemented group sequential methods, predominantly used in phase III to provide confirmatory evidence of efficacy, for which there is both ethical need and regulatory precedent. In addition, some modifications to double-blind trials in the absence of interim information do not, generally, raise concerns over the inflation of type I error or the reliability of the data ultimately generated. A personal perspective, which is shared by other EU regulatory statisticians, is that the data from the majority of trials that make major design modifications, e.g. changing inclusion/exclusion criteria or the randomisation ratio (including the special case of withdrawing a treatment arm) based on unblinded interim information, will not provide data sufficiently reliable to be regarded as confirmatory [35]. This, however, does not rule out the use of some design adaptions in early phase clinical development and, in particular, in the investigation of dose. As stated above, dose selection, in particular with regards to the choice of doses selected for a programme of confirmatory studies, is a frequent risk of the sponsor and not the regulator. Although choice of dose can be of crucial importance to the determination of a license, there is therefore scope for greater flexibility in the design of studies exploring dose-response and the consequent reliability of the data on which the sponsor's conclusions are based.

The 'flexible' designs of greatest interest to the sponsor are those that can provide quality evidence in a manner more timely and using fewer patients than might be the case using a 'standard' design. These would include trials employing adaptive randomisation, trials adding or withdrawing treatment arms (which can be considered as a special case of the former with the randomisation proportion set to zero) and phase II/III combinations. Other adaptions, including major modifications to trial inclusion/exclusion criteria or changes in endpoints, might be avoided by sponsors even in this dose-finding phase of development. While these trials can be properly handled from a statistical point of view [36, 37], the interpretation of the global null-hypothesis (the intersection of the individual null hypothesis) is at best complicated and at worst impossible. Establishing the homogeneity of the two (or more) phases of the trial is also complicated.

By way of explanation, the following is an example of a dose-finding trial where the use of a novel method was beneficial.

2.5.5.2 The ASTIN study

The ASTIN study [38] employed a sequential design within a Bayesian framework. The sequential nature of the study design allowed for accumulating data to influence the future conduct of the study and target the resources (by adapting the proportion of patients randomised to each treatment arm) in a manner considered more optimal than simple random allocation. The Bayesian nature of the design was used to formulate a framework within which assessments of the likelihood of futility or demonstration of efficacy could be made. These are both appealing aspects. The interesting design feature with regards to the trial being 'flexible' is the use of adaptive allocation for each patient to one of the 15 active treatment groups or placebo.

The reader is referred to the publication describing the study for full details of the trial design. In summary, patients were randomised either to placebo (at least 15 % of patients over the course of the trial) or the estimated optimal dose as given in the latest information about the dose-response. The optimal dose was that which minimised the expected variance of the response at the ED95 (the minimal dose for achieving near-maximal efficacy). A total of 966 patients were randomised and treated with between 20 and 40 patients on 12 of the treatment arms and between 80 and 150 on the three highest doses. Just fewer than 250 patients were treated on placebo. The trial ultimately provided good evidence of an insufficient effect via a relatively flat dose-response across the dose range examined. Although many aspects of this trial could be discussed, the feature of greatest interest is that the novel approach of allocation to treatment permitted more doses to be included in the study, thus allowing conclusions to be drawn with some precision across a wide range of doses. It is reported that the 'standard' design would have required 1080 patients to have a similar power to detect the same targeted effect size including just three dose groups. This is not quite a fair comparison as ASTIN stopped early (a design feature that could have been incorporated under a frequentist framework); nevertheless, the advantages of this flexible approach, in terms of efficient use of patients, are clear. A word of caution, however, is needed as the conduct of this type of sequential monitoring is not feasible in all indications. Here, in acute stroke, a surrogate for outcome was defined such that the response could be observed (relatively) quickly, enabling the information to be used for patients subsequently recruited. This would not be an option in all therapeutic indications.

The completed study, given the demonstration of a flat dose-response curve, is unlikely ever to come before any regulatory authority as part of a regulatory submission. Nevertheless, it is worth commenting that, from the information about the study contained in the publication, the study design would seem, in my opinion, to be acceptable from a regulatory perspective. Hypothesising for a moment that the trial had identified two or three doses worthy of further study, the sponsor would presumably have initiated one or more phase III trials confirming the benefit of the chosen dose(s). This would be likely to form the basis of an acceptable submission. It is noted again that the sponsor has not attempted to define precisely the response to a given dose, but to define precisely the dose or range of doses likely to give a particular response.

Many related examples can be found under the framework of the continual re-assessment method (or its close relations) [39, 40] in dose-finding trials relating to cytotoxics. This approach is welcomed as a vast improvement over the standard '3 + 3' design [41, 42]. A lot of literature is available explaining the benefits of this more flexible approach in this particular indication. As highlighted by ASTIN, these can be generalised readily to certain other indications.

2.5.5.3 'Adaptive' trials as evidence of efficacy

It is clear that there is a place in the dose-finding phase of drug development for these 'adaptive' designs. An outstanding question is whether the trials offer the data that are just as reliable as data from a 'standard' design. This is considered from two angles. The sponsor will wish to make robust decisions on dose to enhance the likelihood of success in phase III and beyond. The EU regulator will often not have the opportunity to participate in the choice of dose but will be concerned with overall evidence for efficacy. The question is therefore whether trials with flexible designs can be used a supportive evidence of efficacy. The regulatory concern on this front is that accumulating data form the basis for changes to the ongoing trial conduct. This is not generally welcomed in confirmatory studies, where data from interim analyses should be carefully guarded from the sponsor and where modifications to the trial, other than stopping the trial in the event of efficacy being demonstrated or futility, are rare. In short, confirmatory evidence of efficacy should be statistically valid (controlled type I error), should be able to provide correct and readily interpretable estimates of effect with associated confidence limits (or equivalent) and, in the case of flexible designs, should be able to demonstrate that the knowledge of accumulating efficacy data has not influenced the trial results. If these conditions cannot be met, then the evidence of efficacy provided from the 'flexible' design will be given less weight than data from a trial clearly free from such concerns.

Of particular note are so-called phase II/III combination trials. The acceptability from a regulatory perspective of such trials will depend on their objective: in particular, whether the aim of the trial is to provide confirmatory evidence of efficacy or to provide evidence of dose-response plus supportive evidence of efficacy, with confirmatory evidence of efficacy to be verified independently. The latter scenario is the subject of this chapter and such phase II/III combination trials will be welcomed if the result is increased information on dose-response compared with that which might otherwise be available. Providing a single phase II/III combination that first addresses dose and subsequently attempts to provide the only confirmatory evidence of efficacy is unlikely to be accepted.

2.6 Discussion

It is clear that the dose of a pharmaceutical intervention is of paramount importance with regards to the likelihood of observing the desirable benefits of treatment as well as the undesirable risks. It is also clear that, as patients and treatment episodes differ, the population-based approach of clinical trials does not provide complete information on dose-response for any given patient. It is appropriate therefore to address the quantity and quality of data on dose that are required in a regulatory submission. Although it is difficult to give advice on regulatory requirements for the extent of data on dose, some guidance is given in ICH E4 and a good rule of thumb is to provide compelling data on any aspects of the proposed posology that are not widely accepted from the disease under study, previous experience with the medicine in question or biological plausibility. This may not only relate to the dose of the particular intervention but also to the duration of treatment and how dosing might be modified in the event of a response, lack of response or an unacceptable adverse experience. In Europe, specific guidance on requirements for individual development programmes can be obtained via the European Medicines Agency (EMEA) or individual member states. In the USA, the Food and Drug Administration (FDA) perform a similar role.

The benefits of a comprehensive dossier on dose-response may not only be restricted to an increased likelihood of obtaining a positive opinion from the regulator but may assist in achieving the desired posology (SPC, see Section 4.2), and also in achieving a similar licence worldwide. While it is possible that regulators, physicians and sponsor personnel may disagree over interpretation of dose-response data, it is much more likely that they would disagree in the absence of such data. Comprehensive data on dose-response may also help with future variations to the initial licence and in helping regulatory decision making in the event that an unacceptable level of risk is observed postmarketing. If this means that the product can remain on the market rather than face withdrawal or damaging alterations to the product literature, the sponsor may benefit from providing these additional data during the prelicensure phase of the product life-cycle. Importantly, the probability that an individual patient can find a dose that is 'optimal' is increased.

Of course, regulators appreciate that there are costs in terms of time and money in providing any data and that providing information over and above that necessary to obtain an initial product licence will not be appealing. Indeed, it is accepted that in many indications the resource spent on more precise determination of, for example, the optimal treatment duration and the minimum effective dose would be wasted. It is argued, however, that avoiding such costs early in development will, in other situations, be a false economy. Identifying these latter scenarios is far from straightforward and the only solace offered is that regulators in the EU are open to discussions on early phases of drug development in addition to studies intended to provide confirmatory evidence of efficacy (such interactions with FDA occur as a matter of course). The advantages of speaking to the regulator are not only that those reviewing the dossier can comment on what it might need to contain, but the discussions provide an independent view on the data generated up to that point. Frequently, regulators see clinical trial programmes that need the drug to be highly efficacious and with a clear dose-response in order for the programme to be successful. The source of the sponsor's optimism is often not evident and the requests for further data to be generated, while appearing to be a regulator's pedantry, are simply in place to maximise the chances that the potential benefits of a product can be seen.

The choice of clinical trial design highlights nicely the contradiction of minimising cost and maximising information. Section 2.2.5 discussed the issue of dose increases in nonresponders while Section 2.2.6 discussed the confirmation that long-term treatment is worthwhile. Optimal data on both of these issues would be derived from re-randomisations, which add time to the trial duration and potentially warrant an increase in patient numbers. The question for sponsors to address (with the help of the regulator, should the sponsor desire) is whether or not the costs in providing such data are outweighed by the benefits brought in terms of achieving the desired product licence in the event of convincing results. It is likely that Section 4.2 of the SPC will continue to include a greater level of detail as regulatory interest in the wider questions on 'dose' increase. It is expected that regulators will become more and more interested in having data-driven answers to those aspects of the posology that are not self-evident.

The increased importance of statisticians in the pharmaceutical industry coupled with relatively recent developments in clinical trial methodology (at least an increased willingness to try existing methodology) appears to increase the opportunities for sponsors to provide data on dose-response in a more resource-efficient manner. As demonstrated by ASTIN, sufficient outlay 'up-front' might help save money in the future, particularly if it is established that the product in question is likely to be inefficacious or with an unacceptable side-effect profile. In this case the required sample size and cost for phase III could, of course, be zero. Such approaches appear to be welcomed by the regulators, particularly if they lead to a more precise determination of dose-response or the investigation of aspects relating to dose that would otherwise need to be determined in the absence of data. However, it is not only the pharmaceutical industry statisticians and their organisations that should continually strive for improvement. The regulatory statisticians must be open to new ideas and must be strict on applications in which decisions relating to posology are made on the basis of unreliable data, influencing and educating their medical colleagues accordingly.

It is worth ending with a reminder that data on dose-response is not simply a regulatory hurdle to be cleared in order to enter phase III of drug development. Comprehensive data on important aspects of the posology will increase the likelihood of regulatory success and, crucially, increase the likelihood that the product is ultimately beneficial for patients.

References

1. ICH Topic E4 Step 5. Note for guidance on dose response information to support drug registration (CPMP/ICH/378/95), www.emea.eu.int.
2. R. Temple (1996) The clinical pharmacologist in drug regulation: the US perspective. *Br. J. Clin. Pharmacology*, **42**(8), 73–80.
3. A. Breckenridge (1996) A clinical pharmacologist's view of drug toxicity. *Br. J. Clin. Pharmacology*, **42**(1), 59–62.
4. J. DiMasi, R.W. Hansen and H.G. Grabowski (2003) The price of innovation: new estimates of drug development costs. *J. Health Economy*, **22**, 141–85.
5. A.S. Relman and M. Angell (2002) America's other drug problem. *The New Republic*, **16**, 27–41.
6. Public Citizen (2002) *America's Other Drug Problem: A Briefing Book on the Rx Drug Debate*, Public Citizen, Washington DC.
7. J. DiMasi, R.W. Hansen and H.G. Grabowski (2004) Assessing Claims about the cost of new drug development: a critique of the Public Citizen and TB Alliance Reports. www.csdd.tufts.edu.
8. T. Hubbard and J. Love (2004) A new trade framework for global healthcare *R&D*. *PLoS Biology*, **2**(2), 147–150.
9. M.D. Rawlins (2004) Nature Reviews, Drug Discovery April 2004 doi:10.1038/nrd1347.
10. M. Dickson and J.P. Gagnon (2004) Key factors in the rising cost of new drug discovery and development. *Nature Reviews: Drug Discovery*, **3**, 417–29.
11. www.emea.eu.int for reports of CHMP deliberations.
12. ICH Topic E4 Step 5. Note for guidance on population exposure, The extent of population exposure to assess clinical safety (CPMP/ICH/375/95) www.emea.eu.int.
13. House of Commons Health Committee (2005) The influence of the pharmaceutical industry. Fourth report of session 2004–5. Stationery Office, London.
14. Directive 2001/83/EC of the European Parliament and of the Council of 6 November 2001 on the Community code relating to medicinal products for human use. Official Journal L 311, 28/11/2001 P. 0067 – 0128, 2001.
15. Directive 2002/98/EC of the European Parliament and of the Council of 27 January 2003 setting standards of quality processing storage safety for the collection, testing, distribution of human blood and blood components and amending Directive 2001/83/EC. Official Journal L 033, 08/02/2003 P. 0030 – 0040, 2003.

16. Commission Directive 2003/63/EC of 25 June 2003 amending Directive 2001/83/EC of the European Parliament and of the 'C.

17. Directive 2004/24/EC of the European Parliament and Directive 2001/83/EC on the Community code relating to medicinal products for human use of the Council of 31 March 2004 and amending as regards traditional herbal medicinal products. Official Journal L 136, 30/04/2004 P. 0085 – 0090, 2004.

18. Directive 2004/27/EC of the European Parliament and of the Council of 31 March 2004 and amending Directive 2001/83/EC on the Community code relating to medicinal products for human use. Official Journal L 136, 30/04/2004 P. 0034 – 0057, 2004.

19. CHMP/2330/99 Points to Consider on 'a, www.emea.eu.int.

20. J. Wittes (1994) Introduction: from clinical trials to clinical practice – four papers from a plenary session. *Controlled Clin. Trials*, **15**, 5–6.

21. H. Bloomfield Rubins (1994) From clinical trials to clinical practice – generalizing from participant to patient. *Controlled Clin. Trials*, **15**, 7–10.

22. C.E. Davis (1994) Generalizing from clinical trials. *Controlled Clin. Trials*, **15**, 11–14.

23. K.R. Bailey (1994) Generalizing the results of randomized clinical trials. *Controlled Clin. Trials*, **15**, 15–23.

24. D. Cowan and J. Wittes (1994) Intercept studies, clinical trials and cluster experiments: to whom can we extrapolate? *Controlled Clin. Trials*, **15**, 24–9.

25. S.J. Senn, J. Lillienthal, F. Patalano and D. Till (1997) An incomplete block cross-over in asthma: a case study in collaboration, in *Cross-over Clinical Trials* (eds J. Vollmar and L. Hothorn), Fischer, Stuttgart, pp. 3–26.

26. D. Machin, S. Day and S. Green (eds) (2004) *Textbook of Clinical Trials*, John Wiley & Sons, Ltd, Chichester and New York.

27. C. Redman and T. Colton (eds) (2001) *Biostatistics in Clinical Trials*, John Wiley & Sons, Ltd, Chichester and New York.

28. D.A. Grimes and K.F. Schulz (2005) Multiplicity in randomised trials. I: endpoints and treatments. *Lancet*, **365**, 1591–5.

29. D.A. Grimes and K.F. Schulz (2005) Multiplicity in randomised trials. II: subgroup and interim analyses. *Lancet*, **365**, 1657–61.

30. ICH Topic E9 Step 4. Note for guidance on statistical principles for clinical trials (CPMP/ICH/363/96), www.emea.eu.int.

31. S. Senn (ed.) (2002) *Cross-over Trials in Clinical Research*, John Wiley & Sons, Ltd, Chichester and New York.

32. S.J. Senn, J. Lillienthal, F. Patalano and D. Till (1997) An incomplete blocks cross-over in asthma: a case study in collaboration, in *Cross-over Clinical Trials* (eds J. Vollmar and L. Hothorn), Fischer, Stuttgart, 3–26.

33. CHMP/EWP/240/95. Note for guidance on fixed combination medicinal products, www.emea.eu.int.

34. R.H. Myers and D.C. Montgomery (eds) (1995) *Response Surface Methodology*, John Wiley & Sons, Ltd, New York.

35. Note for guidance on methodological issues in confirmatory clinical trials with flexible design and analysis plan (Manuscript in preparation), www.emea.eu.int.

36. H.H. Muller and H. Schafer (2004) A general statistical principle for changing a design any time during the course of a trial. *Statistics in Medicine*, **23**(16), 2497–508.

37. P. Bauer and K. Kohne (1994) Evaluation of experiments with adaptive interim analyses. *Biometrics*, **50**, 1029–41.

38. M. Krams, K.R. Lees, W. Hacke, A.P. Grieve, J.M. Orgogozo and G.A. Ford (2003) ASTIN Study Investigators. Acute stroke therapy by inhibition of neutrophils (ASTIN): an adaptive dose-response study of UK-279, 276 in acute ischemic stroke. *Stroke*, **34**(11), 2543–8.
39. J. Whitehead, S. Patterson, D. Webber, S. Francis and Y. Zhou (2001) Easy-to-implement, Bayesian methods for dose-escalation studies in healthy volunteers. *Biostatistics*, **2**, 47–61.
40. Y. Zhou and J. Whitehead (2003) Practical implementation of bayesian dose-escalation procedures. *Drug Information J.*, **37**, 45–59.
41. J. O'Quigley and M. Pepe and L. Fisher (1990) Continual reassessment method: a practical design for phase I clinical trials in cancer. *Biometrics*, **46**(1), 33–48.
42. B.E. Storer (1989) Design and analysis of phase I clinical trials. *Biometrics*, **45**(3), 925–37.

Part II
Algorithm-Based Approaches

3

Traditional and modified algorithm-based designs for phase I cancer clinical trials

Weichung Joe Shih and Yong Lin

Department of Biostatistics, School of Public Health, University of Medicine and Dentistry of New Jersey, Piscataway, New Jersey, USA, and Division of Biometrics, The Cancer Institute of New Jersey, University of Medicine and Dentistry of New Jersey, New Brunswick, New Jersey, USA

3.1 Introduction

As stated before, the main goals of a phase I cancer clinical trial are to find the maximum tolerated dose (MTD) of a drug for a specific mode of administration and to characterize the most frequent and dose-limiting toxicities (DLT) [1]. The highest possible dose is sought, since the benefit of the new treatment is believed to increase with dose. The MTD is often defined as the highest dose level at which some target (say γ) per cent of patients experience DLT. The recommended phase II dose level is usually either the MTD or one dose level below the MTD [2].

Prior to the enrollment of patients in a trial, the notion of dose-limiting toxicity is specifically defined. Usually in the United States, the NCI (National Cancer Institute) common toxicity criteria is used. The DLT is defined as a group of toxicities of grade 3 or higher, depending on the haematologic and nonhaematologic toxicities, where the

Statistical Methods for Dose-Finding Experiments Edited by S. Chevret
© 2006 John Wiley & Sons, Ltd

grades are defined as follows: grade 0, no toxicity; grade 1, mild toxicity; grade 2, moderate toxicity; grade 3, severe toxicity; and grade 4, life-threatening toxicity.

Phase I cancer clinical trial designs begin with the selection of a starting dose based on animal studies, usually one-tenth of the lethal dose in mice or one-third toxic low dose in dogs, or based on the information from individual drugs if a combination of several drugs that have toxicity information are used in the trial. The subsequent dose levels in algorithm-based designs usually follow a modified Fibonacci scheme, such as the dose sequence 1.0, 2.0, 3.3, 5.0, 7.0, 9.0, 12.0, 16.0 (dose increments of 100 %, 65 %, 52 %, 40 %, 29 %, 33 %, 33 %), with early doses based on large dose increments that get smaller for higher doses [3].

Despite the fact that the traditional method for dose escalation has been criticized for its tendency to include too many patients at suboptimal dose levels and give a poor estimate of the MTD [4,5], it is still widely used in practice because of its algorithm-based simplicity in logistics for the clinical investigators to carry out, compared to, say, the various model-based CRMs (continual reassessment methods) [4,5].

Lin and Shih [6,7] discussed statistical properties of the traditional and modified algorithm-based designs in a general setting: $A + B$ designs with or without dose de-escalation, which include the popular traditional $3 + 3$ design as a special case. In this chapter we summarize and give examples to illustrate the key statistical properties of these traditional and modified $A + B$ designs. The statistical properties include: (a) the probability of a dose being chosen as the MTD (maximum tolerated dose); (b) the expected number of patients at each dose level; (c) the attained target toxicity level (the expected dose-limiting toxicity at the MTD found through the algorithm-based design); (d) the expected number of toxicity at each dose level; (e) the expected overall toxicity in a trial. Exact formulae for the corresponding statistical quantities are derived, and a computer program to calculate these statistical quantities is provided in the authors' web site at http://www2.umdnj.edu/~linyo. These statistical properties describe the operating characteristics of these designs, and are important for clinicians who use these algorithm-based designs for their phase I cancer clinical trials to gain insights of the design before starting the trial.

3.2   Notation and convention

In the sequel, A, B, C, D, E and F are integers. We use the notation A/B to mean 'A toxicity incidences out of B patients' and $> A/B$ to mean 'more than A toxicity incidences out of B patients'. Similarly, the notation $A/B + \leq C/D$ means 'A toxicity incidences in the first cohort of B patients and no more than C toxicity incidences in the second cohort or both cohorts of D patients' (depending on the specific design). We will also follow the convention that if the lower bound is greater than the upper bound in a summation or product sign, the corresponding summation or product term will not be included in the formula or equation. For example, $\sum_{i=2}^{1} a(i)$ or $\prod_{i=1}^{0} b(i)$ will be deleted.

For designs where the starting dose is the lowest dose level in the study protocol, we assume that there are n predefined doses with increasing levels of $i = 1$ to n.

For designs where the starting dose is somewhere in the middle of the planned dose levels, we assume that there are $m + n$ predefined doses with increasing levels of $i = -m, \ldots, -2, -1, 1, 2, \ldots, n$. Let p_i be the probability of observing an incidence of DLT at dose level i.

For the algorithm-based designs described here, if dose-escalation is still indicated at the highest dose level n, then the MTD is at or above the highest dose level. If the trial stops at the lowest dose, then the MTD is below the lowest dose level. In either of these two cases, the MTD is not determined from the trial.

3.3   Traditional algorithm-based designs

3.3.1   Traditional $A + B$ design without dose de-escalation

The traditional $A + B$ designs without dose de-escalation can be described as follows. Groups of A patients will be entered at dose level i. If $< C/A$ patients have DLT, then the dose will be escalated to the next dose level $i + 1$. If $> D/A$ (where $D \geq C$) patients have DLT, then the previous dose $i - 1$ will be considered the MTD. If $\geq C/A$ but $\leq D/A$ patients have DLT, B more patients will be treated at this dose level i. If no more than E (where $E \geq D$) of the total of $A + B$ patients have DLT, then the dose will be escalated. If more than E of the total of $A + B$ patients have DLT, then the previous dose $i - 1$ will be considered the MTD. Hence this is generally called the '$A + B$' design, for which the traditional '3 + 3' is a special case (see reference [3]). A diagram for the design is shown in Figure 3.1 to assist the understanding.

The traditional $3 + 3$ design without dose de-escalation is a special case of the general $A + B$ design with $A = B = 3$ and $C = D = E = 1$.

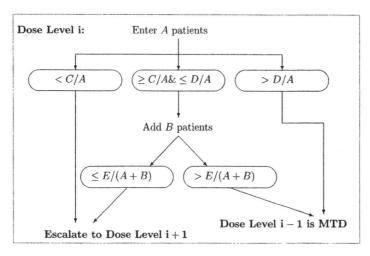

Figure 3.1   Escalation scheme for $A + B$ design without dose de-escalation.

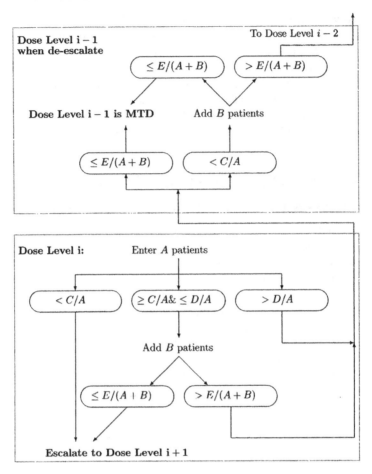

Figure 3.2   Escalation scheme for $A + B$ design with dose de-escalation.

3.3.2   Traditional $A + B$ design with dose de-escalation

The traditional $A + B$ designs with dose de-escalation is basically similar to the previous design, but permits more patients to be treated at a lower dose (i.e. dose de-escalation) when excessive DLT incidences occur at the current dose level. Contrasting Figure 3.2 with Figure 3.1, the dose de-escalation occurs when $> D/A$ (where $D \geq C$) or $> E/(A + B)$ patients have DLT at dose level i; then B more patients will be treated at dose level $i - 1$, provided that only A patients have been previously treated at this prior dose. If more than A patients have already been treated previously, then dose $i - 1$ is the MTD. Of course, the de-escalation may continue to dose level $i - 2$ and so on if necessary.

In summary, for this design, the MTD is the dose level at which $\leq E/(A + B)$ patients experience DLT and $> D/A$ or ($\geq C/A$ and $\leq D/A$) $+ > E/(A + B)$

patients treated with the next higher dose have DLT. Again, the traditional $3 + 3$ design with dose de-escalation is a special case of the traditional $A + B$ design with $A = B = 3$ and $C = D = E = 1$.

3.4 Modified algorithm-based designs

Although the traditional $A + B$ design is quite a general family, it still does not include some important variants of the algorithm-based designs that we often encountered in many phase I cancer clinical trials. As pointed out in reference [8], '...phase I trials should consider alternative designs that increase a patient's chance to receive a therapeutic dose of an agent and also provide a better dose estimate for phase II trials'. Lin and Shih [7] introduced modifications of the traditional $A + B$ design and derived exact formulae for the important operating characteristics of these designs. These modified designs provide clinicians much needed alternatives to the traditional design.

Notice that in the traditional $A + B$ design, the previous lower dose level is always declared as the MTD. The current dose has no chance at all to be declared as the MTD, which is conservative and is a waste of the already scarce information for phase I cancer trials. Hence the first modification is to allow the investigator to declare a current dose level as the MTD (named the 'M1 $A + B$ design'). Next, in the traditional $A + B$ design, the starting dose is always the lowest dose level in the study protocol, which is also conservative. The second modification is, in addition to the above M1, to start somewhere in the middle of the prespecified dose levels with escalation or de-escalation in the sequence of treatment (named the 'M2 $A + B$ design'). This design has the advantage of reaching the MTD faster, and when the starting dose is too toxic, the dose can be de-escalated to avoid stopping the trial or halting it for protocol amendment. The third modification is to have a two-stage process. In the first stage, only one or two patients are treated per dose level in an increasing dose scheme until the first sign of toxicity incidence (either minor or DLT) is observed, at which time the second stage will begin. (The reason for defining either minor or DLT as the endpoint here is because the starting dose in these trials, for which this design is particularly useful, is often very conservative.) In the second stage, the M1 $A + B$ design is applied with possible dose de-escalation. This is named the 'M3 $A + B$ design' (see Section 3.4.3 for a precise definition of the design).

3.4.1 M1 $A + B$ design

3.4.1.1 M1 $A + B$ design without dose de-escalation

In this design, groups of A patients will be entered at dose level i. If $< C/A$ patients have DLT, then the dose will be escalated to the next dose level $i + 1$. If $> D/A$ (where $D \geq C$) patients have DLT, then the previous dose $i - 1$ will be considered the MTD. If $\geq C/A$ but $\leq D/A$ patients have DLT, B more patients will be treated

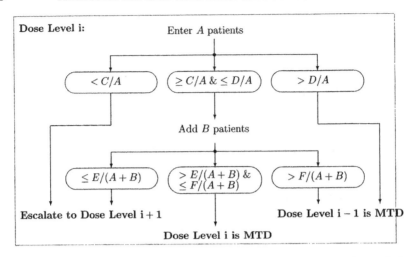

Figure 3.3   Escalation scheme for M1 $A + B$ design without dose de-escalation.

at this dose level i. If no more than E (where $E \geq D$) of the total of $A + B$ patients have DLT, then the dose will be escalated. If more than E but no more than F (where $F \geq E$) of the total of $A + B$ patients have DLT, then the current dose i will be considered the MTD; otherwise the previous dose $i - 1$ will be considered the MTD. A diagram for the design is shown in Figure 3.3 to assist the understanding.

The traditional $A + B$ design without dose de-escalation in Section 3.3.1 is a special case here with $E = F$.

3.4.1.2   M1 $A + B$ design with dose de-escalation

The M1 $A + B$ design with dose de-escalation is basically similar to the previous design, but permits more patients to be treated at a lower dose (i.e. dose de-escalation) when excessive DLT incidences occur at the current dose level. Contrasting Figure 3.4 with Figure 3.3, the dose de-escalation occurs when $> D/A$ (where $D \geq C$) or $> F/(A + B)$ patients have DLT at dose level i; then B more patients will be treated at dose level $i - 1$, provided that only A patients have been previously treated at this prior dose. If more than A patients have already been treated previously, then dose $i - 1$ is the MTD. Of course, the de-escalation may continue to dose level $i - 2$ and so on if necessary.

In summary, for this design, the MTD is the dose level at which ($\geq C/A$ and $\leq D/A$) + ($> E/(A + B)$ and $\leq F/(A + B)$) patients have DLT, or $\leq E/(A + B)$ patients have DLT, but at the next higher dose level $> D/A$ or ($\geq C/A$ and $\leq D/A$) + $> F/(A + B)$ patients have DLT.

The traditional $A + B$ design with dose de-escalation in Section 3.3.2 is a special case here with $E = F$.

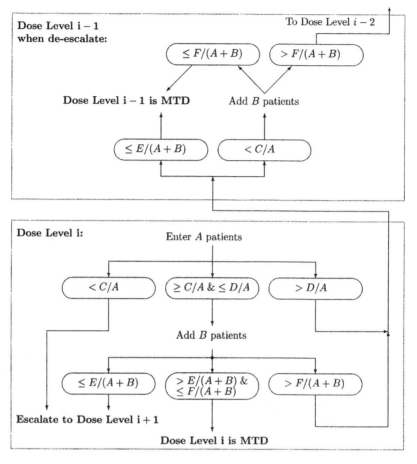

Figure 3.4   Escalation scheme for M1 $A + B$ or M2 $A + B$ design with dose de-escalation.

3.4.2   M2 $A + B$ design

The M2 $A + B$ design (with dose de-escalation and the starting dose is not the lowest dose) is almost the same as the M1 $A + B$ design with dose de-escalation at any dose level $i > 0$, as shown in Figure 3.4, except that it de-escalates from the starting dose (dose level 1). Figure 3.5 shows the diagram of the design at a dose level $i < 0$.

It is important to note that in all the designs with dose de-escalation, we require that in order for a dose to be declared as the MTD, there have to be $A + B$ patients already treated at the dose level. This will make the estimation of the toxicity rate at the MTD more reliable. In many phase I studies, more patients will be entered at the dose level declared as the MTD to improve the estimation of the toxicity rate at the MTD.

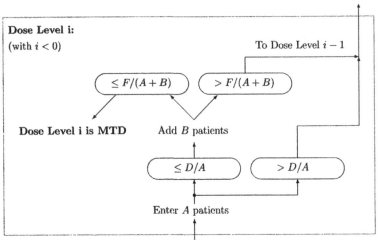

Figure 3.5 De-escalation scheme for M2 $A + B$ design with dose de-escalation when the starting dose is not the lowest dose.

3.4.3   M3 $A + B$ design

The goal of this design is to reach the MTD as quickly as possible when there is a low toxicity at the (very conservative, low) starting dose. The design uses only a cohort size of a ($a = 1$ or 2) until the first sign of toxicity occurs (either a minor toxicity or DLT) and then changes to the M1 $A + B$ design. In the following sections, we assume that the probabilities of toxicity (either minor or DLT) at each dose level to be

$$q_1, q_2, \ldots, q_n,$$

where $q_i \geq p_i$ for $i = 1, 2, \ldots, n$. We also assume that the first sign of toxicity occurs at dose level k, where $1 \leq k \leq n$.

3.4.3.1   M3 $A + B$ design without dose de-escalation

The escalation scheme at dose level k for this design without dose de-escalation is depicted in Figure 3.6. (The escalation scheme at dose level $> k$ for this design follows the previous Figure 3.3.)

3.4.3.2   M3 $A + B$ design with dose de-escalation

The de-escalation scheme at dose level $< k$ for this design is depicted in Figure 3.7, while the escalation scheme at dose level k follows Figure 3.6 and the escalation scheme at dose level $> k$ follows Figure 3.4.

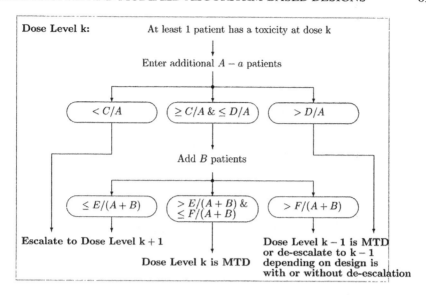

Figure 3.6   Escalation scheme for M3 $A + B$ design.

3.5   Probability of a dose being chosen as the MTD

In this section, we present the probability of a dose being chosen as the MTD for the modified design. The details of the proofs or derivations can be found in reference [7].

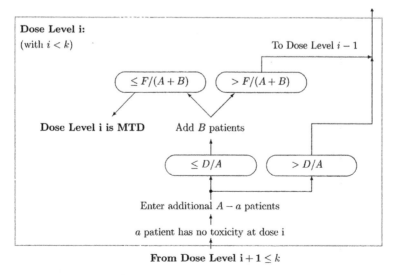

Figure 3.7   De-escalation scheme for M3 $A + B$ design.

3.5.1   M1 $A + B$ design

3.5.1.1   M1 $A + B$ without dose de-escalation

For $1 \leq j \leq n$, let

$$P_0^j = \sum_{k=0}^{C-1} \binom{A}{k} p_j^k (1 - p_j)^{A-k},$$

$$Q_0^j = \sum_{k=C}^{D} \sum_{m=0}^{E-k} \binom{A}{k} p_j^k (1 - p_j)^{A-k} \binom{B}{m} p_j^m (1 - p_j)^{B-m}$$

and

$$R_0^j = \sum_{k=C}^{D} \sum_{m=E-k+1}^{F-k} \binom{A}{k} p_j^k (1 - p_j)^{A-k} \binom{B}{m} p_j^m (1 - p_j)^{B-m}.$$

Then, for $1 \leq i < n$,

$$P(\text{MTD} = \text{dose } i) = \left[\prod_{j=1}^{i-1} \left(P_0^j + Q_0^j \right) \right] \left[R_0^i + \left(P_0^i + Q_0^i \right) \right.$$
$$\left. \left(1 - P_0^{i+1} - Q_0^{i+1} - R_0^{i+1} \right) \right],$$

$$P(\text{MTD} = \text{dose } n) = \left[\prod_{j=1}^{n-1} \left(P_0^j + Q_0^j \right) \right] R_0^n,$$

$$P(\text{MTD} < \text{dose} 1) = 1 - P_0^1 - Q_0^1 - R_0^1$$

and

$$P(\text{MTD} > \text{dose } n) = \prod_{j=1}^{n} \left(P_0^j + Q_0^j \right).$$

3.5.1.2   M1 $A + B$ design with dose de-escalation

For $1 \leq j \leq n$, let P_0^j, Q_0^j and R_0^j be defined as in Section 3.5.1.1. In addition, let

$$P_1^j = \sum_{k=C}^{D} \binom{A}{k} p_j^k (1 - p_j)^{A-k},$$

$$Q_1^j = \sum_{k=0}^{C-1} \sum_{m=0}^{F-k} \binom{A}{k} p_j^k (1 - p_j)^{A-k} \binom{B}{m} p_j^m (1 - p_j)^{B-m}$$

and

$$Q_2^j = \sum_{k=0}^{C-1} \sum_{m=F+1-k}^{B} \binom{A}{k} p_j^k (1 - p_j)^{A-k} \binom{B}{m} p_j^m (1 - p_j)^{B-m}.$$

Then, for $1 \leq i \leq n$,

$$P(\text{MTD} = \text{dose } i) = R_0^i \prod_{j=1}^{i-1} (P_0^j + Q_0^j) + \sum_{k=i+1}^{n} \left[\prod_{j=1}^{i-1} \left(P_0^j + Q_0^j \right) \right] (Q_0^i + Q_1^i)$$

$$\times \left(\prod_{j=i+1}^{k-1} Q_2^j \right) (1 - P_0^k - Q_0^k - R_0^k),$$

$$P(\text{MTD} < \text{dose } 1) = \sum_{k=1}^{n} \left(\prod_{j=1}^{k-1} Q_2^j \right) (1 - P_0^k - Q_0^k - R_0^k)$$

and

$$P(\text{MTD} > \text{dose } n) = \prod_{j=1}^{n} \left(P_0^j + Q_0^j \right).$$

3.5.2 M2 $A + B$ design

In addition to the definitions in the previous section, let

$$\tilde{Q}_2^j = \sum_{k=0}^{D} \sum_{m=F+1-k}^{B} \binom{A}{k} p_j^k (1 - p_j)^{A-k} \binom{B}{m} p_j^m (1 - p_j)^{B-m},$$

$$\tilde{Q}_3^j = \sum_{k=0}^{D} \sum_{m=0}^{F-k} \binom{A}{k} p_j^k (1 - p_j)^{A-k} \binom{B}{m} p_j^m (1 - p_j)^{B-m}.$$

Then, for $1 \leq i \leq n$, we have

$$P(\text{MTD} = \text{dose } i) = R_0^i \prod_{j=1}^{i-1} \left(P_0^j + Q_0^j \right) + \sum_{k=i+1}^{n} \left[\prod_{j=1}^{i-1} (P_0^j + Q_0^j) \right]$$

$$\times (Q_0^i + Q_1^i) \left(\prod_{j=i+1}^{k-1} Q_2^j \right) (1 - P_0^k - Q_0^k - R_0^k)$$

and

$$P(\text{MTD} > \text{dose } n) = \prod_{j=1}^{n} (P_0^j + Q_0^j).$$

These are the same as those in the M1 $A + B$ design with dose de-escalation. For the dose level i with $-m \leq i \leq -1$, we have

$$P(\text{MTD} = \text{dose } i) = \sum_{k=1}^{n} \tilde{Q}_3^i \prod_{j=i+1}^{-1} (1 - \tilde{Q}_3^j) \left(\prod_{j=1}^{k-1} Q_2^j \right) (1 - P_0^k - Q_0^k - R_0^k)$$

and

$$P(\text{MTD} < \text{dose} - m) = \sum_{k=1}^{n} \prod_{j=-m}^{-1} \left(1 - \widetilde{Q}_3^j\right) \left(\prod_{j=1}^{k-1} Q_2^j\right) \left(1 - P_0^k - Q_0^k - R_0^k\right).$$

3.5.3   M3 $A + B$ design

3.5.3.1   M3 $A + B$ design without dose de-escalation

Furthermore, in this section, for $1 \leq j \leq n$, $\gamma \geq 0$ and $a \geq 0$, we let

$$P_{0,a}^{j,\gamma} = \sum_{k=0}^{C-\gamma-1} \binom{A-a}{k} p_j^k (1 - p_j)^{A-a-k},$$

$$Q_{0,a}^{j,\gamma} = \sum_{k=C-\gamma}^{D-\gamma} \sum_{m=0}^{E-\gamma-k} \binom{A-a}{k} p_j^k (1 - p_j)^{A-a-k} \binom{B}{m} p_j^m (1 - p_j)^{B-m},$$

$$R_{0,a}^{j,\gamma} = \sum_{k=C-\gamma}^{D-\gamma} \sum_{m=E-\gamma-k+1}^{F-\gamma-k} \binom{A-a}{k} p_j^k (1 - p_j)^{A-a-k} \binom{B}{m} p_j^m (1 - p_j)^{B-m},$$

$$S_a^j = \sum_{\alpha+\beta+\gamma=a, \beta+\gamma\geq 1} \binom{a}{\alpha\,\beta\,\gamma} (1 - q_j)^\alpha (q_j - p_j)^\beta p_j^\gamma \left(1 - P_{0,a}^{j,\gamma} - Q_{0,a}^{j,\gamma} - R_{0,a}^{j,\gamma}\right),$$

$$T_a^j = \sum_{\alpha+\beta+\gamma=a, \beta+\gamma\geq 1} \binom{a}{\alpha\,\beta\,\gamma} (1 - q_j)^\alpha (q_j - p_j)^\beta p_j^\gamma \left(P_{0,a}^{j,\gamma} + Q_{0,a}^{j,\gamma}\right)$$

and

$$U_a^j = \sum_{\alpha+\beta+\gamma=a, \beta+\gamma\geq 1} \binom{a}{\alpha\,\beta\,\gamma} (1 - q_j)^\alpha (q_j - p_j)^\beta p_j^\gamma R_{0,a}^{j,\gamma}.$$

Then, for $1 \leq i < n$,

$$P(\text{MTD} = \text{dose } i)$$

$$= \sum_{m=1}^{i-1} \prod_{j=1}^{m-1} (1 - q_j)^a T_a^m \prod_{j=m+1}^{i-1} \left(P_0^j + Q_0^j\right) \left[R_0^i + \left(P_0^i + Q_0^i\right)\right.$$

$$\times \left(1 - P_0^{i+1} - Q_0^{i+1} - R_0^{i+1}\right)\right] + \prod_{j=1}^{i-1} (1 - q_j)^a$$

$$\times \left[U_a^i + T_a^i \left(1 - P_0^{i+1} - Q_0^{i+1} - R_0^{i+1}\right)\right] + \prod_{j=1}^{i} (1 - q_j)^a S_a^{i+1},$$

$P(\text{MTD} = \text{dose } n)$

$$= \sum_{m=1}^{n-1} \prod_{j=1}^{m-1} (1 - q_j)^a T_a^m \prod_{j=m+1}^{i-1} \left(P_0^j + Q_0^j\right) R_0^n + \prod_{j=1}^{n-1} (1 - q_j)^a U_a^n,$$

$$P(\text{MTD} < \text{dose1}) = S_a^1$$

and

$$P(\text{MTD} > \text{dose} n) = \sum_{m=1}^{n} \prod_{j=1}^{m-1} (1 - q_j)^a T_a^m \prod_{j=m+1}^{n} \left(P_0^j + Q_0^j\right) + \prod_{j=1}^{n} (1 - q_j)^a.$$

3.5.3.2 M3 $A + B$ design with dose de-escalation

In this section, for $1 \leq j \leq n$, $\gamma \geq 0$ and $a \geq 0$, we further define

$$P_{1,a}^{j,\gamma} = \sum_{k=C-\gamma}^{D-\gamma} \binom{A-a}{k} p_j^k (1 - p_j)^{A-a-k},$$

$$Q_{1,a}^{j,\gamma} = \sum_{k=0}^{C-\gamma-1} \sum_{m=0}^{F-\gamma-k} \binom{A-a}{k} p_j^k (1 - p_j)^{A-a-k} \binom{B}{m} p_j^m (1 - p_j)^{B-m},$$

$$Q_{2,a}^{j,\gamma} = \sum_{k=0}^{C-\gamma-1} \sum_{m=F-\gamma+1-k}^{B} \binom{A-a}{k} p_j^k (1 - p_j)^{A-a-k} \binom{B}{m} p_j^m (1 - p_j)^{B-m},$$

$$\tilde{Q}_{2,a}^{j,\gamma} = \sum_{k=0}^{D-\gamma} \sum_{m=F-\gamma+1-k}^{B} \binom{A-a}{k} p_j^k (1 - p_j)^{A-a-k} \binom{B}{m} p_j^m (1 - p_j)^{B-m},$$

$$\tilde{Q}_{3,a}^{j,\gamma} = \sum_{k=0}^{D-\gamma} \sum_{m=0}^{F-\gamma-k} \binom{A-a}{k} p_j^k (1 - p_j)^{A-a-k} \binom{B}{m} p_j^m (1 - p_j)^{B-m},$$

$$V_a^j = \sum_{\alpha+\beta+\gamma=a,\ \beta+\gamma\geq1} \binom{a}{\alpha\ \beta\ \gamma} (1 - q_j)^\alpha (q_j - p_j)^\beta p_j^\gamma Q_{2,a}^{j,\gamma}$$

and

$$W_a^j = \sum_{\alpha+\beta+\gamma=a,\text{and}\ \beta+\gamma\geq1} \binom{a}{\alpha\ \beta\ \gamma} (1 - q_j)^\alpha (q_j - p_j)^\beta p_j^\gamma \left(Q_{0,a}^{j,\gamma} + Q_{1,a}^{j,\gamma}\right).$$

Then, for $1 \leq i \leq n$,

$P(\text{MTD} = \text{dose } i)$

$$= \sum_{k=i+1}^{n} \sum_{m=1}^{i-1} \prod_{j=1}^{m-1} (1 - q_j)^a T_a^m \left[\prod_{j=m+1}^{i-1} (P_0^j + Q_0^j) \right] (Q_0^i + Q_1^i) \left(\prod_{j=i+1}^{k-1} Q_2^j \right)$$

$$\times \left(1 - P_0^k - Q_0^k - R_0^k \right)$$

$$+ \sum_{m=1}^{i-1} \prod_{j=1}^{m-1} (1 - q_j)^a T_a^m \left[\prod_{j=m+1}^{i-1} (P_0^j + Q_0^j) \right] R_0^i$$

$$+ \sum_{k=i+1}^{n} \prod_{j=1}^{i-1} (1 - q_j)^a W_a^i \left(\prod_{j=i+1}^{k-1} Q_2^j \right) \left(1 - P_0^k - Q_0^k - R_0^k \right) + \prod_{j=1}^{i-1} (1 - q_j)^a U_a^i$$

$$+ \sum_{k=i+1}^{n} \sum_{m=i+1}^{k} \prod_{j=1}^{m-1} (1 - q_j)^a \widetilde{Q}_{3,a}^{i,0} \left[\prod_{j=i+1}^{m-1} \left(1 - \widetilde{Q}_{3,a}^{j,0} \right) \right] V_a^m \left(\prod_{j=m+1}^{k-1} Q_2^j \right)$$

$$\times \left(1 - P_0^k - Q_0^k - R_0^k \right)$$

$$+ \sum_{k=i+1}^{n} \prod_{j=1}^{k-1} (1 - q_j)^a \widetilde{Q}_{3,a}^{i,0} \left[\prod_{j=i+1}^{k-1} \left(1 - \widetilde{Q}_{3,a}^{j,0} \right) \right] S_a^k,$$

$P(\text{MTD} < \text{dose } 1)$

$$= \sum_{k=1}^{n} \sum_{m=1}^{k-1} \prod_{j=1}^{m-1} \left[(1 - q_j)^a \left(1 - \widetilde{Q}_{3,a}^{j,0} \right) \right] V_a^m \left(\prod_{j=m+1}^{k-1} Q_2^j \right) \left(1 - P_0^k - Q_0^k - R_0^k \right)$$

$$+ \sum_{k=1}^{n} \prod_{j=1}^{k-1} \left[(1 - q_j)^a \left(1 - \widetilde{Q}_{3,a}^{j,0} \right) \right] S_a^k$$

and

$$P(\text{MTD} > \text{dose } n) = \sum_{m=1}^{n} \prod_{j=1}^{m-1} (1 - q_j)^a T_a^m \prod_{j=m+1}^{n} (P_0^j + Q_0^j) + \prod_{j=1}^{n} (1 - q_j)^a.$$

3.6 Expected number of patients treated at each dose level

In planning a clinical trial, it is important to know the number of patients needed in the trial. However, for a sequential design, it is not possible to know in advance the exact number of patients in the trial. However, by knowing the probability of toxicity at each dose level, we can find the expected number of patients to be treated at each dose level and hence the expected number of patients in the trial.

In this section, for convenience, we will use the notation MTD = dose $n + 1$ to mean MTD > dose n, MTD = dose 0 to mean MTD < dose 1 and MTD = dose $-m - 1$ to mean MTD < dose $-m$.

3.6.1 M1 $A + B$ design

3.6.1.1 M1 $A + B$ design without dose de-escalation

For $1 \leq j \leq n$, let X_j be the number of patients to be treated at dose level j. Then

$$E(X_j) = \sum_{i=0}^{n+1} \sum_{s=i}^{i+1} E(X_j \mid \text{MTD} = \text{ dose } i \text{ and stop at dose } s)$$

$$\times P(\text{MTD} = \text{dose } i \text{ and stop at dose } s),$$

where, for $0 \leq i \leq n+1$ and $s = i$ or $i+1$,

$E(X_j \mid \text{MTD} = \text{dose } i\text{ and stop at dose } s)$

$$= \begin{cases} \dfrac{AP_0^j + (A+B)Q_0^j}{P_0^j + Q_0^j} & \text{if } j < i = s \leq n \text{ or} \\ & \qquad j \leq i = s - 1 < n \text{ or} \\ & \qquad j \leq i = s = n+1; \\ A + B & \text{if } j = i = s \leq n; \\ \dfrac{A\left(1 - P_0^j - P_1^j\right) + (A+B)\left(P_1^j - Q_0^j - R_0^j\right)}{1 - P_0^j - Q_0^j - R_0^j} & \text{if } j = i+1 = s \leq n; \\ 0 & \text{otherwise} \end{cases}$$

and

$P(\text{MTD} = \text{dose } i \text{ and stop at dose } s)$

$$= \begin{cases} \prod_{j=1}^{i-1}\left(P_0^j + Q_0^j\right)R_0^i & \text{if } i = s \leq n+1; \\ \prod_{j=1}^{i}\left(P_0^j + Q_0^j\right)\left(1 - P_0^{i+1} - Q_0^{i+1} - R_0^{i+1}\right) & \text{if } i = s - 1 < n, \end{cases}$$

where we set $R_0^{n+1} = 1$.

3.6.1.2 M1 $A + B$ design with dose de-escalation

For $1 \leq j \leq n$,

$$E(X_j) = \sum_{i=0}^{n} \sum_{k=i}^{n} E(X_j \mid \text{MTD} = \text{dose } i \text{ and stop escalation at dose } k)$$

$$\times P(\text{MTD} = \text{dose } i \text{ and stop escalation at dose } k)$$

$$+ E(X_j \mid \text{MTD} > \text{dose } n)P(\text{MTD} > \text{dose } n),$$

where, for $0 \leq i \leq n$ and $i \leq k \leq n$,

$E(X_j \mid \text{MTD} = \text{dose } i \text{ and stop escalation at dose } k)$

$$
= \begin{cases}
\dfrac{AP_0^j + (A+B)Q_0^j}{P_0^j + Q_0^j} & \text{if } j < i\,; \\[2mm]
A+B & \text{if } i \le j < k\,; \\[2mm]
\dfrac{A\left(1 - P_0^j - P_1^j\right) + (A+B)\left(P_1^j - Q_0^j - R_0^j\right)}{1 - P_0^j - Q_0^j - R_0^j} & \text{if } i < j = k\,; \\[2mm]
0 & \text{otherwise}\,,
\end{cases}
$$

$$
E(X_j \mid \text{MTD} > \text{dose } n) = \frac{AP_0^j + (A+B)Q_0^j}{P_0^j + Q_0^j}
$$

and

$P(\text{MTD} = \text{dose } i \text{ and stop escalation at dose } k)$

$$
= \begin{cases}
\left(\prod_{j=1}^{i-1}\left(P_0^j + Q_0^j\right)\right)\left(Q_0^i + Q_1^i\right)\left(\prod_{j=i+1}^{k-1} Q_2^j\right) \\
\quad \times \left(1 - P_0^k - Q_0^k - R_0^k\right), & \text{if } 1 \le i < k\,; \\[2mm]
R_0^i \prod_{j=1}^{i-1}\left(P_0^j + Q_0^j\right) & \text{if } i = k\,; \\[2mm]
\left(\prod_{j=1}^{k-1} Q_2^j\right)\left(1 - P_0^k - Q_0^k - R_0^k\right) & \text{if } i = 0 < k\,.
\end{cases}
$$

3.6.2 M2 $A + B$ design

For $j = -m, \ldots, -2, -1, 1, 2, \ldots, n$,

$$
\begin{aligned}
E(X_j) = {}& \sum_{i=-m-1}^{-1} \sum_{k=1}^{n} E(X_j \mid \text{MTD} = \text{dose } i \text{ and stop escalation at dose } k) \\
& \quad \times P(\text{MTD} = \text{dose } i \text{ and stop escalation at dose } k) \\
& + \sum_{i=1}^{n} \sum_{k=i}^{n} E(X_j \mid \text{MTD} = \text{dose } i \text{ and stop escalation at dose } k) \\
& \quad \times P(\text{MTD} = \text{dose } i \text{ and stop escalation at dose } k) \\
& + E(X_j \mid \text{MTD} > \text{dose } n) P(\text{MTD} > \text{dose } n)\,,
\end{aligned}
$$

where, for $-m \le j \le -1$, $-m-1 \le i \le n$ and $\max(1, i) \le k \le n$,

$E(X_j \mid \text{MTD} = \text{dose } i \text{ and stop escalation at dose } k)$

$$
= \begin{cases}
0 & \text{if } j < i\,; \\[2mm]
A+B & \text{if } j = i\,; \\[2mm]
\dfrac{A\left(1 - \widetilde{Q}_2^j - \widetilde{Q}_3^j\right) + (A+B)\widetilde{Q}_2^j}{1 - \widetilde{Q}_3^j} & \text{if } j > i\,,
\end{cases}
$$

for $1 \leq j \leq n$, $-m - 1 \leq i \leq n$ and $\max(1, i) \leq k \leq n$,

$E\left(X_j \mid \text{MTD} = \text{dose } i \text{ and stop escalation at dose } k\right)$

$$
= \begin{cases}
\dfrac{A P_0^j + (A + B) Q_0^j}{P_0^j + Q_0^j} & \text{if } j < i\,; \\[2ex]
A + B & \text{if } i \leq j < k\,; \\[2ex]
\dfrac{A(1 - P_0^j - P_1^j) + (A + B)(P_1^j - Q_0^j - R_0^j)}{1 - P_0^j - Q_0^j - R_0^j} & \text{if } j = k > i\,; \\[2ex]
0 & \text{otherwise}\,,
\end{cases}
$$

$$
E(X_j \mid \text{MTD} > \text{dose } n) = \dfrac{A P_0^j + (A + B) Q_0^j}{P_0^j + Q_0^j}
$$

and for $-m - 1 \leq i \leq n$ and $\max(1, i) \leq k \leq n$,

$P\,(\text{MTD} = \text{dose } i \text{ and stop escalation at dose } k)$

$$
= \begin{cases}
R_0^i \prod_{j=1}^{i-1} \left(P_0^j + Q_0^j\right) & \text{if } 1 \leq i = k\,; \\[2ex]
\left(\prod_{j=1}^{i-1} \left(P_0^j + Q_0^j\right)\right)\left(Q_0^i + Q_1^i\right)\left(\prod_{j=i+1}^{k-1} Q_2^j\right) \\
\quad \times \left(1 - P_0^k - Q_0^k - R_0^k\right) & \text{if } 1 \leq i < k\,; \\[2ex]
\widetilde{Q}_3^i \prod_{j=i+1}^{-1} \left(1 - \widetilde{Q}_3^j\right)\left(\prod_{j=1}^{k-1} Q_2^j\right) \\
\quad \times \left(1 - P_0^k - Q_0^k - R_0^k\right) & \text{if } -m \leq i < 0\,; \\[2ex]
\prod_{j=-m}^{-1} \left(1 - \widetilde{Q}_3^j\right)\left(\prod_{j=1}^{k-1} Q_2^j\right) \\
\quad \times \left(1 - P_0^k - Q_0^k - R_0^k\right) & \text{if } i = -m - 1.
\end{cases}
$$

3.6.3 M3 $A + B$ design

3.6.3.1 M3 $A + B$ design without dose de-escalation

For $1 \leq j \leq n$,

$$
E(X_j) = \sum_{i=0}^{n+1} \sum_{s=i}^{i+1} \sum_{m=1}^{s} E(X_j \mid \text{MTD} = \text{dose } i, \text{ stop at dose } s \text{ and first sign of toxicity at dose } m)
$$

$$
\times P(\text{MTD} = \text{dose } i, \text{ stop at dose } s \text{ and first sign of toxicity at dose } m).
$$

Let

$$
\widetilde{P}_0^j = \sum_{\alpha + \beta + \gamma = a,\ \beta + \gamma \geq 1} \begin{pmatrix} a \\ \alpha\ \beta\ \gamma \end{pmatrix} (1 - q_j)^\alpha (q_j - p_j)^\beta p_j^\gamma P_{0,a}^{j,\gamma},
$$

$$
\widetilde{Q}_0^j = \sum_{\alpha + \beta + \gamma = a,\ \beta + \gamma \geq 1} \begin{pmatrix} a \\ \alpha\ \beta\ \gamma \end{pmatrix} (1 - q_j)^\alpha (q_j - p_j)^\beta p_j^\gamma Q_{0,a}^{j,\gamma},
$$

$$\tilde{R}_0^j = \sum_{\alpha+\beta+\gamma=a,\ \beta+\gamma\geq 1} \begin{pmatrix} a \\ \alpha\ \beta\ \gamma \end{pmatrix} (1-q_j)^\alpha (q_j - p_j)^\beta p_j^\gamma R_{0,a}^{j,\gamma},$$

$$\tilde{P}_1^j = \sum_{\alpha+\beta+\gamma=a,\ \beta+\gamma\geq 1} \begin{pmatrix} a \\ \alpha\ \beta\ \gamma \end{pmatrix} (1-q_j)^\alpha (q_j - p_j)^\beta p_j^\gamma P_{1,a}^{j,\gamma}.$$

Then, for $0 \leq i \leq n+1$, $s = i$ or $i+1$ and $1 \leq m \leq n+1$,

$E(X_j \mid \text{MTD} = \text{dose } i, \text{stop at dose } s \text{ and first sign of toxicity at dose } m)$

$$= \begin{cases} a & \text{if } j < m \leq n+1; \\[2mm] \dfrac{A\tilde{P}_0^j + (A+B)\tilde{Q}_0^j}{\tilde{P}_0^j + \tilde{Q}_0^j} & \text{if } m = j < i = s \leq n+1 \text{ or} \\ & \quad m = j \leq i = s - 1 < n; \\[2mm] A+B & \text{if } m = j \leq i = s \leq n; \\[2mm] \dfrac{A\left(1-\tilde{P}_0^j - \tilde{P}_1^j\right) + (A+B)\left(\tilde{P}_1^j - \tilde{Q}_0^j - \tilde{R}_0^j\right)}{1 - \tilde{P}_0^j - \tilde{Q}_0^j - \tilde{R}_0^j} & \text{if } m = j = i+1 = s \leq n; \\[2mm] \dfrac{A\left(1 - P_0^j - P_1^j\right) + (A+B)\left(P_1^j - Q_0^j - R_0^j\right)}{1 - P_0^j - Q_0^j - R_0^j} & \text{if } m \leq i < j = i+1 = s \leq n; \\[2mm] \dfrac{AP_0^j + (A+B)Q_0^j}{P_0^j + Q_0^j} & \text{if } m < j < i = s \leq n+1 \text{ or} \\ & \quad m < j \leq i = s - 1 < n; \\[2mm] 0 & \text{otherwise}, \end{cases}$$

and

$P\left(\text{MTD} = \text{dose } i, \text{ stop at dose } s \text{ and first sign of toxicity at dose } m\right)$

$$= \begin{cases} \prod_{j=1}^{m-1}(1-q_j)^a T_a^m \prod_{j=m+1}^{i-1}\left(P_0^j + Q_0^j\right) R_0^i & \text{if } m < i = s \leq n+1; \\[2mm] \prod_{j=1}^{i-1}(1-q_j)^a U_a^i & \text{if } m = i = s \leq n+1; \\[2mm] \prod_{j=1}^{m-1}(1-q_j)^a T_a^m \prod_{j=m+1}^{i}\left(P_0^j + Q_0^j\right) \\ \quad \times \left(1 - P_0^{i+1} - Q_0^{i+1} - R_0^{i+1}\right) & \text{if } m < i = s - 1 < n; \\[2mm] \prod_{j=1}^{i-1}(1-q_j)^a T_a^i \left(1 - P_0^{i+1} - Q_0^{i+1} - R_0^{i+1}\right) & \text{if } m = i = s - 1 < n; \\[2mm] \prod_{j=1}^{i}(1-q_j)^a S_a^{i+1} & \text{if } m = i+1 = s \leq n, \end{cases}$$

where we set $R_0^{n+1} = 1$ and $U_a^{n+1} = 1$.

3.6.3.2 M3 $A + B$ design with dose de-escalation

For $1 \leq j \leq n$,

$$
E(X_j) = \sum_{i=0}^{n+1} \sum_{k=i}^{n+1} \sum_{m=1}^{k} E(X_j \mid \text{MTD} = \text{dose } i, \text{ first sign of toxicity at}
$$
$$
\text{dose } m \text{ and stop escalation at dose } k)
$$
$$
\times P(\text{MTD} = \text{dose } i, \text{ first sign of toxicity at dose } m
$$
$$
\text{and stop escalation at dose } k)
$$

where, for $1 \leq m \leq n + 1, 0 \leq i \leq n + 1$ and $i \leq k \leq n + 1$,

$E\left(X_j \mid \text{MTD} = \text{dose } i, \text{ first sign of toxicity at dose } m \text{ and stop escalation}\right.$
$\left. \text{at dose } k\right)$

$$
= \begin{cases}
a & \text{if } j < \min(m, i); \\[2ex]
\dfrac{A\widetilde{P}_0^j + (A + B)\widetilde{Q}_0^j}{\widetilde{P}_0^j + \widetilde{Q}_0^j} & \begin{array}{l} \text{if } j = m < i \leq k \leq n \text{ or} \\ \quad j = m < i = k = n + 1; \end{array} \\[3ex]
\dfrac{AP_0^j + (A + B)Q_0^j}{P_0^j + Q_0^j} & \begin{array}{l} \text{if } m < j < i \leq k \leq n \text{ or} \\ \quad m < j < i = k = n + 1; \end{array} \\[3ex]
A + B & \begin{array}{l} \text{if } m < i = j \leq k \leq n \text{ or} \\ \quad m < i < j < k \leq n \text{ or} \\ \quad m = i \leq j < k \leq n \text{ or} \\ \quad m = i = j = k \leq n \text{ or} \\ \quad i = j < m \leq k \leq n \text{ or} \\ \quad 0 \leq i < m \leq j < k \leq n; \end{array} \\[5ex]
\dfrac{A\left(1 - P_0^j - P_1^j\right) + (A + B)\left(P_1^j - Q_0^j - R_0^j\right)}{1 - P_0^j - Q_0^j - R_0^j} & \begin{array}{l} \text{if } m \leq i < j = \leq n \text{ or} \\ \quad 0 \leq i < m < j = k \leq n; \end{array} \\[3ex]
\dfrac{A\left(1 - \widetilde{Q}_{2,a}^{j,0} - \widetilde{Q}_{3,a}^{j,0}\right) + (A + B)\widetilde{Q}_{2,a}^{j,0}}{1 - \widetilde{Q}_{3,a}^{j,0}} & \text{if } 0 \leq i < j < m \leq k \leq n; \\[3ex]
\dfrac{A\left(1 - \widetilde{P}_0^j - \widetilde{P}_1^j\right) + (A + B)\left(\widetilde{P}_1^j - \widetilde{Q}_0^j - \widetilde{R}_0^j\right)}{1 - \widetilde{P}_0^j - \widetilde{Q}_0^j - \widetilde{R}_0^j} & \text{if } 0 \leq i < m = j = k \leq n; \\[3ex]
0 & \text{otherwise}
\end{cases}
$$

and

$P(\text{MTD} = \text{dose } i, \text{ first sign of toxicity at dose } m \text{ and stop escalation at dose } k)$

$$
=
\begin{cases}
\prod_{j=1}^{m-1}(1-q_j)^a T_a^m \left(\prod_{j=m+1}^{i-1}\left(P_0^j + Q_0^j\right)\right)\left(Q_0^i + Q_1^i\right) & \\
\quad \times \left(\prod_{j=i+1}^{k-1} Q_2^j\right)\left(1 - P_0^k - Q_0^k - R_0^k\right) & \text{if } m < i < k \le n; \\
\prod_{j=1}^{m-1}(1-q_j)^a T_a^m \left(\prod_{j=m+1}^{i-1}\left(P_0^j + Q_0^j\right)\right) R_0^i & \text{if } m < i = k \le n+1; \\
\prod_{j=1}^{i-1}(1-q_j)^a W_a^i \left(\prod_{j=i+1}^{k-1} Q_2^j\right)\left(1 - P_0^k - Q_0^k - R_0^k\right) & \text{if } m = i < k \le n; \\
\prod_{j=1}^{i-1}(1-q_j)^a U_a^i & \text{if } m = i = k \le n+1; \\
\prod_{j=1}^{m-1}(1-q_j)^a \widetilde{Q}_{3,a}^{i,0} \left(\prod_{j=i+1}^{m-1}\left(1 - \widetilde{Q}_{3,a}^{j,0}\right)\right) V_a^m & \\
\quad \times \left(\prod_{j=m+1}^{k-1} Q_2^j\right)\left(1 - P_0^k - Q_0^k - R_0^k\right) & \text{if } 0 \le i < m < k \le n; \\
\prod_{j=1}^{k-1}(1-q_j)^a \widetilde{Q}_{3,a}^{i,0} \left(\prod_{j=i+1}^{k-1}\left(1 - \widetilde{Q}_{3,a}^{j,0}\right)\right) S_a^k & \text{if } 0 \le i < m = k \le n.
\end{cases}
$$

For convenience, we set $\widetilde{Q}_{3,a}^{0,0} = 1$, $R_0^{n+1} = 1$ and $U_a^{n+1} = 1$.

3.7 Other statistical properties

Once we find the probability of a dose being chosen as the MTD (Section 3.5) and the expected number of patients treated at each dose level (Section 3.6), other important statistical properties can be found easily, as shown in reference [6] when the starting dose is the lowest dose level. For the case when the starting dose is not the lowest dose level, the quantities can be found in the following.

The attained target toxicity level (ATTL) is the expected dose-limiting toxicity at the MTD found through the algorithm-based design:

$$
\begin{aligned}
\text{ATTL} &= E(\text{DLT at MTD}|\text{dose} - m \le \text{MTD} \le \text{dose } n) \\
&= \frac{\sum_{i=-m}^{-1} p_i P(\text{MTD} = \text{dose } i) + \sum_{i=1}^{n} p_i P(\text{MTD} = \text{dose } i)}{\sum_{i=-m}^{-1} P(\text{MTD} = \text{dose } i) + \sum_{i=1}^{n} P(\text{MTD} = \text{dose } i)}.
\end{aligned}
$$

Note that the ATTL depends heavily on the algorithm-based design used in a trial, and does not necessarily reach the target level γ, as seen in the examples in the next section.

For $-m \le j \le n$ and $j \ne 0$, let Y_j be the number of DLT at dose j and X_j be the number of patients treated at dose level j. Then the expected number of toxicity at dose level j is

$$
E(Y_j) = E(X_j)P(\text{DLT at dose } j) = p_j E(X_j)
$$

and the expected overall DLT in a trial equals

$$
\sum_{-m \le j \le n, j \ne 0} E(X_j)P(\text{DLT at dose } j) = \sum_{-m \le j \le n, j \ne 0} p_j E(X_j).
$$

3.8   Examples

We give three real examples to illustrate the modified $A + B$ designs: (1) an 'M1 $A + B$' design without dose de-escalation and the current dose can be defined as the MTD, where $A = 3$ and $B = 2$; (2) an 'M2 $A + B$' design with dose de-escalation and the starting dose is not the lowest dose level, where $A = B = 3$; and (3) an 'M3 $A + B$' design without dose de-escalation, where $A = B = 3$.

3.8.1   Example 1: M1 3 + 2 design without dose de-escalation

This is a phase I trial to determine the MTD of oral capecitabine and trimetrexate in patients with metastatic or recurrent cancer [9]. The dosing regimen is defined in the top portion of Table 3.1. The dose escalation strategy follows the M1 3 + 2 design without dose de-escalation and with $C = D = E = 1$ and $F = 2$.

The MTD is the dosing regimen that $0/3$ or $1/5$ patient experience DLT and at least $2/3$ or $3/5$ patients treated with the next higher dosing regimen have had DLT, or is the dosing regimen that $2/5$ patients have DLT. Note that if the escalation occurs at the last dosing regimen, or at least $2/3$ or $3/5$ patients treated with the first dosing regimen have had DLT, then the MTD is not determined from the trial.

Table 3.1 gives three different scenarios for the probabilities of DLT at the dosing regimens. In the first scenario, we assume low DLT at dosing regimen 1 and high DLT at the last dosing regimen. In the second scenario, we assume low DLT at all dosing regimens. In the third scenario, we assume high DLT at dosing regimen 1.

Based on the three scenarios of probabilities of DLT, the probability that a dosing regimen will be declared as the MTD is calculated and summarized in Table 3.1. Also included in Table 3.1 is the expected number of patients, the expected number of DLT incidences at each dosing regimen and the target toxicity level (i.e. the probability of toxicity at the MTD, if MTD is determined in the given dosing regimens). Table 3.1 shows that it is most likely that the fourth dosing regimen (Trimetrexate 60 mg/m^2/dose daily Monday to Friday, Capecitabine 1000 mg/m^2/dose twice a day Tuesday to Saturday) will be declared as the MTD for the first two toxicity model scenarios and the first dosing regimen (Trimetrexate 20 mg/m^2/dose daily Monday to Friday, Capecitabine 1000 mg/m^2/dose twice a day Tuesday to Saturday) will be declared as the MTD for the third toxicity model scenario. Table 3.1 also shows that, on average, we expect to treat 10 to 16 patients and observe 2 or 3 incidences of DLT (about 14.9 to 25.9 %) under the three toxicity model scenarios.

3.8.2   Example 2: M2 3 + 3 design with dose de-escalation

This trial is a phase I study of intraperitoneal Gemcitabine combined with intravenous Paclitaxel and Carboplatin in women with optimally debulked epithelial ovarian cancer, primary peritoneal carcinoma and primary fallopian tube cancer [10]. It is designed to determine the MTD of the combination therapy. With a fixed Paclitaxel dose

Table 3.1 Probability that a dosing regimen will be declared as the MTD, expected number of patients and expected number of DLT incidences at each dosing regimen in Example 1.

Dosing regimen	1	2	3	4	5	Total
Trimetrexate (mg/m^2)	20	40	60	60	60	
Schedule	Mon–Fri	Mon–Fri	Mon–Fri	Mon–Fri	Mon–Fri	
Capecitabine (mg/m^2)/BID	750	750	750	1000	1250	
schedule	Tues–Sat	Tues–Sat	Tues–Sat	Tues–Sat	Tues–Sat	
First scenario[a]						
Probability of DLT	0.10	0.15	0.20	0.30	0.50	
Probability that the dose is declared as MTD	0.107	0.171	0.249	0.308	0.062	
Expected number of patients	3.5	3.4	3.0	2.3	1.2	13.4
Expected number of toxicity incidences	0.35	0.51	0.59	0.69	0.62	2.77
Second scenario[b]						
Probability of DLT	0.05	0.10	0.15	0.20	0.30	
Probability that the dose is declared as MTD	0.043	0.105	0.167	0.244	0.108	
Expected number of patients	3.3	3.4	3.3	2.9	2.3	15.2
Expected number of toxicity incidences	0.16	0.34	0.50	0.58	0.68	2.26
Third scenario[c]						
Probability of DLT	0.20	0.25	0.30	0.35	0.40	
Probability that the dose is declared as MTD	0.261	0.248	0.186	0.111	0.027	
Expected number of patients	3.8	2.9	1.9	1.1	0.5	10.2
Expected number of toxicity incidences	0.75	0.73	0.58	0.38	0.20	2.64

[a] P(MTD < regimen 1) = 0.030, P(MTD > regimen 5) = 0.073, ATTL = 23.4 %, expected overall toxicity rate = 20.7 % for first scenario.
[b] P(MTD < regimen 1) = 0.008, P(MTD > regimen 5) = 0.326, ATTL = 17.8 %, expected overall toxicity rate = 14.9 % for second scenario.
[c] P(MTD < regimen 1) = 0.119, P(MTD > regimen 5) = 0.048, ATTL = 26.4 %, expected overall toxicity rate = 25.9 % for third scenario.

of 175 mg/m^2, the fixed Carboplatin dose of an AUC (area under the curve) of 5.5 and the starting Gemcitabine dose of 70 mg/m^2, the dose level of the Gemcitabine follows a modified Fibonacci sequence (see the top portion of Table 3.2).

The dose sequencing follows the M2 3 + 3 design with the starting dose at dose level 1 (the second lowest dose level) and the current dose level can be declared as the MTD with $C = D = E = 1$ and $F = 2$. The MTD is the dose level that 0/6 (or 0/3 if at dose level 1) or 1/6 patients experience DLT, and at least 2/3 or 3/6 patients treated with the next higher dose have had DLT, or the dose level that 2/6 patients has DLT.

Note that if dose-escalation is still indicated at the last (i.e. the highest) dose level 5, then the MTD is at or above the last dose level. If the trial stops at the dose level -1 (at least 2 out of 3 patients or at least 3 out of 6 patients have DLT at the dose level -1), then the MTD is below the dose level -1. In either of the above cases, the MTD is not determined from the trial.

Table 3.2 gives three different scenarios for the probabilities of DLT at the dose levels. In the first scenario, we assume linear dose–DLT rates such that the rate is 5 % at dose level -1 and 50 % at dose level 5. In the second scenario, we assume linear dose–DLT rates such that the rate is 15 % at dose level 1 and 50 % at dose level 5. In the third scenario, the dose–DLT rates are calculated from a two-parameter logistic model such that the rate is 3 % at dose level -1 and 50 % at dose level 5.

Based on the three scenarios of probabilities of DLT, the probability that a dose level will be declared as the MTD is calculated in Table 3.2. Table 3.2 shows that it is most likely that the 230 mg/m^2 dose (dose level 3) will be declared as the MTD under the first toxicity model scenario. For the second scenario, 140 mg/m^2 (dose level 2) is likely to be declared as MTD. For the third scenario, 350 mg/m^2 (dose level 4) is likely to be the MTD. There is less than a 10 % chance that the MTD cannot be determined from this M2 3 + 3 design in all the scenarios (<3.2 %, 2.2 % and <8.3 % for the first, second and third scenarios respectively).

Table 3.2 also summarizes the expected number of patients and the expected number of toxicity incidences at each dose level. Table 3.2 shows that, on average, we expect to treat 10 to 16 patients and observe 2 or 3 incidences of DLT ($= 15.6$–22.5 %) under the three toxicity model scenarios.

3.8.3 Example 3: M3 3 + 3 design without dose de-escalation

This is a phase I study of L-000021649 for patients with solid tumors or acute myelogenous leukemia [11]. The dose levels are listed in the top portion of Table 3.3, where the starting dose of 48 mg/m^2 is considered far below the MTD. The dose escalation strategy follows M3 3 + 3 design without dose de-escalation (with $a = 1, C = D = E = 1$ and $F = 2$). Starting from dose level 1, one patient will be entered at each dose level and the dose will be escalated to the next level (with no

Table 3.2 Probability that a dose level will be declared as the MTD, expected number of patients and expected number of DLT incidences at each dose level for Example 2.

Dose level	−1	1	2	3	4	5	Total
Dose (mg/m²)	35	70	140	230	350	490	
Dose multiplier	0.5	1	2	3.3	5	7	
% of increment from starting dose	−50	0	100	65	52	40	
First scenario[a]							
Probability of DLT	0.05	0.08	0.15	0.24	0.36	0.50	
Probability that the dose is declared as MTD	0.022	0.117	0.257	0.336	0.212	0.025	
Expected number of patients	0.234	3.551	3.489	2.884	1.750	0.588	12.496
Expected number of toxicity incidences	0.012	0.284	0.523	0.692	0.630	0.294	2.435
Second scenario[b]							
Probability of DLT	0.12	0.15	0.21	0.28	0.38	0.50	
Probability that the dose is declared as MTD	0.077	0.235	0.280	0.246	0.125	0.014	
Expected number of patients	0.524	3.636	2.982	2.068	1.094	0.337	10.641
Expected number of toxicity incidences	0.063	0.545	0.626	0.579	0.416	0.168	2.398
Third scenario[c]							
Probability of DLT	0.03	0.04	0.06	0.12	0.26	0.50	
Probability that the dose is declared as MTD	0.005	0.024	0.073	0.275	0.474	0.067	
Expected number of patients	0.296	3.290	3.393	3.660	3.316	1.564	15.519
Expected number of toxicity incidences	0.009	0.132	0.204	0.439	0.862	0.782	2.427

[a] $P(\text{MTD} < 35 \text{ mg/m}^2) < 0.001$, $P(\text{MTD} \geq 490\text{mg/m}^2) = 0.031$, ATTL $= 22.6$ %, expected overall toxicity rate $= 19.5$ % for first scenario.
[b] $P(\text{MTD} < 35 \text{ mg/m}^2) = 0.004$, $P(\text{MTD} \geq 490\text{mg/m}^2) = 0.018$, ATTL $= 23.2$ %, expected overall toxicity rate $= 22.5$ % for second scenario.
[c] $P(\text{MTD} < 35 \text{ mg/m}^2) < 0.001$, $P(\text{MTD} \geq 490\text{mg/m}^2) = 0.082$, ATTL $= 21.3$ %, expected overall toxicity rate $= 15.6$ % for third scenario.

Table 3.3 Probability that a dose level will be declared as the MTD, expected number of patients and expected number of toxicity incidences at each dose level for M3 3 + 3 design without dose de-escalation.

Dose level	1	2	3	4	5	6	7	8	Total
Dose(mg/m^2)	48	96	140	200	280	390	540	760	
First scenario[a]									
Probability of toxicity[b]	0.004	0.006	0.008	0.012	0.021	0.045	0.121	0.400	
Probability of DLT	0.002	0.003	0.004	0.006	0.011	0.026	0.076	0.300	
Probability of dose is declared as MTD	<0.001	<0.001	<0.001	<0.001	0.002	0.015	0.178	0.046	
Expected number of patients	1.014	1.029	1.048	1.078	1.134	1.265	1.614	1.468	9.649
Expected number of DLT incidences	0.002	0.003	0.004	0.006	0.012	0.033	0.123	0.440	0.624
Second scenario[c]									
Probability of toxicity	0.004	0.007	0.011	0.020	0.047	0.140	0.454	0.900	
Probability of DLT	0.002	0.003	0.005	0.008	0.017	0.046	0.163	0.600	
Probability of dose is declared as MTD	<0.001	<0.001	<0.001	0.001	0.006	0.081	0.745	0.063	
Expected number of patients	1.014	1.031	1.059	1.107	1.227	1.583	2.593	2.857	12.471
Expected number of DLT incidences	0.002	0.003	0.005	0.009	0.021	0.073	0.423	1.714	2.250

(Continued)

Table 3.3 (Continued)

Dose level	1	2	3	4	5	6	7	8	Total
Third scenario[d]									
Probability of toxicity	0.020	0.028	0.039	0.059	0.102	0.205	0.439	0.800	
Probability of DLT	0.010	0.014	0.018	0.026	0.043	0.084	0.195	0.500	
Probability of dose is declared as MTD	0.001	0.001	0.002	0.006	0.024	0.129	0.570	0.091	
Expected number of patients	1.070	1.137	1.223	1.355	1.582	1.997	2.566	2.448	13.377
Expected number of DLT incidences	0.011	0.016	0.022	0.035	0.068	0.168	0.500	1.224	2.044

[a] $P(\text{MTD} < 48 \text{ mg/m}^2) < 0.001$, $P(\text{MTD} > 760 \text{mg/m}^2) = 0.758$, ATTL $= 11.5\%$, expected overall toxicity rate $= 6.5\%$ for first scenario.
[b] Includes both minor toxicity and DLT.
[c] $P(\text{MTD} < 48 \text{ mg/m}^2) < 0.001$, $P(\text{MTD} > 760 \text{mg/m}^2) = 0.104$, ATTL $= 18.2\%$, expected overall toxicity rate $= 18.0\%$ for second scenario.
[d] $P(\text{MTD} < 48 \text{ mg/m}^2) < 0.001$, $P(\text{MTD} > 760 \text{ mg/m}^2) = 0.175$, ATTL $= 20.5\%$, expected overall toxicity rate $= 15.3\%$ for third scenario.

sign of toxicity) until the first sign of toxicity (minor or DLT) occurred. After that the dose-escalation scheme follows the corresponding M1 3 + 3 design.

Table 3.3 gives three different scenarios for the probabilities of toxicity (minor toxicity or DLT, and DLT only separately) at each dose level. We assume that the dose–toxicity relationship and the dose–DLT relationship follow two-parameter logistic models in these scenarios. For the first scenario, we assume a low toxicity (0.4 %) at the first dose level. For the second scenario, we assume a high toxicity (90 %) at the last dose (level 8). For the third scenario, we assume a moderate toxicity (2 %) at the first dose level.

Based on the third scenario of probabilities of toxicities and DLTs, the probability that a dose will be declared as the MTD is calculated and summarized in Table 3.3 together with the expected number of patients, the expected number of toxicity incidences at each dose level and the target toxicity level. Table 3.3 shows that it is most likely that the seventh dose level (540 mg/m^2) will be declared as the MTD for the second and third scenarios, and that it is most likely that the trial cannot determine the MTD for the first scenario. The target toxicity levels are 11.5 %, 18.2 % and 20.5 % for the three scenarios respectively. Table 3.3 also shows that, on average, we expect to treat 9 to 14 patients and observe no more than 3 incidences of DLT (about 6.5 %–18.0 %) under the three toxicity model scenarios.

For comparison, in Table 3.4 we have also calculated the probability that a dose will be declared as the MTD, and the expected number of patients and expected toxicity incidences at each dose level respectively, when using the traditional 3 + 3 design without dose de-escalation, based on the same three dose–toxicity scenarios in Table 3.3. We obtain similar conclusions for the probability of a dose being declared as the MTD, but the target toxicity levels are 7.0 %, 13.3 % and 14.6 % for the three scenarios respectively, which are lower than the 'M3 3 + 3' design, because more patients would be treated at suboptimal dose levels.

Furthermore, from Table 3.4 we see that, on average, we expect to treat 25 to 27 patients and observe about 2 or 3 incidences of DLT under the three toxicity model scenarios, while using the 'M3 3 + 3' design we need only treat 9 to 14 patients. Therefore, under these three scenarios, the 'M3 3 + 3' design requires only less than half of the expected total number of patients as the traditional 3 + 3 design, while both have similar conclusions for probabilities for a dose being declared as the MTD.

3.9 Discussion

Although there is no single universally accepted standard method for phase I cancer clinical trials, the algorithm-based designs are certainly still the most commonly used method. In this note we have reviewed the traditional and modified $A + B$ designs. When there are only a few dose levels in a trial (especially for trials with the complicated combinations of drugs or schedules), the M1 $A + B$ design will make full use of all the available dose levels in the trial when the last dose level has an appropriate toxicity rate and may be declared as the MTD. Using the M2 $A + B$ design by adding several dose levels below the starting dose level avoids stopping or

Table 3.4 Probability that a dose level will be declared as the MTD, expected number of patients and expected number of toxicity incidences at each dose level for traditional 3 + 3 design without dose de-escalation

Dose level	1	2	3	4	5	6	7	8	Total
Dose (mg/m²)	48	96	140	200	280	390	540	760	
First scenario[a]									
Probability of DLT	0.002	0.003	0.004	0.006	0.011	0.026	0.076	0.300	
Probability of dose declared as MTD	<0.001	<0.001	<0.001	0.001	0.008	0.057	0.472	0.000	
Expected number of patients	3.018	3.027	3.035	3.052	3.094	3.215	3.549	4.034	26.025
Expected number of toxicity incidences	0.006	0.009	0.012	0.018	0.034	0.084	0.270	1.210	1.643
Second scenario[b]									
Probability of DLT	0.002	0.003	0.005	0.008	0.017	0.046	0.163	0.600	
Probability of dose declared as MTD	<0.001	<0.001	0.001	0.003	0.023	0.207	0.703	0.000	
Expected number of patients	3.018	3.027	3.044	3.069	3.144	3.361	3.918	2.959	25.542
Expected number of toxicity incidences	0.006	0.009	0.015	0.025	0.053	0.155	0.639	1.776	2.677
Third scenario[c]									
Probability of DLT	0.010	0.014	0.018	0.026	0.043	0.084	0.195	0.500	
Probability of dose declared as MTD	0.002	0.004	0.008	0.020	0.067	0.252	0.536	0.000	
Expected number of patients	3.088	3.119	3.145	3.199	3.305	3.509	3.720	2.668	25.753
Expected number of toxicity incidences	0.031	0.044	0.057	0.083	0.142	0.295	0.725	1.334	2.711

[a] $P(\text{MTD} < 48 \text{ mg/m}^2)$ <0.001, $P(\text{MTD} > 760 \text{ mg/m}^2)$ = 0.461, ATTL = 7.0 %, expected overall toxicity rate = 6.3 % for first scenario.
[b] $P(\text{MTD} < 48 \text{ mg/m}^2)$ <0.001, $P(\text{MTD} > 760 \text{ mg/m}^2)$ = 0.063, ATTL = 13.3 %, expected overall toxicity rate = 10.5 % for second scenario.
[c] $P(\text{MTD} < 48 \text{ mg/m}^2)$ <0.001, $P(\text{MTD} > 760 \text{ mg/m}^2)$ = 0.111, ATTL = 14.6 %, expected overall toxicity rate = 10.5 % for third scenario.

halting the trial for protocol amendment when the starting dose is too toxic. Another situation for the M2 $A + B$ or M3 $A + B$ designs to be useful is when we suspect the toxicity rate of the starting dose is too low. In order to reach the MTD as quickly as possible, the M2 $A + B$ design begins the trial at a higher dose level that may have the appropriate toxicity rate and leave room for dose de-escalation, while the M3 $A + B$ design follows the dose levels with smaller cohorts until reaching a certain toxicity and then switches to the M1 $A + B$ design.

All the statistical properties discussed in this note are based on the toxicity rate at each dose level selected for the trial. Of course the exact dose–toxicity curve is not known in advance, but the clinicians should have some knowledge, no matter how weak that knowledge may be, of the drug toxicity based on similar trials or other sources of information. (Otherwise, it would be very difficult for the investigator to justify the dose levels selected for testing.) We suggest that several possible scenarios of the toxicity rate at given dose levels should be contemplated during the study planning stage. The statistical properties should help investigators to gain insights of the design before starting the trial.

Acknowledgments

The authors would like to thank Drs W. Hait, J. Aisner, E. Rubin and E. Poplin at the Cancer Institute of New Jersey (CINJ) for their helpful comments. This paper is supported through the NIH Cancer Center Support Grant 2P30 CA 72720-04.

References

1. S.K. Carter (1987) The phase I study, in *Fundamentals of Cancer Chemotherapy* (eds K.K. Hellmann and S.K. Carter), McGraw-Hill, New York, pp. 285–300.
2. S.F. Dent and E.A. Eisenhauer (1996) Phase I trial design: are new methodologies being put into practice? *Ann. Oncology*, **7**(6), 561–6.
3. L. Edler (1990) Statistical requirements of phase I studies. *Onkologie*, **13**(2), 90–5.
4. J.M. Heyd and B. Carlin (1999) Adaptive design improvements in the continual reassessment method for phase I studies. *Statistics in Medicine*, **18**(11), 1307–21.
5. J. O'Quigley, M. Pepe and L. Fisher (1990) Continual reassessment method: a practical design for phase I clinical trials in cancer. *Biometrics*, **46**(1), 33–48.
6. Y. Lin and W.J. Shih (2001) Statistical properties of the traditional algorithm-based designs for phase I cancer clinical trials. *Biostatistics*, **2**(2), 203–15.
7. Y. Lin and W.J. Shih (2004) Statistical properties of the modified algorithm-based designs for phase I cancer clinical trials. Technical report, Department of Biostatistics, University of Medicine and Dentistry of New Jersey.
8. T.L. Smith, J.J. Lee, H.M. Kantarjian, S.S. Legha and M.N. Raber (1996) Design and results of phase I cancer clinical trials: three-year experience at M.D. Anderson Cancer Center. *J. Clin. Oncology*, **14**(1), 287–95.
9. E. Poplin, E. Rubin, B. Kamen and J. Bertino (2004) A phase I study of oral capecitabine, trimetrexate and leucovorin (TRI-X) in patients with metastatic or recurrent cancer. Technical report, Clinical trial protocol of the Cancer Institute of New Jersey.

10. D. Gibbon, E. Rubin and J. Aisner (2001) A Phase I trial for the combination IV pacli-taxel and carboplatin with escalating doses of intraperitoneal gemcitabine in patients with epithelial ovarian cancer. Technical report, Clinical trial protocol of the Cancer Institute of New Jersey.

11. M. Wojtowicz, Y. Elsayed, D. Schaar and E. Rubin (2003) A phase I study of the novel kinase insert-domain-containing receptor (KDR) and fms-like tyrosine kinase-3 (flt-3) inhibitor, L-000021649 in patients with advanced hematologic and non-hematologic ma-lignancies. Technical report, Clinical trial protocol of the Cancer Institute of New Jersey.

4

Accelerated titration designs

Janet Dancey

Investigational Drug Branch, CTEP, DCTD, NCI, Bethesda, Maryland, USA

Boris Freidlin and Larry Rubinstein

Biometric Research Branch, DCTD, NCI, Bethesda, Maryland, USA

4.1   Introduction

A decade ago, investigators in oncology had a clear interest in modifications to the standard phase I design to make it more efficient, to treat fewer patients at nontoxic dose levels (which may be less efficacious) and to increase the precision of phase II dose recommendations. This was the conclusion of the 1996 Joint Meeting of the US National Cancer Institute and the European Organization for the Research and Treatment of Cancer [1, 2]. At approximately the same time, a review of the recent phase I oncology literature revealed that few investigators were making use of the innovative phase I trial designs developed over the previous decade [3], which were meant to accomplish these very objectives.

Approximately five years previous to this, Sheiner and coworkers published a series of papers in which they argued for the use of dose-response models in the analysis of phase I trials [4–6]. Standard practice in oncology trials, among other fields, was to analyze the dose-toxicity relationship only in terms of the population as a whole, and to analyze it separately for each dose. Rarely were attempts made to fit a dose-toxicity model to the phase I data that accounted for interpatient and intrapatient variability

Statistical Methods for Dose-Finding Experiments   Edited by S. Chevret
© 2006 John Wiley & Sons, Ltd

separately, accommodated the possibility of cumulative toxicity and allowed for the construction of dose-toxicity curves for the sensitive as well as the typical patients. In addition, Sheiner argued for the use of intrapatient dose escalation, to maximize the possibility of individual patients receiving efficacious doses and to increase the accuracy of the analysis of the phase I data. This was not commonly practised in oncology phase I trials.

In response to the above, Simon *et al.* [7] developed a family of 'accelerated titration designs' and proposed the use of an accompanying dose-toxicity model, based on the work of Sheiner and coworkers [4, 5]. The main distinguishing features of these designs are (a) a rapid initial escalation phase, (b) intrapatient dose escalation and (c) the ability to analyze trial results using a dose-toxicity model that incorporates parameters for intrapatient and interpatient variation in toxicity and cumulative toxicity. The distinguishing features of the model are its simplicity and the incorporation of separate variables for interpatient and intrapatient variability, as well as for the possibility of cumulative toxicity.

4.2 Design

Simon *et al.* [7] proposed a family of accelerated titration dose-escalation designs. In their formulation all designs use 40 % dose-escalation steps. The dose-escalation/ de-escalation rules are based on definitions of dose-limiting toxicity (DLT) and of 'moderate' toxicity. These definitions may be protocol specific. For example, Simon *et al.* used any grade 2 toxicity that was considered to be treatment related as moderate toxicity. For purposes of comparison, they designated the standard phase I design (with 40 % escalation steps in place of the standard modified Fibonacci escalation) as 'design 1'. They then introduced accelerated designs designated as 'design 2', 'design 3' or 'design 4'.

Design 1 dictates that patients are dose escalated in cohorts of three until DLT is observed. One instance of DLT leads to treatment of three additional patients at the current dose level (with escalation continuing if no additional DLT is observed). Two instances of DLT, at a dose level, leads to a halt in dose escalation, with the prior dose level declared the MTD so long as six patients have been treated at that level, with one instance of DLT (de-escalation continues until such a dose level is determined).

Design 2 starts with an accelerated phase that uses single-patient cohorts per dose level. When the first instance of first-course DLT is observed or the second instance of first-course moderate toxicity is observed, the cohort for the current dose level is expanded to three patients and the trial reverts to use of design 1 for further cohorts.

Design 3 is similar to design 2 except that double-dose steps are used during the accelerated phase. Two 40 % dose steps correspond to approximately a doubling of the actual dose. The accelerated phase ends, as with design 2, when the first instance of first-course DLT or the second instance of first-course moderate toxicity is observed. After that, design 1 is used for further patients.

Design 4 is similar to design 3, except for the criterion that is used for triggering the end of the accelerated phase. With designs 2 and 3, the accelerated phase ends with the first-course instance of DLT or second instance of first-course moderate toxicity. With design 4, the trigger is the first instance of any-course DLT or the second instance of any-course intermediate toxicity. In addition, when the first instance of moderate toxicity is observed, two additional patients must have been treated at that dose, or a higher dose (during any course), without experiencing moderate or worse toxicity, in order that the accelerated phase continues. This may require the treatment of one or two additional patients at that dose. Hence, design 4 may stop the accelerated phase earlier than design 3.

Table 4.1 summarizes the characteristics of the four dose escalation designs.

Table 4.1   Summary of the four dose-escalation designs and the two intrapatient dose-escalation options.

Design	Description
1	Cohorts of 3 new patients per dose level. If 1 of 3 patients experiences DLT in first course, expand to 6 patients
2	Cohorts of 1 patient per dose level. When first instance of first-course DLT is observed, or second instance of first-course grade 2 toxicity of any type, expand cohort for current dose level and revert to use of design 1 for all further cohorts
3	Same as design 2, except that double-dose steps are used during initial accelerated stage of trial (both for between-patient and within-patient escalation)
4	Cohort of 1 new patient per dose level and double-dose steps are used during the initial accelerated stage of the trial. When the first instance of DLT is observed at any course, or the second instance of any-course grade 2 toxicity of any type, expand cohort for current dose level and revert to use of design 1 for all further cohorts. When the first instance of moderate toxicity is observed, two additional patients must have been treated at that dose, or a higher dose (during any course), without experiencing moderate or worse toxicity, in order that the accelerated phase continues

Escalation	Description
A	No within-patient dose escalation. De-escalate if grade 3 or worse toxicity at previous course
B	Escalate if grade 0–1 toxicity at previous course. De-escalate if grade 3 or worse toxicity at previous course

4.2.1   Intrapatient dose-escalation

In order to maximize each patient's chance to be treated at a potentially active dose, the accelerated titration design allows intrapatient dose-escalation for a patient who remains on study and has no evidence of toxicity at the current dose. Specifically, the dose for the next course is escalated if less than moderate toxicity was observed for the patient during the current course. If moderate toxicity occurred, then the dose stays the same for the next course for that patient. If DLT occurred, then the patient generally goes off-study, but if not, then the dose is reduced. For design 2, single-dose steps are used for intrapatient dose changes. For designs 3 and 4, double-dose steps are used for intrapatient dose changes during the accelerated stage, and single-dose steps subsequently.

All four designs may be used with and without intrapatient dose-escalation. Simon *et al.* [7] compared the performance of the four designs, with and without intrapatient dose-escalation, in terms of toxicity, potential efficacy (reduction of treatment at doses below the MTD) and trial length. Table 4.1 also summarizes the two intrapatient dose-escalation options.

4.3   Evaluation of performance

Simon *et al.* [7] fit the above model to data from 20 phase I trials (involving 9 distinct agents). Only three of the trials showed any evidence of cumulative toxicity ($\alpha > 0$). The estimates of α for the other trials were zero or very close to zero. The trials varied substantially in the other parameters and thus provide a broad range of experience for evaluation of the accelerated titration designs.

Simon *et al.* [7] evaluated the performance of the accelerated titration designs by simulating phase I data based on the 20 sets of parameters estimated from the 20 real trials that they studied. For each of the 20 sets of parameters, they generated data for 1000 phase I trials and applied each of their designs to the simulated data. Figure 4.1 shows the average number of patients per trial utilized by each of the designs. For each design, the average is taken over the same 20 000 simulated datasets generated from the sets of parameters derived from the 20 actual trials analyzed. Results for eight designs are shown. Designs 1 to 4 are as described above. The designs labeled with B utilize intrapatient dose-escalation if the toxicity in the previous course is less than intermediate. Designs labeled with A do not permit intrapatient dose-escalation.

Design 1A corresponds to the standard design, although it does not use Fibonacci dose steps. Design 1B is the standard design augmented to permit intrapatient dose-escalation. As can be seen in Figure 4.1, the average number of patients is much greater for the standard design 1A or 1B than for any of the accelerated titration designs. The average number of patients is somewhat less for designs 3 and 4 that use double-dose steps compared to design 2. Although the average differences are not great, the differences for individual trials can be; i.e. for a trial in which the starting dose is very low relative to the dose at which intermediate toxicity is expected, designs 2 and 3 will require substantially fewer patients.

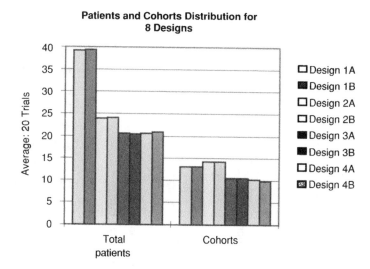

Figure 4.1   Average number of patients and number of cohorts for the eight designs.

Figure 4.1 also shows the average number of patient cohorts utilized by each design. The average is lowest for designs 3 and 4, which use double-dose steps. Although the difference in average number of cohorts is not large, the difference in average time to complete the trials will be much shorter for designs 2 to 4 if patients are not instantaneously available, since the accelerated phase of those designs requires only one patient per cohort.

Figure 4.2 shows the average number of patients experiencing each level of toxicity as their worst toxicity during their treatment on the trial. With the standard design, an average of 23 patients experience less than intermediate toxicity (labeled 'no toxicity' in the figure). These patients are undertreated. For design 2B the average number of undertreated patients is about eight and for designs 3B and 4B the number is less than five. This major reduction in the number of undertreated patients is achieved with very small increases in the average number of patients experiencing DLT or unacceptable toxicity with the accelerated titration designs. Figure 4.3 shows the average percentage of patients experiencing each level of toxicity as their worst toxicity during their treatment on the trial.

The accelerated titration designs without intrapatient dose-escalation, 2A, 3A and 4A, performed quite well with regard to reduction in average number of patients and reduction of number of undertreated patients. However, they do not provide patients accrued early in the trial a full opportunity to be treated at a therapeutic dose. They are also less effective in situations where interpatient variability in susceptibility to toxicity is large.

These designs may be attractive, however, when there is concern about cumulative toxicity. It is worth noting in this regard that analysis of the 20 phase I trials used

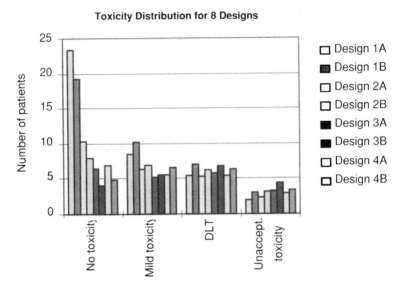

Figure 4.2   Average number of patients with worst toxicity at each toxicity level, for the eight designs.

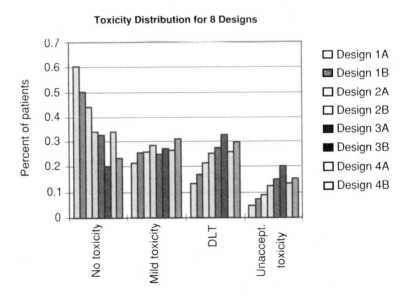

Figure 4.3   Average percentage of patients with worst toxicity at each toxicity level, for the eight designs.

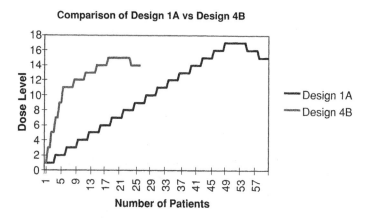

Figure 4.4   Diagram of the comparative performances of design 1A and design 4B, in terms of patients required to reach each dose level and to define the MTD.

for evaluation of these designs revealed no evidence of ill effects from intrapatient dose-escalation and lead the investigators to conclude that 'cumulative toxicity does not appear to be a valid reason to prohibit intra-patient dose escalation, as it occurs rarely' [1].

To illustrate further the efficiency of the accelerated designs in comparison with the standard, we give in Figure 4.4 a simulated comparison of the performance of design 4B versus design 1A for a particular dose-toxicity model. The accelerated design completes the trial with less than half the number of patients required by the standard. More dramatically, due to the single-patient cohorts and two-step escalations, it requires only one patient for every six of the standard design to escalate through the portion of the dose-toxicity curve where DLT is unlikely. Of course, if the initial dose of the trial is not defined so conservatively, the comparison is not so extreme.

4.4   Model-based analysis

By using a model for the statistical distribution of toxicity, based on current and previous doses, a graded toxicity scale, based on the unobserved continuous variable associated with toxicity and multicourse treatment results, the accelerated titration designs allow for an efficient approach to analysis of phase I data. The model used in Simon *et al.* [7] was based on measuring the worst toxicity experience for each patient during each course of treatment; i.e. the model does not consider separate toxicity for each organ system, but takes the maximum over all organ systems and records that worst toxicity separately for each course of treatment for each patient. The model was designed to represent different levels of worst toxicity. The toxicity experienced in a particular course was determined by the current dose administered and the total

Table 4.2   Summary of the dose-toxicity model
for both the unobserved continuous toxicity
variable and the observed toxicity grade level.

Model relating toxicity to dose
$Y_{ij} = \log(d_{ij} + \alpha D_i) + \beta_i + \varepsilon_{ij}$
d_{ij} = dose for the ith patient in course j
α = cumulative toxicity parameter
D_{ij} = cumulative dose up to course j
β_i = interpatient random effect, $N(0, \sigma_\beta^2)$
ε_{ij} = intrapatient random effect, $N(0, \sigma_\varepsilon^2)$

$Y_{ij} < K_1$	grade 0–1 toxicity
$K_1 < Y_{ij} < K_2$	grade 2 toxicity
$K_2 < Y_{ij} < K_3$	grade 3 toxicity
$Y_{ij} > K_3$	grade 4 toxicity

dose administered in the previous courses. The model incorporated parameters for
both intrapatient and interpatient variability, and for cumulative toxicity.

Suppose that the ith patient receives dose d_{ij} during dose j and received a total
dose D_{ij} for courses prior to j. Let α represent the effect of cumulative toxicity
($\alpha = 0$ indicates no effect of cumulative toxicity). The random variable β_i represents
interpatient variability in the toxic effects; β_i is taken to be normally distributed
with mean zero and variance σ_β^2. The random variable ε_{ij} represents intrapatient
variability in the toxic response; ε_{ij} is taken to be normally distributed with mean
zero and variance σ_ε^2. These terms and random variables determine the unobserved
magnitude y_{ij} of the worst toxicity for patient i in course j, according to the formula

$$y_{ij} = \log(d_{ij} + \alpha D_{ij}) + \beta_i + \varepsilon_{ij}.$$

In addition to the three parameters α, σ_β^2 and σ_ε^2, there are also several parameters
for converting value y_{ij} into a graded level of toxicity. Values of y_{ij} less than K_1
correspond to less then moderate toxicity values between K_1 and K_2 correspond to
moderate toxicity, values between K_2 and K_3 correspond to dose-limiting toxicity and
values greater than K_3 correspond to life-threatening toxicity. If one does not wish
to distinguish DLT from life-threatening toxicity, then only K_1 and K_2 are needed.
Therefore there are five or six parameters to be estimated from the data. Table 4.2
summarizes the characteristics of the model. This model is a generalization of the K_{max}
model of Sheiner, Beal and Sambol [5] and of the model of Chou and Talalay [8, 9].

Given the data of the grade of toxicity (worst over organ systems) for each
course of each patient, the method of maximum likelihood is used to estimate
the model parameters. Splus software for fitting the parameters is available at
http://linus.nci.nih.gov/brb. That website also contains an Excel macro for managing

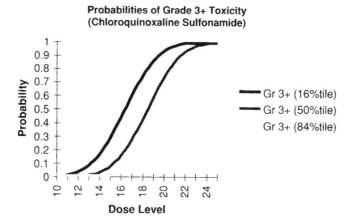

Figure 4.5   Probabilities of grade 3+ toxicity at various dose levels for the mean patient and the patients one standard deviation above and below the mean.

dose assignments to patients during accelerated titration design trials. The macro assists investigators in quality controlling the dose assignment and provides a convenient way of recording dose assignments in a systematic manner that makes the data available for subsequent analysis.

Figure 4.5 illustrates the power of the model-based analysis to construct a dose-toxicity curve, not only for the typical patient (50th percentile) but also for the patient who falls one standard deviation below the typical in terms of increased susceptibility to toxicity (16th percentile). The standard approach to defining the MTD is based on the probability of toxicity at a given dose for the population as a whole, which often roughly corresponds to the probability of toxicity for the typical patient. With this approach, the initial phase II dose would be set, for Figure 4.5, at dose level 16 or 17, to keep the probability of DLT below 30%. However, the model-based analysis reveals that such a dose level results in at least a 40–60% likelihood of DLT for a nontrivial subgroup of the patient population (those at the 16th percentile or below). This might suggest that a more prudent approach would be to define a lower initial phase II dose, to accommodate the susceptibility of this subgroup.

Figure 4.6 illustrates the power of the model-based analysis to construct comparative dose-toxicity curves for the different levels of toxicity. For example, the analysis suggests that the dose-toxicity curves for grade 2 versus grade 3 toxicity are separated by approximately four dose levels. This indicates that for a given patient, as well as for the population as a whole, DLT is likely to occur approximately four dose levels beyond moderate toxicity, suggesting that accelerated dose-escalation is likely to be safe, both for the population and for a given individual. Even though the dose-toxicity curve for DLT is relatively steep, it is well separated from the curve for moderate toxicity.

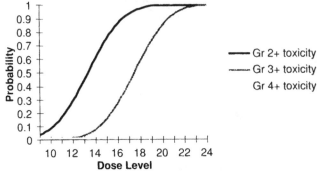

Figure 4.6 Probabilities of grade 2+, grade 3+ and grade 4+ toxicity at various dose levels for the mean patient.

Sheiner and coworkers [4,5] proposed the use of dose-toxicity models for phase I trials a decade ago. They are still rarely used, despite their potential for facilitating the definition of a phase II starting dose.

4.5 Clinical applications

First-in-man phase I trial designs of oncology agents share the following characteristics: selection of a 'safe' starting dose, sequential dose-escalation in cohorts of patients and determination of a recommended dose based on a prespecified primary endpoint, usually the occurrence of unacceptable toxicity in a defined number of patients treated at a given dose level. Optimal phase I designs result in the identification of a dose for further evaluation in a manner that is both safe and efficient. Higher starting doses, fewer patients per dose level and large escalation steps require fewer patients overall. However, safety is enhanced by lower starting doses, more patients per dose level to ensure safety of the dose and smaller dosing increments. Phase I designs must strike a balance between these elements. Accelerated titration designs proposed by Simon *et al.* [7] use the following modifications to enhance efficiency: as few as one patient per level are enrolled and initial dose-escalation steps are larger (e.g. 100 % increments in the absence of toxicity). The number of patients per dose level increases to three, once toxicity of a minimum degree (e.g. second instance of grade 2; first instance of DLT) has been seen in at least one patient. Thereafter a minimum of three patients in each cohort are recruited, expanding to six in the event that one of three has a DLT in the protocol prescribed observation period (usually one cycle or 4–8 weeks of chronic therapy) and the dose-escalation increments are reduced.

To assess the use and utility of the accelerated titration designs in the evaluation of novel oncology therapeutics, we conducted a literature search using the ISI Web of Knowledge Database (Thomson ISI, Thomson Corporation, Philadelphia, Pennsylvania) in May and August 2005. All articles in the database that cited the original paper by Simon et al. [7] were retrieved and reviewed. In total, 106 publications were identified. Articles that focused on statistical methodology of phase I studies (10), were not of phase I studies (4), that evaluated combinations of agents (12), were review articles (34), or of phase I studies that did not use the Simon et al. [7] accelerated titration designs (10), were not included in our review. In total, 36 publications of phase I trials of novel cancer therapeutics were identified. From the trial publications, the following details were abstracted: agent/class, schedule, type of design, study-specific modifications to the design (e.g. patients/cohort and dose-escalation increments during the accelerated phase, rules for terminating the accelerated phase, dose-escalation increments following termination of the accelerated phase, dose levels evaluated and the number of dose levels evaluated during the accelerated phase and subsequently). A summary of these trials are provided in Tables 4:3 and 4.4.

From the results of our review a number of observations can be made regarding the utilization of the designs. Firstly, the classes of agents selected for evaluation using an accelerated titration design favor agents that belong to chemical classes that have been previously studied or to biological agents not associated with significant risk of severe, irreversible organ toxicity. This is not surprising, as agents with these characteristics would engender a level of comfort regarding the safety of using an accelerated titration design. Secondly, designs 3 and 4, which utilize single-patient cohorts and 100 % dose-escalations, are the most commonly used. Thirdly, almost half of the studies do not utilize intrapatient dose-escalation. Fourthly, the most common modifications to the designs are those determining the dose-escalation increments following termination of the accelerated phase and/or modifications to rules for terminating the accelerated phase. Most trials with modifications in the dose increments following termination of the accelerated phase stipulated dose increments of 15–30 % rather than 40 %. A few utilized higher-dose increments (50–67 %) and a few reverted to a modified Fibonacci escalation schema. Rules for terminating the accelerated phase included the first occurrence of any toxicity, or the achievement of a prespecified dose (e.g. mouse equivalent MTD). Given the frequency and nature of these modifications, it appears that investigators retain concerns regarding the safety of the accelerated titration design dose-escalation increments and termination rules.

To assess the efficiency and safety of the accelerated designs, the numbers of patients and dose levels, overall and during the accelerated phase, were evaluated across the 36 studies. Patients treated above the ultimately recommended phase II dose (RP2D) were identified. If a patient was treated at a dose level prescribed by the accelerated phase dose increase and that dose exceeded the RP2D, then the dose level was considered to have exceeded the recommended dose due to the accelerated phase rules. Similarly, patients that died on the study due to obvious or suspected treatment-related toxicity were identified. Those fatalities which occurred at doses prescribed during the accelerated phase of the study were classified as deaths during

Table 4.3   Phase I trials using accelerated titration design.

Author/reference	Agent	Schedule	Design	Intra patient dose-escalation	Recommended dose
LoRusso et al. [10]	5-Fluoro-pyrimidinone	Orally daily for 5 days every 4 weeks	4B	Yes	625 mg/m^2/day orally for 5 days every 4 weeks
Goetz et al. [11]	17-(Allylamino)-17-demethoxygeldanamycin	IV weekly × 3 every 4 weeks	2B	Yes	308 mg/m^2 weekly × 3 every 4 weeks
Grem et al. [12]	17-(Allylamino)-17-demethoxygeldanamycin	1 hour is IV infusion daily for 5 days every 3 weeks	2B	Yes	40 mg/m^2 daily × 5 every 3 weeks
Sessa et al. [13]	BBR3464, cationic triplatinum complex	IV daily × 5 every 3 weeks	4B	Yes	0.12 mg/m^2/day × 5 every 3 weeks
Mross et al. [14]	BBR3576, aza-anthrapyrazole	IV infusion every 4 weeks	4A	No	150 mg/m^2 every 4 weeks
Plummer et al. [15]	BMS-184476, taxane analog	IV weekly × 3 every 4 weeks, later amended to weekly × 2 every 21 days	4B	Yes	50 mg/m^2/week × 2 every 21 days
Mani et al. [16]	BMS-247550, derivative of Epothilone B	1 hour IV infusion every 3 weeks	Modified 4B	Yes	40 mg/m^2 every 3 weeks
Abraham et al. [17]	BMS-247550, derivative of Epothilone B	1 hour IV infusion daily × 5 every 21 days	Modified 3B	Yes	6 mg/m^2/day × 5 every 21 days
Gadgeel et al. [18]	BMS-247550, derivative of Epothilone B	1 hour IV infusion every 21 days	Modified 2B	Yes	40 mg/m^2 every 21 days

Reference	Agent	Schedule	Design	Intrapatient	Dose
Undevia et al. [19]	CEP-2563, receptor tyrosine kinase inhibitor	1 hour IV daily × 5 every 21 days	Modified 3B	Yes	256 mg/m²/day × 5 every 21 days
Hovstadius et al. [20]	CHS 828, cyanoguanidine	orally once daily × 5 days every 4 weeks	4B	Yes	20 mg once daily for 5 days (100 mg/cycle) every 4 weeks
Rudek et al. [21]	COL-3, matrix metalloproteinase inhibitor	orally daily	4A	No	36 mg/m²/d without sunblock
Syed et al. [22]	COL-3, matrix metalloproteinase inhibitor	Orally daily	2A	No	50 mg/m²/day
Rustin et al. [23]	Combretastatin A4 phosphate, ubulin targeting agent	IV × 5 for 2 weeks every 3 weeks	Modified 4B	Yes	52–68 mg/m² × 5 for 2 weeks every 3 weeks
Chatterjee et al. [24]	DRF-1042, camptothecin analog	Orally daily × 5 for 2 weeks every 3 weeks	Modified 3B	Yes	80 mg/m² × 5 for 2 weeks every 3 weeks
Villalona-Calero et al. [25]	Ecteinascidin-743, tetrahydroisoquinoline alkaloid	IV daily × 5 every 3 weeks	Modified 3A	No	325 g/m²/day daily × 5
Ko et al. [26]	EMD 273066 (huKS-IL2) immunocytokine	IV daily × 3 every 4 weeks	Modified 4A	No	6.4 mg/m²/day × 3 every 4 weeks
Goel et al. [27]	GEM231, oligonucleotide to type I regulatory subunit of protein kinase A	3 day (1 patient) or a 5 day continuous IV infusion	Modified 4A	No	120 mg/m²/day × 5 days
Chen et al. [28]	GEM231, oligonucleotide to type I regulatory subunit of protein kinase A	2 hour IV infusions twice weekly	Modified 4A	No	240 mg/m² twice weekly

(Continued)

Table 4.3   (*Continued*)

Author/ reference	Agent	Schedule	Design	Intra patient dose-escalation	Recommended dose
Borchmann et al. [29]	H22xKi-4, bispecific anti-CD30 and CD64 monoclonal antibody	IV days 1, 3, 5, 7–21 days	4B	Yes	80 mg/m² per cycle
Gadgeel et al. [30]	KRN5500, spicamycin derivative	1 hour IV daily × 5 every 3 weeks	2B	Yes	4.3 mg/m²/day × 5 every 3 weeks
Schoemaker et al. [31]	MAG-CPT, polymer conjugate of camptothecin	IV infusion over 3 days every 4 weeks	Modified 2A	No	68 mg/m²/day for 3 days every 4 weeks
Matsumura et al. [32]	MCC-465, doxorubicin PEG immunoliposome	1 hour IV infusion every 3 weeks	ATD planned	No	32.5 mg/m² every 3 weeks
Clive et al. [33]	Antagonist G substance P analog	IV every 3 weeks until the target maximum plasma concentration of 10 μM then weekly	Modified 4A	No	400 mg/m² weekly 6 hour IV infusion
Matsumura et al. [34]	NK911, micelle encapsulated doxorubicin	IV every 3 weeks	Modified 3A	No	50 mg/m² every 3 weeks
de Jonge et al. [35]	PNU-159548, alkylcycline	IV every 3 weeks (2 studies)	Modified 4B	Yes	12 and 14 mg/m² IV every 3 weeks in HP and MP patients
Lockhart et al. [36]	PNU-166196A, brostallicin, a nonalkylating DNA minor groove binder	IV weekly × 3 every 4 weeks	Modified 3B	Yes	2.4 mg/m²/week

Reference	Drug	Schedule	Design		Starting dose
Ten Tije et al. [37]	PNU-166196A, brostallicin, a nonalkylating DNA minor groove binder	IV every 3 weeks	3B	Yes	10 mg/m²/3 weeks
Dupont et al. [38]	Ro 31-7453, oral cell-cycle inhibitor	Two Schedules: once or twice daily × 5 every 21 days	3A	No	560 mg/m² every 21 days or flat dose of 1000 mg daily for 4 days for both schedules
Salazar et al. [39]	Ro 31-7453, oral cell-cycle inhibitor	Two schedules orally every 12 hours for 7 days or 14 days every 4 weeks	4A	No	200 mg/m² bid for 7 days; 125 mg/m² bid for 14 days
Wadler et al. [40]	Triapine, ribonucleotide reductase inhibitor	96 hour continuous IV infusion every 3 weeks or every 2 weeks	4B	Yes	120 mg/m²/d every 2 weeks
Murren et al. [41]	Triapine, ribonucleotide reductase inhibitor	2 hour IV daily × 5 days every 4 weeks or every 2 weeks	Began as modified Fibonacci then 4B	Yes	96 mg/m² by 2 hour IV infusion daily for 5 days every 2 weeks
Jones et al. [42]	Tazarotene, acetylenic retinoid	Orally daily	Modified 3A	No	25.2 mg/day
Al-Batran et al. [43]	Trofosfamide	Orally in 3 doses per day for 3 weeks	1B	Yes	125 mg/m² administered in 3 doses per day every 3 weeks
Dees et al. [44]	UCN-01, tyrosine kinase inhibitor	1–3 hour IV infusion every 4 weeks	4A	No	95 mg/m² over 3 hours
Goh et al. [45]	ZD9331, thymidylate synthase inhibitor	IV for 5 days every 21 days	3A	No	25 mg/day

Table 4.4 Summary of phase I studies using accelerated titration design.

			36
Trials (n)			36
Patients (n)			911

	Type		Trials (n)
Design	1		1
	2		6
	3		10
	4		18
	Unknown		1
Intrapatient dose-escalation			
	Yes		20
	No		16
Modifications	Yes		15
	No		11
Types of modifications		Dose-escalation during the accelerated phase	3
		Patients/cohort during the accelerated phase	2
		Rules for termination of accelerated phase	8
		Dose-escalation following accelerated phase	19

	During accelerated phase		For study	
	Median	Range	Median	Range
Patients/study (n)	5	0–15	22	7–74
Dose levels (n)	3	0–12	6	3–15
Fold dose range			16	2–320
Patients treated				
Above RP2D	0	0–6	6	0–28
Dose levels				
Above RP2D	0	0–1 (4 of 36 studies had a dose level that exceeded the RP2D during the ATD)	1	0–3
Deaths due to toxicity	0	0–1 (1 patient across all studies died due to toxicities)	0 (13 patients across all studies died due to toxicities)	0–3

the accelerated phase. As summarized in Table 4.4, the accelerated titration designs, as used in these studies, rarely resulted in dose escalation beyond the recommended phase II dose. Only 4 of 36 exceeded the recommended phase II dose during the accelerated titration phase and only 1 death from toxicity occurred during the accelerated titration phase, among the 911 patients enrolled in these studies. (It should be noted, however, that the use of acceleration may have contributed, in some trials, to exceeding the RP2D by a greater number of doses, or for a greater number of patients, than would otherwise have happened. Thus, the use of acceleration in these trials may have increased the overall number of patients treated above the RP2D, even beyond the acceleration phase itself, and thus contributed to a greater death rate from toxicity.) Based on its utilization in these selected studies, the accelerated titration design appears to provide an enhanced efficiency with acceptable safety. However, there are a number of issues investigators might consider prior to selecting an accelerated titration design to evaluate a novel agent in a first-in-man phase I clinical trial.

The use of minimum one-patient cohorts and larger dose-escalation steps may be advantageous under the following circumstances: (a) the agent is of a chemical class that has been widely studied; (b) the agent is predicted to have minimal interpatient variability in pharmacokinetics; (c) the agent's anticipated toxicity is unlikely to be severe or irreversible and is amenable to close monitoring and supportive interventions. Examples of agents most amenable to evaluation using a phase I accelerated titration design might be the following: a new formulation of a previously studied agent (e.g. liposomal formulation of paclitaxel), a biological agent with minimal toxicity based on animal models (e.g. antibody or small molecule inhibitor of a receptor tyrosine kinase inhibitor) or an agent for which significant interspecies variability in preclinical toxicology has led to a very conservative starting dose in a human phase I study. Under these circumstances, the increased efficiency and presumed safety of an accelerated design might make it preferable.

Conversely, there are situations where an accelerated titration design may not provide the optimal balance between safety and efficiency as either larger numbers of patients/dose cohort and/or smaller dose increments would be preferable. Agents associated with steep dose-response curves for toxicity, severe irreversible toxicity, unexplained mortality in animal toxicology studies or large variability in doses or plasma drug levels eliciting effects may require alternative designs to balance safety and efficiency optimally. For example, larger patient numbers/dose cohorts may be preferred if there is anticipated wide interpatient variability in toxic effects due to pharmacokinetic or pharmacogenomic differences between patients. For this circumstance, larger patient numbers per dose level is appropriate since decisions about the safety of a given dose may require more than a single patient's experience. Similarly, when a pharmacokinetic or a pharmacodynamic endpoint, rather than toxicity, is the primary endpoint, larger numbers of patients per dose level are recommended due to anticipated interpatient variability in these endpoints. With either situation, the use of an accelerated titration design with single-patient cohorts may not be optimal.

There are also situations where small dose-escalation increments may be advisable. For example, if the agent is predicted to have severe, irreversible or potentially fatal organ toxicity based on animal toxicology, particularly if associated with a steep dose-response curve for toxicity, relatively small changes in dose/concentration may lead from minimal toxicity to severe toxicity, and thus smaller dose-escalation increments are preferable to ensure safety.

Approaches to enhancing the proportion of patients in a phase I trial receiving 'therapeutic' dose levels includes not only limiting enrolment on lower dose levels but also allowing dose-escalation within individual patients. Intrapatient dose-escalation provides two advantages: it improves the likelihood of benefit from the agent for the individual patient and it increases the experience at higher dose levels. Accelerated titration designs proposed by Simon *et al.* [7] allow intrapatient dose escalation if no toxicity > grade 1 was seen in the first cycle at the assigned dose level. While it did not appreciably shorten the study duration, it did allow more patients to be treated at or near the recommended phase II dose and increased the number of cycles evaluated at the higher dose levels.

Although the rationale supporting intrapatient dose-escalation is appealing, it does not seem to be widely applied. Thus, despite the appeal of escalating patients to higher doses than they were assigned initially, should safety criteria be met, some issues remain with its routine application in phase I protocols. Many phase I protocols continue to be written prohibiting intrapatient escalation since it is believed to have a minimal impact on trial efficiency while bringing with it concerns about practical issues regarding the 'rules' for implementing dose-escalation and safety. Studies that have allowed intrapatient escalation within their protocols have generally allowed dose-escalation to occur after the patient has been evaluated at the current dose level for the duration of the observation period and where the patient has had minimal/no toxicity. Less commonly used are rules that require not only that the patient has not had significant toxicity but also that the next higher dose level has been evaluated in one or more new patients – a more stringent and cumbersome criterion that may be favored to enhance safety and also to distinguish between acute versus cumulative toxic events. Although experience with intrapatient dose-escalation within phase I studies is limited, to date its use within phase I studies using an accelerated titration design did not appear to compromise patient safety or complicate the interpretation of the study results. Of note, within a given protocol, it is important to require a minimum number of newly recruited patients at each dose level and to base further dose-escalation decisions upon the behavior of the drug in these individuals.

4.6 Conclusions

Accelerated titration designs can dramatically reduce the number of patients accrued to a phase I trial, in comparison to the standard phase I design. They can also substantially shorten the duration of the phase I trial. With intrapatient dose-escalation and application of a dose-toxicity model, they provide much greater information than the standard design and analysis with regard to cumulative toxicity, interpatient and intrapatient variability, steepness of the dose-toxicity curve and separation of the dose-toxicity curves for the varying toxicity levels. They also provide all patients entered in the trial a maximum opportunity to be treated at a therapeutic dose.

Despite this, we find that the designs are not widely used, which is likely to be due to the conservativeness of investigators. Even when they are used, they are often used with an initial dose set much more conservatively than would be done for the standard design and without use of intrapatient dose-escalation, thereby reducing their effectiveness. A recent comprehensive review of the risk-benefit relationship for phase I trials conducted over the past decade reveals an overall toxicity death rate of only 0.005 [46]. An accompanying editorial [47] argues that such a low toxicity death rate, in the context of treatment for an often rapidly fatal disease, suggests that phase I trials may be conducted in an overly cautious fashion. Appropriate utilization of designs such as the accelerated titration designs might increase the potential for benefit in phase I trials, with little increase in risk.

References

1. S.G. Arbuck (1996) Workshop on phase I study design. Ninth NCI/EORTC New Drug Development Symposium, Amsterdam, March 12, 1996. *Ann. Oncology*, **7**(6), 567–73.
2. E.A. Eisenhauer, P.J. O'Dwyer, M. Christian and J.S. Humphrey (2000). Phase I clinical trial design in cancer drug development. *J. Clin. Oncology*, **18**(3), 684–92.
3. S.F. Dent and E.A. Eisenhauer (1996) Phase I trial design: are new methodologies being put into practice? *Ann. Oncology*, **7**(6), 561–6.
4. L.B. Sheiner (1990) Implications of an alternative approach to dose-response trials. *J. Acquired Immune Deficiency Syndrome*, **3**(Suppl. 2), 20–6.
5. L.B. Sheiner, S.L. Beal and N.C. Sambol (1989) Study designs for dose-ranging. *Clin. Pharmacology Theory*, **46**(1), 63–77.
6. L.B. Sheiner, Y. Hashimoto and S.L. Beal (1991) A simulation study comparing designs for dose ranging. *Statistics in Medicine*, **10**(3), 303–21 March.
7. R. Simon, B. Freidlin, L. Rubinstein, S.G. Arbuck, J. Collins and M.C. Christian (1997) Accelerated titration designs for phase I clinical trials in oncology. *J. Natl Cancer Inst.*, **89**(15), 1138–47.
8. T.C. Chou and P. Talalay (1981) Generalized equations for the analysis of inhibitions of Michaelis–Menten and higher-order kinetic systems with two or more mutually exclusive and nonexclusive inhibitors. *Eur. J. Biochemistry*, **115**(1), 207–16.
9. T.C. Chou and P. Talalay (1984) Quantitative analysis of dose–effect relationships: the combined effects of multiple drugs or enzyme inhibitors. *Adv. Enzyme Regulation*, **22**, 27–55.
10. P.M. LoRusso, S. Prakash, A. Wozniak, L. Flaherty, M. Zalupski, A. Shields, H. Sands, R. Parchment and B. Jasti (2002) Phase I clinical trial of 5-fluoropyrimidinone (5FP), an oral prodrug of 5-fluorouracil (5FU). *Investigational New Drugs*, **20**(1), 63–71.
11. M.P. Goetz, D. Toft, J. Reid, M. Ames, B. Stensgard, S. Safgren, A.A. Adjei, J. Sloan, P. Atherton, V. Vasile, S. Salazaar, A. Adjei, G. Croghan and C. Erlichman (2005) Phase I

trial of 17-allylamino-17-demethoxygeldanamycin in patients with advanced cancer *J. Clin. Oncology*, **23**(6), 1078–87.

12. J.L. Grem, G. Morrison, X.D. Guo, E. Agnew, C.H. Takimoto, R. Thomas, E. Szabo, L. Grochow, F. Grollman, J.M. Hamilton, L. Neckers and R.H. Wilson (2005) Phase I and pharmacologic study of 17-(allylamino)-17-demethoxygeldanamycin in adult patients with solid tumors. *J. Clin. Oncology*, **23**(9), 1885–93.

13. C. Sessa, G. Capri, L. Gianni, F. Peccatori, G. Grasselli, J. Bauer, M. Zucchetti, L. Viganò, A. Gatti, C. Minoia, P. Liati, S. Van den Bosch, A. Bernareggi, G. Camboni and S. Marsoni (2000) Clinical and pharmacological phase I study with accelerated titration design of a daily times five schedule of BBR3464, a novel cationic triplatinum complex. *Ann. Oncology*, **11**(8), 977–83.

14. K. Mross, M.E. Scheulen, T. Licht, C. Unger, H. Richly, A.C. Stern, K. Kutz, M.G. Camboni, P. Barbieri, E. Verdi, B. Vincenzi and A. Bernareggi (2004) Phase I clinical and pharmacokinetic study of BBR 3576, a novel aza-anthrapyrazole, administered i.v. every 4 weeks in patients with advanced solid tumors: a phase I study group trial of the Central European Society of Anticancer-Drug Research (CESAR). *Anticancer Drugs*, **15**(1), 15–22.

15. R. Plummer, M. Ghielmini, P. Calvert, M. Voi, J. Renard, G. Gallant, E. Gupta, H. Calvert and C. Sessa (2002) Phase I and pharmacokinetic study of the new taxane analog BMS-184476 given weekly in patients with advanced malignancies. *Clin. Cancer Res.*, **8**(9), 2788–97.

16. S. Mani, H. McDaid, A. Hamilton, H. Hochster, M.B. Cohen, D. Khabelle, T. Griffin, D.E. Lebwohl, L. Liebes, F. Muggia and S.B. Horwitz (2004) Phase I clinical and pharmacokinetic study of BMS-247550, a novel derivative of epothilone B, in solid tumors. *Clin. Cancer Res.*, **10**(4), 1289–98.

17. J. Abraham, M. Agrawal, S. Bakke, A. Rutt, M. Edgerly, F.M. Balis, B. Widemann, L. Davis, B. Damle, D. Sonnichsen, D. Lebwohl, S. Bates, H. Kotz and T. Fojo (2003) Phase I trial and pharmacokinetic study of BMS-247550, an epothilone B analog, administered intravenously on a daily schedule for five days. *J. Clin. Oncology*, **21**(9), 1866–73.

18. S.M. Gadgeel, A. Wozniak, R.R. Boinpally, R. Wiegand, L.K. Heilbrun, V. Jain, R. Parchment, D. Colevas, M.B. Cohen and P.M. LoRusso (2005) Phase I clinical trial of BMS-247550, a derivative of epothilone B, using accelerated titration 2B design. *Clin. Cancer Res.*, **11**(17), 6233–9.

19. S.D. Undevia, N.J. Vogelzang, A.M. Mauer, L. Janisch, S. Mani and M.J. Ratain (2004) Phase I clinical trial of CEP-2563 dihydrochloride, a receptor tyrosine kinase inhibitor, in patients with refractory solid tumors. *Invest. New Drugs*, **22**(4), 449–58.

20. P. Hovstadius, R. Larsson, E. Jonsson, T. Skov, A.M. Kissmeyer, K. Krasilnikoff, J. Bergh, M.O. Karlsson, A. Lönnebo and J. Ahlgren (2002) A phase I study of CHS 828 in patients with solid tumor malignancy. *Clin. Cancer Res.*, **8**(9), 2843–50.

21. M.A. Rudek, W.D. Figg, V. Dyer, W. Dahut, M.L. Turner, S.M. Steinberg, D.J. Liewehr, D.R. Kohler, J.M. Pluda and E. Reed (2001) Phase I clinical trial of oral COL-3, a matrix metalloproteinase inhibitor, in patients with refractory metastatic cancer. *J. Clin. Oncology*, **19**(2), 584–92.

22. S. Syed, C. Takimoto, M. Hidalgo, J. Rizzo, J.G. Kuhn, L.A. Hammond, G. Schwartz, A. Tolcher, A. Patnaik, S.G. Eckhardt and E.K. Rowinsky (2004) A phase I and pharmacokinetic study of Col-3 (Metastat), an oral tetracycline derivative with potent matrix metalloproteinase and antitumor properties. *Clin. Cancer Res.*, **10**(19), 6512–21.

23. G.J. Rustin, S.M. Galbraith, H. Anderson, M. Stratford, L.K. Folkes, L. Sena, L. Gumbrell and P.M. Price (2003) Phase I clinical trial of weekly combretastatin A4 phosphate: clinical and pharmacokinetic results. *J. Clin. Oncology*, **21**(15), 2815–22.

24. A. Chatterjee, R. Digumarti, R.N. Mamidi, K. Katneni, V.V. Upreti, A. Surath, M.L. Srinivas, S. Uppalapati, S. Jiwatani, S. Subramaniam and N.R. Srinivas (2004) Safety, tolerability, pharmacokinetics, and pharmacodynamics of an orally active novel camptothecin analog, DRF-1042, in refractory cancer patients in a phase I dose escalation study. *J. Clin. Pharmacology*, **44**(7), 723–36.

25. M.A. Villalona-Calero, S.G. Eckhardt, G. Weiss, M. Hidalgo, J.H. Beijnen, C. van Kesteren, H. Rosing, E. Campbell, M. Kraynak, L. Lopez-Lazaro, C. Guzman, D.D. Von Hoff, J. Jimeno and E.K. Rowinsky (2002) A phase I and pharmacokinetic study of ecteinascidin-743 on a daily × 5 schedule in patients with solid malignancies. *Clin. Cancer Res.*, **8**(1), 75–85.

26. Y.J. Ko, G.J. Bubley, R. Weber, C. Redfern, D.P. Gold, L. Finke, A. Kovar, T. Dahl and S.D. Gillies (2004) Safety, pharmacokinetics, and biological pharmacodynamics of the immunocytokine EMD 273066 (huKS-IL2): results of a phase I trial in patients with prostate cancer. *J. Immunotherapy*, **27**(3), 232–9.

27. S. Goel, K. Desai, A. Bulgaru, A. Fields, G. Goldberg, S. Agrawal, R. Martin, M. Grindel and S. Mani (2003) A safety study of a mixed-backbone oligonucleotide (GEM231) targeting the type I regulatory subunit alpha of protein kinase A using a continuous infusion schedule in patients with refractory solid tumors. *Clin. Cancer Res.*, **9**(11), 4069–76.

28. H.X. Chen, J.L. Marshall, E. Ness, R.R. Martin, B. Dvorchik, N. Rizvi, J. Marquis, M. McKinlay, W. Dahut and M.J. Hawkins (2000) A safety and pharmacokinetic study of a mixed-backbone oligonucleotide (GEM231) targeting the type I protein kinase A by two-hour infusions in patients with refractory solid tumors. *Clin. Cancer Res.*, **6**(4), 1259–66.

29. P. Borchmann, R. Schnell, I. Fuss, O. Manzke, T. Davis, L.D. Lewis, D. Behnke, C. Wickenhauser, P. Schiller, V. Diehl and A. Engert (2002) Phase I trial of the novel bispecific molecule H22 × Ki-4 in patients with refractory Hodgkin lymphoma. *Blood*, **100**(9), 3101–7.

30. S.M. Gadgeel, R.R. Boinpally, L.K. Heilbrun, A. Wozniak, V. Jain, B. Redman, M. Zalupski, R. Wiegand, R. Parchment and P.M. LoRusso (2003) A phase I clinical trial of spicamycin derivative KRN5500 (NSC 650426) using a phase I accelerated titration '2B' design. *Investigational New Drugs*, **21**(1), 63–74.

31. N.E. Schoemaker, C. van Kesteren, H. Rosing, S. Jansen, M. Swart, J. Lieverst, D. Fraier, M. Breda, C. Pellizzoni, R. Spinelli, M. Grazia Porro, J.H. Beijnen, J.H. Schellens and W.W. ten Bokkel Huinink (2002) A phase I and pharmacokinetic study of MAG-CPT, a water-soluble polymer conjugate of camptothecin. *Br. J. Cancer*, **87**(6), 608–14.

32. Y. Matsumura, M. Gotoh, K. Muro, Y. Yamada, K. Shirao, Y. Shimada, M. Okuwa, S. Matsumoto, Y. Miyata, H. Ohkura, K. Chin, S. Baba, T. Yamao, A. Kannami, Y. Takamatsu, K. Ito and K. Takahashi (2004) Phase I and pharmacokinetic study of MCC-465, a doxorubicin (DXR) encapsulated in PEG immunoliposome, in patients with metastatic stomach cancer. *Ann. Oncology*, **15**(3), 517–25.

33. S. Clive, D.J. Webb, A. MacLellan, A. Young, B. Byrne, L. Robson, J.F. Smyth and D.I. Jodrell (2001) Forearm blood flow and local responses to peptide vasodilators: a novel pharmacodynamic measure in the phase I trial of antagonist G, a neuropeptide growth factor antagonist. *Clin. Cancer Res.*, **7**(10), 3071–8.

34. Y. Matsumura, T. Hamaguchi, T. Ura, K. Muro, Y. Yamada, Y. Shimada, K. Shirao, T. Okusaka, H. Ueno, M. Ikeda and N. Watanabe (2004) Phase I clinical trial and pharmacokinetic evaluation of NK911, a micelle-encapsulated doxorubicin. *Br. J. Cancer*, **91**(10), 1775–81.

35. M.J. de Jonge, J. Verweij, A. van der Gaast, O. Valota, O. Mora, A.S. Planting, M.A. Mantel, S.V. Bosch, M.J. Lechuga, F. Fiorentini, D. Hess and C. Sessa (2002) Phase I and pharmacokinetic studies of PNU-159548, a novel alkycycline, administered intravenously to patients with advanced solid tumours. *Eur. J. Cancer*, **38**(18), 2407–15.

36. A.C. Lockhart, M. Howard, K.R. Hande, B.J. Roth, J.D. Berlin, F. Vreeland, A. Campbell, E. Fontana, F. Fiorentini, C. Fowst, V.A. Paty, O. Lankford and M.L. Rothenberg (2004) A phase I dose-escalation and pharmacokinetic study of brostallicin (PNU-166196A), a novel DNA minor groove binder, in adult patients with advanced solid tumors. *Clin. Cancer Res.*, **10**(2), 468–75.

37. A.J. Ten Tije, J. Verweij, A. Sparreboom, A. Van Der Gaast, C. Fowst, F. Fiorentini, J. Tursi, A. Antonellini, M. Mantel, C.M. Hartman, G. Stoter, A.S. Planting and M.J. De Jonge (2003) Phase I and pharmacokinetic study of brostallicin (PNU-166196), a new DNA minor-groove binder, administered intravenously every 3 weeks to adult patients with metastatic cancer. *Clin. Cancer Res.*, **9**(8), 2957–64.

38. J. Dupont, B. Bienvenu, C. Aghajanian, S. Pezzulli, P. Sabbatini, P. Vongphrachanh, C. Chang, C. Perkell, K. Ng, S. Passe, L. Breimer, J. Zhi, M. DeMario, D. Spriggs and S.L. Soignet (2004) Phase I and pharmacokinetic study of the novel oral cell-cycle inhibitor Ro 31-7453 in patients with advanced solid tumors. *J. Clin. Oncology*, **22**(16), 3366–74.

39. R. Salazar, D. Bissett, C. Twelves, L. Breimer, M. DeMario, S. Campbell, J. Zhi, S. Ritland and J. Cassidy (2004) A phase I clinical and pharmacokinetic study of Ro 31-7453 given as a 7- or 14-day oral twice daily schedule every 4 weeks in patients with solid tumors. *Clin. Cancer Res.*, **10**(13), 4374–82.

40. S. Wadler, D. Makower, C. Clairmont, P. Lambert, K. Fehn and M. Sznol (2004) Phase I and pharmacokinetic study of the ribonucleotide reductase inhibitor, 3-aminopyridine-2-carboxaldehyde thiosemicarbazone, administered by 96-hour intravenous continuous infusion. *J. Clin. Oncology*, **22**(9), 1553–63.

41. J. Murren, M. Modiano, C. Clairmont, P. Lambert, N. Savaraj, T. Doyle and M. Sznol (2003) Phase I and pharmacokinetic study of triapine, a potent ribonucleotide reductase inhibitor, administered daily for five days in patients with advanced solid tumors. *Clin. Cancer Res.*, **9**(11), 4092–100.

42. P.H. Jones, R.D. Burnett, I. Fainaru, P. Nadolny, P. Walker, Z. Yu, D. Tang-Liu, T.S. Ganesan, D.C. Talbot, A.L. Harris and G.J. Rustin (2003) A phase 1 study of tazarotene in adults with advanced cancer. *Br. J. Cancer*, **89**(5), 808–15.

43. S.E. Al-Batran, A. Atmaca, F. Bert, D. Jäger, C. Frisch, A. Neumann, J. Orth, A. Knuth and E. Jäger (2004) Dose escalation study for defining the maximum tolerated dose of continuous oral trofosfamide in pretreated patients with metastatic lung cancer. *Onkologie*, **27**(6), 534–8.

44. E.C. Dees, S.D. Baker, S. O'Reilly, M.A. Rudek, S.B. Davidson, C. Aylesworth, K. Elza-Brown, M.A. Carducci and R.C. Donehower (2004) A phase I and pharmacokinetic study of short infusions of UCN-01 in patients with refractory solid tumors. *Clin. Cancer Res.*, **11**(2 Pt 1), 664–71.

45. B.C. Goh, M.J. Ratain, D. Bertucci, R. Smith, S. Mani, N.J. Vogelzang, R.L. Schilsky, M. Hutchison, M. Smith, S. Averbuch and E. Douglass (2001) Phase I study of ZD9331 on short daily intravenous bolus infusion for 5 days every 3 weeks with fixed dosing recommendations. *J. Clin. Oncology*, **19**(5), 1476–84.

46. E. Horstmann, M.S. McCabe, L. Grochow, S. Yamamoto, L. Rubinstein, T. Budd, D. Shoemaker, E.J. Emanuel and C. Grady (2005) Risks and benefits of phase 1 oncology trials, 1991 through 2002. *N. Engl. J. Medicine*, **352**(9), 895–904.

47. R. Kurzrock and R.S. Benjamin (2005) Risks and benefits of phase 1 oncology trials, revisited. *N. Engl. J. Medicine*, **352**(9), 930–2.

5

Group up-and-down designs in toxicity studies

Anastasia Ivanova and Nancy Flournoy

Department of Biostatistics, The University of North Carolina at Chapel Hill, North Carolina, USA
Department of Statistics, University of Missouri-Columbia, Columbia, Missouri, USA

5.1 Introduction

The literature on up-and-down designs is vast as these procedures have been developed for many different types of applications including, for example, psychology, biophysics and adaptive testing. The first ones of which we are aware are by Wilson and Worchester [1, 2]. We focus on up-and-down designs that have been developed for phase I and phase I/II clinical trials and for acute toxicity studies, and make no claim of covering the development of up-and-down procedures for other applications.

For phase I clinical trials, the goal is to estimate a dose $\mu_{100\Gamma}$ with prescribed probability of toxicity Γ. Although quite a misnomer, $\mu_{100\Gamma}$ is often called the maximum tolerated dose. For phase I studies, Γ typically ranges from 0.1 to 0.35. For efficacy studies the outcome of interest is therapeutic response and Γ is usually above 0.5. For acute toxicity studies designed to determine labeling requirements for pesticides, cosmetics and other consumer products, the goal is to estimate μ_{50}, sometimes with a confidence interval. For acute toxicity studies relevant to endangered

Statistical Methods for Dose-Finding Experiments Edited by S. Chevret
© 2006 John Wiley & Sons, Ltd

species, Γ is much less than 0.1. For phase I/II studies, the goal is to estimate the dose with the highest probability of success, which is defined as efficacy without toxicity. We briefly mention some up-and-down designs for these more complex situations.

In an up-and-down procedure, a subject's treatment is never more than one level higher or lower than the dose given to the previous subject. Many ad hoc up-and-down procedures have been proposed. See, for example, Wetherill and Glazebrook [3] and Korn *et al.* [4]. We focus on simple up-and-down procedures that perform in a predictable manner without requiring a parametric specification of the probability of response as a function of dose. The most common such up-and-down procedures are first-order Markovian procedures in which the rule for allocating the next dose depends only on the current treatment and its recent outcomes. Advantages of Markovian procedures include their simplicity, the availability of a well–known theory (finite and asymptotic) for analysis and their relatively fast speed of convergence so that asymptotic theory applies to moderate sample sizes. Non–Markovian procedures, while abundant, are studied by simulation.

Let $d, d \in \Re$, denote the dose on a log scale. Let $D = \{d_1, \ldots, d_K\}$ be the set of allowable ordered doses. Let $F(d)$ denote the probability of toxicity at dose d. We assume that $F(d)$ is an increasing function of d. The group up-and-down design is described in Section 2. In Sections 3 and 4, we describe fully sequential first-order Markovian procedures, which are random walk procedures. In Section 3, we describe some applications of the classical up-and-down design for estimating μ_{50} and in Section 4, we generalize this classical procedure to a fully sequential procedure that clusters observations around an arbitrary $\mu_{100\Gamma}$. In Section 5, we discuss start-up rules. Methods of estimating $\mu_{100\Gamma}$ are taken up in Section 6. In Section 7, we assume that the probability of success, efficacy without toxicity, is a unimodal function of dose and review up-and-down procedures for estimating the dose with the maximum success probability.

5.2 Group up-and-down designs for phase I clinical trials

The group up-and-down design of Tsutakawa [5, 6] has been studied in a more general context by Gezmu and Flournoy [7]. The goal is to find a dose $\mu_{100\Gamma}$ with a probability of toxicity Γ. Subjects are treated in cohorts of size s. Let $R(d_j)$ be the number of toxic responses in the most recent cohort assigned to dose d_j. Then, conditional on d_j, $R(d_j)$ has a binomial distribution with parameters s and $F_j \equiv F(d_j)$. Let c_L and c_U be two integers such that $0 \le c_L < c_U \le s$. The group up-and-down design is defined as follows.

Given that a cohort of s subjects has been treated at dose d_j, $j = 2, \ldots, K - 1$, the next cohort of s subjects is assigned to dose:

1. d_{j-1} if $R(d_j) \geq c_U$;

2. d_{j+1} if $R(d_j) \leq c_L$;

3. d_j if $c_L < R(d_j) < c_U$.

Applying this rule when treatment has been given at $j = 1$ or K would cause treatments to be assigned outside of the preset range of D with positive probability. Thus for $j = 1$ or K, when the rule would cause a treatment to be outside of the range of D, the current treatment is repeated instead. We denote this design by $UD(s, c_L, c_U)$.

Let q_j be the probability of decreasing the dose from d_j; p_j denotes the probability of increasing the dose from d_j; and r_j is the probability of repeating the dose at d_j. Then

$$q_j = \sum_{i=c_U}^{s} \binom{s}{i} F_j^i \left(1 - F_j\right)^{s-i},$$

$$p_j = \sum_{i=0}^{c_L} \binom{s}{i} F_j^i \left(1 - F_j\right)^{s-i} \quad \text{and} \quad r_j = 1 - p_j - q_j.$$

These elements comprise the transition probability matrix for $UD(s, c_L, c_U)$, which is

$$\mathbf{P} = \begin{pmatrix} r_1 & p_1 & 0 & \cdots & & \cdots & 0 \\ q_2 & r_2 & p_2 & 0 & \ddots & & \vdots \\ 0 & q_3 & r_3 & p_3 & \ddots & & \vdots \\ \vdots & \ddots & \ddots & \ddots & \ddots & & \vdots \\ \vdots & & \ddots & \ddots & q_{K-1} & r_{K-1} & p_{K-1} \\ 0 & \cdots & & \cdots & 0 & q_K & r_K \end{pmatrix}.$$

Let $N_j(n)$ be the number of subjects assigned to dose d_j by the time n subjects have been assigned. Then, {if $F(d_j)$} are bounded away from 0 and 1, $(N_1(n)/n, \ldots, N_K(n)/n) \xrightarrow{p} \pi = (\pi_1, \ldots, \pi_K)$ as $n \to \infty$ by the law of large numbers for regular Markov chains. The vector π is called the stationary treatment distribution. The convergence rate to π is exponential, and it is determined by the second largest (in absolute value) eigenvalue of the transition probability matrix $\mathbf{P}$. Gezmu and Flournoy [7] give examples and illustrate the closeness of asymptotic results to the results for sample sizes of 16 or 24. Furthermore, $\sqrt{n}[N_k(n)/n - \pi_k] \xrightarrow{n \to \infty} N\left(0, \sigma_k^2(P)\right)$ by the central limit theorem for regular Markov chains.

Gezmu and Flournoy [7] prove that π is unimodal and illustrate how, given Γ, to choose s, c_L, and c_U so as to cause the treatment mode to be near $\mu_{100\Gamma}$. Let Bin(s, Γ) denote a binomial random variable with parameters s and Γ. Then choosing

s, c_L and c_U so that the equation

$$\Pr\{\mathrm{Bin}(s, \Gamma) \leq c_L\} = \Pr\{\mathrm{Bin}(s, \Gamma) \geq c_U\} \tag{5.1}$$

is approximately true will cluster treatments around $\mu_{100\Gamma}$. The approximation is required because, given Γ, D and practical values of s, there may not be values of $\{c_L, c_U\}$ such that the equation $F(\mu) = \Gamma$ has a solution in D. Note that according to equation (5.1), Γ is such that the probability of increasing the dose from $\mu_{100\Gamma}$ is the same as the probability of decreasing the dose from $\mu_{100\Gamma}$.

To evaluate a prospective $UD(s, c_L, c_U)$ for an experiment you are designing, you will want to determine the expected numbers treated at each dose and the expected number of toxicities for various dose sets and a range of possible response scenarios $\{F(d_j)\}$. Select a dose set D, design parameters $\{s, c_L, c_U\}$ and a set of response scenarios $\{F(d_j)\}$. Compute $\{p_j, q_j, r_j\}$ according to the definition of the group up-and-down design and construct the transition probability matrix $\mathbf{P}$. Using software that performs matrix multiplication, keep multiplying $\mathbf{P}$ times itself until all the rows are identical to each other to as many decimal places as you care about. Suppose this requires $\mathbf{P}$ to be raised to the τth power. Each row vector of the resulting matrix $\mathbf{P}^\tau$ is equal to π to the chosen number of decimal points, i.e $\pi_j = \lim_{n\to\infty} E[N_j(n)/n]$, $j = 1, \ldots, K$. Asymptotically, the expected number of toxicities may now be computed directly as $\sum_{j=0}^{K} \pi_j F(d_j)$.

To explore finite sample performance given a dose set D, design parameters $\{s, c_L, c_U\}$ and a hypothetical set of response scenarios $\{F(d_j)\}$, including the effect of the starting dose and the rate of convergence, compute

$$E_i\left[\frac{N_j(n)}{n}\right] = \delta_{ij} + \sum_{m=1}^{n-1} p_{ij}(m),$$

where the index i denotes the level of the initial dose, δ_{ij} is Kronneker's delta and $p_{ij}(\tau)$ is the (i, j)th element of $\mathbf{P}^\tau$. The expected number of toxicities for a finite sample of size n then follows:

$$E[\# \text{ toxicities starting with dose} d_i] = \sum_{j=1}^{K} E_i\left[\frac{N_j(n)}{n}\right] F(d_j).$$

Gezmu and Flournoy [7] illustrate for sample sizes 16 and 24 that, when $\{s, c_L, c_U\}$ are selected according to equation (5.1), treatments cluster around $\mu_{100\Gamma}$, even when the initial treatment is far from $\mu_{100\Gamma}$. Table 5.1 gives the values of Γ that are the solution of equation (5.1) for all possible values c_L and c_U for group sizes $s = 2, 3, 4, 5$ and 6. To cluster treatments around some unknown dose $\mu_{100\Gamma}$, find the values close to Γ in the tables, and choose one of the corresponding combinations of s, c_L, and c_U. For example, if one wants to estimate μ_{20}, $UD(3, 0, 1)$, $UD(5, 0, 2)$ and $UD(6, 0, 2)$ are good choices.

The so-called 'standard design', or '3 + 3 design', described by Korn et al. [4] can be viewed as a truncated mixture of two group up-and-down designs. According to the 3 + 3 design, subjects are assigned in groups of 3, starting with the lowest dose. If no toxicity is observed, the dose is increased. If one toxicity is observed, 3 more subjects

Table 5.1 Γ values for $UD(s, c_L, c_U)$, for $s = 2, 3, 4, 5$ and 6.

$c_L \backslash c_U$	1	2
0	0.29	0.50
1		0.71

$c_L \backslash c_U$	1	2	3
0	0.21	0.35	0.50
1		0.50	0.65
2			0.79

$c_L \backslash c_U$	1	2	3	4
0	0.16	0.27	0.38	0.50
1		0.39	0.50	0.62
2			0.61	0.73
3				0.84

$c_L \backslash c_U$	1	2	3	4	5
0	0.13	0.22	0.29	0.38	0.50
1		0.31	0.41	0.50	0.61
2			0.50	0.59	0.70
3				0.69	0.78
4					0.87

$c_L \backslash c_U$	1	2	3	4	5	6
0	0.11	0.18	0.25	0.33	0.41	0.50
1		0.26	0.34	0.42	0.50	0.59
2			0.42	0.50	0.58	0.67
3				0.58	0.66	0.75
4					0.74	0.82
5						0.89

are assigned to that dose. If 0 or 1 toxicities are observed among 6 subjects, the dose is increased; otherwise, the dose in decreased. This design can be constructed as a combination of $UD(s = 3, c_L = 0, c_U = 2)$ and $UD(s = 6, c_L = 1, c_U = 2)$, with a changeover rule and a stopping rule. Reiner, Paoletti and O'Quigley [8] analyzed this design and concluded that 'the risk of choosing an incorrect level is large'. Group up-and-down designs constructed as we have described using equation (5.1) provide an effective alternative.

5.3   Designs for acute toxicity studies

Von Békésy [9], Dixon and Mood [10] and subsequently many others studied a procedure in which the treatment increases one level following a nontoxic response and decreases one level if toxicity is observed. Actually, they were not studying toxicity, but biophysical reactions and explosives respectively. However, we follow others in adapting their procedure to the problem of acute toxicity testing. This is the $UD(1, 0, 1)$ design, which has became popular in some bench laboratory settings. It was found to perform well with small sample sizes for estimating μ_{50}, which is useful for classifying toxic substances for labeling purposes.

Animal laboratories resisted adopting the $UD(1, 0, 1)$, claiming that it was too burdensome to handle animals individually, until toxicologists at Proctor and Gamble began experimenting with the procedure. Enthusiastic reports by Bruce [11, 12] and Yam, Reer and Bruce [13] stimulated the application of this procedure and it was presented to the European Union Ministry of Public Health and the Environment, with start-up and stopping rules, for consideration by Bonnyns, Delcour and Vral [14].

In the United States, Proctor and Gamble scientists worked with the Environmental Protection Agency (EPA) to bring $UD(1, 0, 1)$, with starting and stopping rules, to the Interagency Coordinating Committee on the Validation of Alternative Methods (ICCVAM) for evaluation. ICCVAM's mission is to facilitate development, validation and regulatory acceptance of new and revised regulatory test methods that reduce, refine and replace the use of animals in testing while maintaining and promoting scientific quality and the protection of human health animal health and the environment. Members of ICCVAM include the Agency for Toxic Substances and Disease Registry, the Consumer Product Safety Commission, the Departments of Agriculture, Defense, Energy, Interior, Transportation, the EPA, the Food and Drug Administration, the National Cancer Institute, National Institute of Environmental Health Sciences, National Institute of Occupational Safety and Health, the National Institutes of Health (Offices of Scientific Affairs and Laboratory Animal Welfare), the National Library of Medicine and the Occupational Safety and Health Administration.

ICCVAM convened a working group to draft guidelines for use of the up-and-down method, including start-up and stopping rules, for applications spread across the purviews of the committee's members. The 2001 final report, following revisions incorporating suggestions made by a peer panel and a public meeting, is cited in the references along with the background review document. The EPA organized training sessions and on-line aids for toxicologists. Concerns about the burden of handling individual animals were not borne out, and the up-and-down method has reportedly become the method of choice for acute oral toxicity testing among chemical toxicologists.

Chemical toxicologists appear unaware that μ_{50} could be well estimated by $UD(3, 1, 2)$, $UD(3, 0, 3)$, $UD(4, 1, 3)$, $UD(4, 0, 4)$, $UD(5, 2, 3)$, $UD(5, 1, 4)$, $UD(5, 0, 5)$, $UD(6, 2, 4)$, $UD(6, 1, 5)$, $UD(6, 0, 6)$, etc., in addition to $UD(1, 0, 1)$ (see Table 5.1). Trade-offs in such choices between designs are conjectured and illustrated by Gezmu and Flournoy [7].

5.4 Fully sequential designs for phase I clinical trials

In a clinical setting, assigning treatments to subjects one at a time may be natural and/or necessary due to time and logistical constraints. The only fully sequential version of the $UD(s, c_L, c_U)$ is $UD(1, 0, 1)$, which clusters subjects around μ_{50}. Different strategies that make use of a biased coin to shift the mode of the treatment distribution to cluster treatments around an arbitrary $\mu_{100\Gamma}$ have been suggested by Derman [15] and Durham and Flournoy [16, 17], and generalized by Giovagnoli and Pintacuda [18].

Giovagnoli and Pintacuda [18] show that Durham and Flournoy's 1994 [16] procedure (hereafter called BCD) is optimal within a general class of random walk designs that use additional randomization to cluster treatments around $\mu_{100\Gamma}$, in the sense that π is most peaked around $\mu_{100\Gamma}$. Here we describe the BCD for $\Gamma \leq 0.5$ (see Durham and Flournoy [16] for the analogous procedure for $\Gamma \geq 0.5$).

Let a coin have probability of heads $b = \Gamma/(1 - \Gamma), 0 \leq b \leq 0.5$. Given a subject has been treated at dose d_j, $j = 2, \ldots, K - 1$, the next subject is assigned to dose:

1. d_{j-1} if the last response was toxic;

2. d_{j+1} if the last response was not toxic and the biased coin toss results in heads;

3. d_j otherwise.

Similarly to the group up-and-down design, appropriate adjustments are made at the lowest and highest doses. For the biased coin design, the probability to decrease the dose from d_j is $q_j = F_j$, the probability to increase the dose is $p_j = b \left(1 - F_j\right)$ and the probability to repeat the dose at d_j is $r_j = 1 - p_j - q_j$.

An expository review of BCD with illustrations is given by Durham, Flournoy and Rosenberger [19]. They compared the BCD with the continual reassessment method [20]. However, in spite of the attractive operating characteristics and the simplicity of the BCD, it is not widely used because researchers do not like the idea of randomizing dose assignments in a dose-finding experiment. To avoid this criticism, Ivanova et al. [21] introduced moving average up-and-down designs [$MA(s, c_L, c_U)$]. $MA(s, c_L, c_U)$ assumes that treatment assignments are fully sequential, but the decision to increase, decrease or leave the treatment level for the next subject is based on the outcomes of the last s subjects that were treated at the dose assigned to the most recent subject.

For moving average up-and-down design MA (s, c_L, c_U), let $R(d_j)$ be the number of toxic responses among the most recent s subjects that were assigned to receive dose d_j. The next subject is assigned to dose

1. d_{j-1} if $R(d_j) \geq c_U$;
2. d_{j+1} if $R(d_j) \leq c_L$;
3. d_j if $c_L < R(d_j) < c_U$.

Note that the probability q_j to decrease the dose from d_j, the probability p_j to increase the dose and the probability r_j to repeat the dose at d_j for $MA(s, c_L, c_U)$ are the same as for the corresponding $UD(s, c_L, c_U)$. Because $MA(s, c_L, c_U)$ uses nonconsecutive prior responses instead of a new group of subjects, it does not induce a finite Markov chain. However, Ivanova *et al.* [21] pointed out that the stationary distribution of the $MA(s, c_L, c_U)$ design exists and is the same as the stationary distribution for the $UD(s, c_L, c_U)$. Ivanova *et al.* [21] also show by simulations that the $MA(s, c_L, c_U)$ procedure performs better on average than the BCD.

Once the requisite numbers (c_U) of failures are observed, it is intuitively desirable to curtail the group size and begin again at the next lower dose without examining the total subjects at the current dose. Gezmu [22] proposed a curtailed version of the fully sequential $UD(s, 0, 1)$ in which subjects are assigned to the same dose until either toxicity is seen or s consecutive non-toxic responses are observed, whichever comes first. A dose is decreased as soon as toxicity is observed and increased if s nontoxic responses are observed. Ivanova [23] calls this design the k-in-a-row design. In simulations, they showed that its performance is alright, but one needs to be very cautious when considering its adoption. Because of the curtailment, the stationary distribution for the k-in-a-row design is not the same as the stationary distribution of $UD(s, 0, 1)$. In fact, it will not even be unimodal if the doses are sparse and the response function changes too rapidly.

5.5 Start-up rules

A start-up rule is often adopted to save resources because the initial dose may be far from $\mu_{100\Gamma}$. A primary design is the core dose-finding procedure chosen for a study, be it an up-and-down design or some other procedure. Start-up rules are important for human studies in which the first dose is often the lowest dose and so it is expected to be far below $\mu_{100\Gamma}$. In contrast, in acute toxicity studies in animals, or *in vitro*, every attempt will be made to start the study close to $\mu_{100\Gamma}$.

In the start-up phase of a study on human subjects in which toxicities are severe, the dose is escalated in subsequent subjects until the first toxicity is seen, after which the primary design is used to determine treatment assignments. We call this procedure the classical start-up rule. For example, Storer [24] suggested that the classical start-up rule precede a $UD(3, 0, 2)$ procedure with the goal of estimating $\mu_{100\Gamma}$.

Korn *et al.* [4] indicated that the first dose where toxicity is seen under the classical start-up is likely to have a toxicity rate higher than 0.33. They suggested treating two subjects at a time in the start-up phase until the first toxicity is observed and then reverting to the primary design. The distribution of the dose where the first toxicity is seen during a start-up with groups of size s depends on s as well as the number of doses and the probability of toxicity at each dose. The larger the group size s, the lower the toxicity rate of the dose where the first toxicity is seen.

Hence, it is logical to choose the group size s for the start-up based on the target toxicity rate Γ. The classical start-up procedure and the one proposed by Korn *et al.* [4] can be viewed as $UD(1, 0, 1)$ and $UD(2, 0, 1)$ procedures, respectively, in which the procedures are stopped when the first toxicity is observed. Because a severe stopping rule is employed, the limiting properties of $UD(s, 0, 1)$ do not apply. However, they can be used as a guideline to determine a reasonable group size s to use in the start-up phase.

Consider the general $UD(s, 0, 1)$ design, in which subjects are assigned in groups of size s and the dose is increased only if no toxicity has been observed in the most recent group; otherwise the dose is decreased. For this procedure,

$$\Pr\{\text{Bin}(s, \Gamma) = 0\} = 1 - \Pr\{\text{Bin}(s, \Gamma) \geq 1\} = (1 - \Gamma)^s.$$

Therefore equation (5.1) reduces to

$$(1 - \Gamma)^s = 1 - (1 - \Gamma)^s$$

with the solution $\Gamma = 1 - 0.5^{1/s}$. For example, $\Gamma = 0.50$, if $s = 1$; $\Gamma = 0.29$, if $s = 2$; $\Gamma = 0.21$, if $s = 3$; $\Gamma = 0.16$, if $s = 4, \ldots$. Solving $\Gamma = 1 - 0.5^{1/s}$ for s, we get $s = \log(0.5) / \log(1 - \Gamma)$, where s is not necessarily integer. Ivanova *et al.* [21] performed a simulation study investigating the distribution of the dose where the first toxicity is seen in the start-up with different group sizes. Let $\lfloor a \rfloor$ denote the largest integer not exceeding a. They concluded that choosing $s = \lfloor \log(0.5) / \log(1 - \Gamma) \rfloor$ is somewhat conservative and recommend choosing $s = \max\{\lfloor \log(0.5) / \log(1 - \Gamma) \rfloor - 1, 1\}$. We now summarize the recommended start-up rule to use in a dose-finding trial estimating $\mu_{100\Gamma}$.

For a recommended start-up rule for clinical toxicity studies, begin at the lowest treatment level. Treat s subjects per dose, where

$$s = \max\{\lfloor \log(0.5) / \log(1 - \Gamma) \rfloor - 1, 1\}.$$

Increase the dose if no toxicity in the group is observed. Stop after the first toxicity and then go down to the next lower dose level and revert to the primary design.

An additional element to consider adding to a start-up rule is the use of a more sparse set of doses. After the first toxicity, the primary design with the finer set of dose levels would be adopted.

5.6   Estimation

The method of estimating the dose $\mu_{100\Gamma}$ at the end of the study is the critical component of any dose-finding procedure. We discuss four estimation procedures: (1) the average of the doses assigned (the empirical mean), (2) the mode of the treatment distribution, (3) the maximum likelihood estimator (MLE) assuming a parametric form for the response function $F(d)$, and finally (4) our recommended estimator based on isotonic regression (cf. Robertson, Wright and Dykstra [25]).

5.6.1   The empirical mean estimator

Brownlee, Hodges and Rosenblatt [26] suggested using the mean of the dose assignments distribution (excluding the first run of toxic or nontoxic responses) as an estimator of μ_{50}. The stationary distribution of treatments from a $UD(s, c_L, c_U)$, a BCD or an $MA(s, c_L, c_U)$ procedure is unimodal. Indeed, if $F(d)$ is logistic, the stationary treatment distribution from the BCD is a mixture of two almost completely overlapping discrete normal distributions (see Durham and Flournoy [16]). Therefore, using the average of the treatment distribution to estimate $\mu_{100\Gamma}$ is a logical suggestion that was made by Durham and Flournoy [16].

5.6.2   The mode of the treatment distribution

Because the treatments from a $UD(s, c_L, c_U)$ or a BCD procedure tend to a unimodal distribution with the mode close to $\mu_{100\Gamma}$, Giovagnoli and Pintacuda [18] suggest using the most frequent treatment as an estimate of $\mu_{100\Gamma}$.

5.6.3   The maximum likelihood estimator (MLE)

The maximum likelihood estimator of $\mu_{100\Gamma}$ is obtained by inverting $\widehat{F}(d) = \Gamma$ and assuming a parametric model for F. Location-scale cumulative distribution functions are common, i.e. $F(d) = H(\alpha + \beta d)$. The logit is preferred in the clinical trial community, the probit is preferred among toxicologists and the extreme value function is preferred by engineers. More complicated models can be used as appropriate for a particular application, so long as the function is increasing over the range of interest.

One well-known problem with the maximum likelihood estimation is that, at the end of the study, the estimator may well not exist. The problem occurs when no toxicities occur at doses lower than the greatest dose at which no toxicities are observed [27]. This problem is not hard to rectify conceptually, but it is a computational hassle. When the maximum likelihood estimate fails to exist, the ICCVAM [28, 29] procedure recommends estimating μ_{50} by the midpoint between the greatest dose at which no toxicities are observed and the lowest dose at which all toxicities occur.

Another proposal for ensuring the existence of the MLEs of α and β and assuming a location-scale model, $F(d) = H(\alpha + \beta d)$, involves augmenting the data by adding several 'observations', with toxic and nontoxic responses. The probability mass of the added observations is distributed over the dose levels in proportion to the actual sample size at each dose. Ivanova *et al.* [21] give an example where two observations are added, one toxic and one nontoxic. If 5, 7 and 3 subjects were assigned to the first three doses, add $10/15$, $14/15$ and $6/15$ of an 'observation' on those doses with $5/15$, $7/15$ and $3/15$ toxicities respectively. Then the MLE of μ is computed based on the augmented data as $\widehat{\mu} = [\Gamma^{-1}(F) - \widehat{\alpha}]/\widehat{\beta}$, where $\widehat{\alpha}$ and $\widehat{\beta}$ are MLEs of α and β.

While these two procedures technically get around the nonexistence problem, they mask the fact that, when the MLEs do not exist, the range of D was much too broad (i.e. the slope of F is unexpectedly steep) and one should seriously consider repeating the experiment with a more compact set of doses.

5.6.4   The isotonic regression-based estimator

The isotonic regression estimator is a special case of the MLE where the only model assumption is monotonicity of the probability of the outcome with dose. The concept behind the isotonic regression-based estimator of $\mu_{100\Gamma}$ is quite simple. It involves two steps: (1) obtain isotonic estimates of $\{F(d_j)\}$ and then (2) interpolate between the doses d_m and d_{m+1}, where m is such that $\widehat{F}(d_m) < \Gamma < \widehat{F}(d_{m+1})$. We now describe these steps in a bit more detail.

Step 1: the pool adjacent violators algorithm (cf. Barlow et al. [30]). First estimate $F(d_j)$ by the empirical toxicity frequencies, i.e. define $\widehat{F}(d_j) = R_j(n)/N_j(n)$ for all $j \in [1, \ldots, K]$ for which $N_j(n) > 0$. If this set is nondecreasing in d_j, go to step 2. If this set is not nondecreasing, adjust them to make them nondecreasing. Specifically, scan the set $\{\widehat{F}(d_j)\}$ sequentially starting with the lowest dose j for which $N_j(n) > 0$. When one encounters an estimator that is lower than the preceding one, average it with the preceding one (and any others that are or have been set, equal to it). This step is worked out in detail for an example by Stylianou and Flournoy [30].

Step 2: interpolate the response function. (Because m is such that $\widehat{F}(d_m) < \Gamma \leq \widehat{F}(d_{m+1})$), we want an estimator of $\mu_{100\Gamma}$ to be in the interval (d_m, d_{m+1}). Stylianou and Flournoy [31] studied simple linear interpolation. Natural alternatives include using the location-scale cumulative distribution functions that typically are used to model $F(d)$. Again, the logistic, probit and extreme value functions are popular in different research communities. Ivanova *et al.* [21] did not find a noteworthy difference between using the logit interpolating function and using simple linear interpolation.

Stylianou (personal communication) reports that the mode of the treatment distribution is a very poor estimator in small to moderately large samples and not meritorious of further investigation. Stylianou and Flournoy [31] came to a similar conclusion regarding the empirical mean estimator. The isotonic estimates of $\{F(d_j)\}$ are nonparametric restricted MLEs and the isotonic estimators of μ_{100r} do not have the nonexistence problem of the parametric MLEs. Recently, Stylianou and Flournoy [31] compared the performance of the isotonic regression estimator, the empirical mean and the MLE along with several others under a logistic model using the BCD procedure. They found that the isotonic regression estimator had superior performance in all the scenarios they studied.

Several papers involving the use of isotonic estimators in more complex toxicity experiments have appeared recently (see, for example, Ivanova and Wang [32] and Paul, Rosenberger and Flournoy [33]).

5.7   Up-and-down designs to find the dose with maximum success probability

Consider an example from reference [34] concerning antiretroviral treatment for children with HIV. Therapeutic response was defined as an adequate viral suppression. Toxicity was defined as any adverse event that leads to treatment discontinuation. The goal is to find the dose that maximizes the probability of adequate viral suppression with no toxicity.

This experiment has three possible outcomes: define $Y = 1$ if toxicity; $Y = 2$ if no efficacy (inadequate suppression) without toxicity; and $Y = 3$ if efficacy (adequate suppression) without toxicity. Then $P\{Y = 1|d\} + P\{Y = 2|d\} + P\{Y = 3|d\} = 1$. The outcome $Y = 3$ is called a *success*.

Define the response functions $F(d) \equiv P\{Y = 1|d\}$ and $G(d) \equiv P\{Y = 2|Y \neq 1, d\}$. Then $H(d) \equiv P\{Y = 3|d\} = [1 - F(d)] \times [1 - G(d)]$ is the probability of success. Li, Durham and Flournoy [35] call this the contingent response model. Rabie and Flournoy [36] show that it is equivalent to the continuation ratio model [37], which is usually written in terms of logistic response functions. The optimal dose is the dose d^* that maximizes $H(d)$. Li, Durham and Flournoy [35] give conditions for $F(d)$ and $G(d)$ which guarantee that $H(d)$ will be unimodal. It is sufficient that $F(d)$ and $1 - G(d)$ be cumulative distribution functions. Assuming that $H(d)$ is unimodal, Li, Durham and Flournoy [38] propose a class of up-and-down designs and claim they will cluster treatments unimodally around the optimal dose. Kpamegan and Flournoy [39] give the stationary treatment distribution that Kpamegan [40] derives and proves it is unimodal for the following special case.

5.7.1   An optimizing up-and-down design

Subjects are assigned in pairs at adjacent doses. The first pair of subjects is treated with doses (d_1, d_2). Suppose the most recent pair of subjects was allocated to doses (d_j, d_{j+1}), $j \in \{1, 2, \ldots, K - 1\}$. The next pair of subjects is assigned to:

1. doses (d_{j-1}, d_j) if a success was observed at d_j and no success at d_{j+1};

2. doses (d_{j+1}, d_{j+2}) if no success was observed at d_j and a success at d_{j+1};

3. doses (d_j, d_{j+1}) otherwise.

Appropriate adjustments are made at the lowest and the highest doses; i.e. the pair is treated at (d_1, d_2) instead of (d_0, d_1) and (d_{K-1}, d_K) instead of (d_K, d_{K+1}) when necessary.

Treatment assignments using this procedure induce a regular Markov chain. Hence convergence is exponentially fast, and again asymptotic results apply to relatively small sample sizes. Kpamegan and Flournoy [39] show that this procedure dramatically outperforms stochastic approximation.

However, if treatments are given in the tails of $H(d)$ where the probability of success is very small, convergence is very slow. Thus if treatments are intentionally started at a low dose, a dose-escalation start-up procedure should be adopted. To address this problem in general, Kpamegan [40] examines randomizing ties; i.e. if both treatments from a pair are either successes or failures, randomly assign the next treatment one level higher or lower. Kpamegan showed that this modification greatly speeds convergence when the initial treatment is in the tails of $H(d)$.

When the two types of failure are distinguishable (toxicity and inadequate suppression in our example), one wants to utilize this information when deciding whether to increase or decrease the dose. The following up-and-down procedure does this.

5.7.2   A balancing up-and-down design

Suppose the most recent subject was allocated to level d_j, $j \in \{1, \ldots, K\}$. Assign the next subject to dose:

1. d_{j-1} if the most recent subject had toxicity;

2. d_j if the most recent subject had efficacy and no toxicity;

3. d_{j+1} if the most recent subject had no efficacy and no toxicity.

Appropriate adjustments are made at the lowest and the highest doses.

Kpamegan and Flournoy [39] and Ivanova et al. [21] point out that Theorem 1 of Durham and Flournoy [16] applied to this design establishes that the mode of the treatment distribution is not connected mathematically to the mode of $H(d)$, and may be quite distant from it. Analogous to equation (5.1), the mode of the treatment distribution is the value of d (approximately due to the discrete dose space) such that $F(d) = G(d)$. In the contingent response model, $H(d)$ is maximized when the 'hazard' functions are equal, i.e. when $[\partial F(d)/\partial d]/[1 - F(d)] = -[\partial G(d)/\partial d]/[1 - G(d)]$. Thus, for example, if the two failure functions are approximately symmetric, the procedure will work. Ivanova [23] described group versions of the balancing design and compared the optimizing, balancing and the designs of O'Quigley, Hughes and Fenton [34].

5.8   Discussion

Up-and-down designs are easy to use and easy to understand by a practitioner. These designs are flexible. To estimate $\mu_{100\Gamma}$ for a toxicity study with any target probability rate Γ, we have presented the group up-and-down design, the biased coin up-and-down design and the moving average up-and-down design. We have described how these designs can be constructed to cluster treatments around $\mu_{100\Gamma}$ for any target probability rate Γ, with subjects assigned one at a time or in groups. We showed how the performance of these procedures can be explored with exact theoretical computations for finite sample sizes; of course, simulations are also helpful.

Group up-and-down designs can be used in dose-finding trials with more complex objectives. We have described the optimizing and the balancing up-and-down procedures for phase I/II clinical trials where the goal is to identify the dose with maximum success probability.

In designing a dose-finding experiment, apart from the parameters in the up-and-down design, the investigator needs to specify the total sample size and the estimation procedure to use upon completion of the trial. Alternatively, a random stopping rule can be used. Our recommendation is not to use a random stopping rule with the group up-and-down design with a small group size s since it negatively affects the performance of the procedure. An adequate sample size can be established by conducting a simulation study. The use of a start-up rule is optional, but typically desirable when intentionally starting from a very low dose.

References

1. E.B. Wilson and J.T. Worcester (1943) The determination of the LD.50 and its sampling error in bio-assay. *Proc. Natl. Academy Sci.*, **29**, 79.
2. E.B. Wilson and J. Worcester (1943) The determination of the LD.50 and its sampling error in bio-assay, II. *Proc. Natl. Academy Sci.*, **29**, 114–20.
3. G.B. Wetherill and K.D. Glazebrook (1986) *Sequential Methods in Statistics*, Chapman and Hall, London and New York.
4. E.L. Korn, D. Midthune, T.T. Chen, L.V. Rubinstein, M.C. Christian and R.M. Simon (1994) A comparison of two phase I trial designs. *Statistics in Medicine*, **13**(18), 1799–806.
5. R.K. Tsutakawa (1967) Random walk design in bioassay. *JASA*, **62**, 842–56.
6. R.K. Tsutakawa (1967) Asymptotic properties of the block up-and-down method in bioassay. *Ann. Math. Statistics*, **38**, 1822–8.
7. M. Gezmu and N. Flournoy (2006) Group up-and-down designs for dose-finding. *J. Statistical Planning and Inference*, **136**, 1749–1764.
8. E. Reiner, X. Paoletti and J. O'Quigley (1999) Operating characteristics of the standard phase I clinical trial design. *Computational Statistics and Data Analysis*, **30**, 303–15.
9. G.V. Von Békésy (1947) A new audiometer, *Acta Otolaryngology (Stockholm)*, **35**, 411–22.
10. W.J. Dixon and A.M. Mood (1954) A method for obtaining and analyzing sensitivity data. *JASA*, **43**, 109–26.
11. R.D. Bruce (1985) An up-and-down procedure for acute toxicity testing, *Fundamentals Appl. Toxicology*, **5**(1), 151–7.
12. R.D. Bruce (1987) A confirmatory study of the up-and-down method for acute oral toxicity testing. *Fundamentals Appl. Toxicology*, **8**(1), 97–100.
13. J. Yam, P.J. Reer and R.D. Bruce (1991) Comparison of the up-and-down method and the fixed-dose procedure for acute oral toxicity testing. *Food Chem. Toxicology*, **29**(4), 259–63.

14. E. Bonnyns, M.P. Delcour and A. Vral (1990) Up-and-down method as an alternative to the EC-method for acute toxicity testing. Technical report, IHE project 2153/88/11, pp. 33, Institute of Hygiene and Epidemiology, Ministry of Health and the Environment, Brussels.
15. C. Derman (1957) Nonparametric up and down experimentation. *Ann. Math. Statistics*, **28**, 795–8.
16. S.D. Durham and N. Flournoy (1994) Random walks for quantile estimation, in *In Statistical Decision Theory and Related Topics V* (eds S.S. Gupta and J.O. Berger), Springer-Verlag, New York, pp. 467–76.
17. S.D. Durham and N. Flournoy (1995) Up-and-down designs. I. Stationary treatment distributions, in *Adaptive Designs. Lecture Notes – Monograph Series 25* (eds N. Flournoy and W.F. Rosenberger), Institute of Mathematical Statistics, Hayward, California, pp. 139–57.
18. A. Giovagnoli and N. Pintacuda (1998) Properties of frequency distributions induced by general 'up-and-down' methods for estimating quantiles. *J. Statistical Planning and Inference*, **74**, 51–63.
19. S.D. Durham, N. Flournoy and W. F. Rosenberger (1997) A Random walks rule for phase I clinical trials. *Biometrics*, **53**(2), 745–60.
20. J. O'Quigley M. Pepe and L. Fisher (1990) Continual reassessment method: a practical design for phase I clinical trials in cancer. *Biometrics*, **46**(1), 33–48.
21. A. Ivanova, A. Montazer-Haghighi, S.G. Mohanty and S.D. Durham (2003) Improved up-and-down designs for phase I trials. *Statistics in Medicine*, **22**(1), 69–82.
22. M. Gezmu (1996) The Geometric up-and-down design for allocating dosage levels, Dissertation, American University.
23. A. Ivanova (2003) A new dose-finding design for bivariate outcomes. *Biometrics*, **59**(4), 1001–7.
24. B.E. Storer (1989) Design and analysis of phase I clinical trials. *Biometrics*, **45**(3), 925–37.
25. T. Robertson, F.T. Wright and R.L. Dykstra (1988) *Ordered Restricted Statistical Inference*, John Wiley & Sons, Inc., New York.
26. K.A. Brownlee, J.L. Hodges and M. Rosenblatt (1953) The up-and-down method with small samples. *JASA*, **48**, 262–77.
27. M.J. Silvapulle (1981) On the existence of maximum likelihood estimators for the binomial response model. *JRSS B*, **43**, 310–13.
28. NIH (2001) Up-and-down procedure background review document, http://iccvam.niehs.nih.gov/docs/docs.htm udp.
29. The revised up-and-down procedure: a test method for determining the acute oral toxicity of chemicals, NIH Publication 02-4501, http://iccvam.niehs.nih.gov/docs/docs.htm udp., 2001.
30. R.E. Barlow, D.J. Bartholomew, J.M. Bremner and H.D. Brunk (1972) *Statistical Inference under Order Restrictions*, John Wiley & Sons, Ltd, London and New York.
31. M. Stylianou and N. Flournoy (2002) Dose finding using the biased coin up-and-down design and isotonic regression. *Biometrics*, **58**(1), 171–7.
32. A. Ivanova and K. Wang (2004) A non-parametric approach to the design and analysis of two-dimensional dose-finding trials. *Statistics in Medicine*, **23**(12), 1861–70.
33. R.K. Paul, W.F. Rosenberger and N. Flournoy (2004) Quantile estimation following non-parametric phase I clinical trials with ordinal response. *Statistics in Medicine*, **23**(16), 2483–95.
34. J.O'Quigley, M.D. Hughes and T. Fenton (2001) Dose-finding designs for HIV studies. *Biometrics*, **57**(4), 1018–29.

35. W. Li, S.D. Durham and N. Flournoy (1995) An adaptive design for maximization of a contingent binary response, in *Adaptive Designs. Lecture Notes – Monograph Series 25* (eds N. Flournoy and W.F. Rosenberger), Institute of Mathematical Statistics, Hayward, California, pp. 179–96.

36. H. Rabie and N. Flournoy (2004) Optimal designs for contingent response models, in *mODa 7 – Advances in Model-Oriented Design and Analysis* (eds A. Di Bucchianico, H. Lauter and H.P. Wynn), Physica-Verlag, Heidelberg and New York, 133–41.

37. A. Agresti (1990) *Categorical Data Analysis*, John Wiley & Sons, Inc., New York.

38. W. Li, S.D. Durham and N. Flournoy (1998) A sequential design for maximizing the probability of a favourable response. *The Can. J. Statistics*, **26**, 479–95.

39. E.E. Kpamegan and N. Flournoy (2001) An optimizing up and down design, in *Optimum Design 2000* (eds A.C. Atkinson, B. Bogacka and A. Zhigljavsky), Kluwer Academic, Dordrecht, The Netherlands.

40. E.E. Kpamegan (2000) An optimizing up-and-down design. Dissertation, Technical report, American University.

Part III
Model-Based Approaches

6

The continual reassessment method

Sylvie Chevret and Sarah Zohar

*Département de Biostatistique et Informatique Médicale, U717 Inserm,
Hôpital Saint-Louis, Paris, France*

6.1 Introduction

The continual reassessment method (CRM) was first proposed by O'Quigley, Pepe and Fisher [1] to challenge the standard designs in cancer studies, in addressing explicitly the concerns raised by the conduct of such trials, namely: (a) ineffectiveness of the treatment at low doses; (b) severe toxic effects expected at high doses; (c) poor knowledge of the dose-toxicity relationship at the trial onset; (d) potential therapeutical benefit for the patient; and (e) need for efficient design with a small number of patients.

The CRM relates to the stochastic approximation methods originated by Robbins and Monro [2]. Rather than a sequential design, it is an adaptative design, in the sense that it uses all of the available data prior to the trial onset and all the data from the trial that have accumulated at the time each dose level is selected for new patients. By contrast, the standard "3 + 3" design has a shorter memory and does not use all of the available data; it only uses the data from the more recent one or two cohorts, while ignoring data from any earlier patient. Actually, it has been demonstrated that standard designs, though still currently used in most phase I trials, have inferior properties compared to the CRM [3, 4].

Statistical Methods for Dose-Finding Experiments   Edited by S. Chevret
© 2006 John Wiley & Sons, Ltd

The CRM addresses practical and ethical concerns within a rigorous mathematical framework. Indeed, it is a model-based design, which aims at estimating the dose associated with some acceptable target toxicity level, expressing the maximum tolerated dose (MTD) as any target percentile of the underlying dose-toxicity curve and assuming a monotically nondecreasing response function. As a model for locating quantiles, the CRM has then been applied to dose-finding for phase II trials, i.e. when the objective is to select, among a fixed number of dose levels, the minimum effective dose (MED).

Though it has long been reported as a Bayesian dose-finding method, this appears restrictive, since maximum likelihood estimates of toxicity probabilities have been derived in the so-called likelihood CRM (CRML) [5, 6]. Moreover, it is more directed towards achieving convergence successively closer to the allocated doses to the target quantile, the MTD, rather than towards obtaining (Bayes or maximum likelihood) estimates of the target quantile [7].

The CRM has gained popularity since its proposal by O'Quigley, Pepe and Fisher [1]. Many variations have been published and discussed in the statistical literature, but there has been little attempt made to make the design considerations accessible to nonstatisticians. As a result, some clinicians or reviewers of clinical trials tend to be wary of the CRM due to safety concerns. This could at least explain why it is still rarely used in dose-finding for phase I trials as compared to standard approaches. This chapter aims at summarizing the main concepts of the CRM, with practical considerations given through illustrative trials.

6.2 The original continual reassessment method (CRM)

The CRM is designed to estimate, out a set of prespecified dose levels, the highest dose with a probability of toxicity closest to a preassigned target called the MTD.

6.2.1 Trial planification

Let Y denote a binary covariate modeling the outcome of interest, mostly the dose-limiting toxicity (DLT). Let p be the targeted toxic probability. By contrast to the standard "$3 + 3$" method, which cannot account for the indication or patient population specific DLT rate, any target toxic probability could be chosen. O'Quigley, Pepe and Fisher first used a target response of $p = 0.20$ [1] and then studied other targets (such as 0.25, 0.30 and 0.35) [3].

Let $d_i (i = 1, \ldots, k)$ denote the various dose levels of the drug regimen to be tested, which is supposed to belong to the portion of the dose-toxicity curve where the MTD is expected. Practical considerations generally result in about six dose levels, though using more or less levels presents no conceptual difficulty. Since the CRM does not rely on the scale in which the doses are expressed, there is no need for equally spaced doses. The only constraint on doses is that they are increasingly ordered in terms of

Table 6.1   Initial dose-response relationship.

Dose levels	d_1	d_2	d_3	d_4	...	d_k
Initial guesses of toxic probability	$p_1 \leq$	$p_2 \leq$	$p_3 \leq$	$p_4 \leq$	$... \leq$	p_k

toxic probabilities, with initial guesses denoted p_i, $i = 1, \ldots, k$. This is exemplified in Table 6.1.

A simple one-parameter mathematical model, $\psi(x_i; \theta) = P(Y = 1|x_i) = E(Y|x_i)$, for a dose-response is assumed, the so-called working model [6], where x_i is a function of doses (Figure 6.1). This parametric model should be flexible enough to approximate the underlying true dose-toxicity relationship in the neighborhood of the targeted toxic probability, p.

O'Quigley, Pepe and Fisher initially [1] used an increasing, convex–concave curve, the hyperbolic tangent function

$$\psi(x_i; \theta) = [(\tanh x_i + 1)/2]^\theta, \tag{6.1}$$

with $\theta > 0$ (though reparametrization whereby θ was replaced by $\exp(\theta)$ is possible [5]). Then, the logistic function was also proposed [3]:

$$\psi(x_i; \theta) = \frac{\exp(a_0 + \theta x_i)}{1 + \exp(a_0 + \theta x_i)}, \tag{6.2}$$

with the intercept, a_0, fixed.

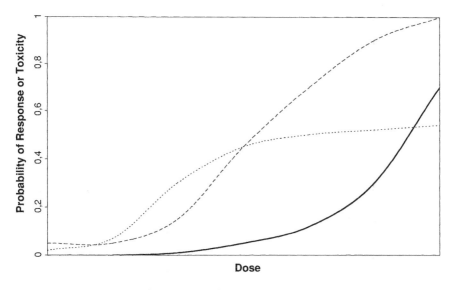

Figure 6.1   Schematic dose-response models.

The logistic regression model, mostly used in bioassays, gives rise to a wide class of sigmoid curves, likely to be appropriate for many dose-response relationships [8]. Other parametric models were also proposed, including power functions, $\psi(x_i; \theta) = p_i^\theta$ or $\psi(x_i; \theta) = p_i^{\exp(\theta)}$ [6].

Whatever the model, the dose levels that we are working with are defined by $x_i = \psi^{-1}(p_i; \theta_0)$ $(i = 1, \ldots, k)$, where θ_0 is our initial guess of the parameter value, θ. In a Bayes framework, since the uncertainty in the model parameter, θ, is expressed through a prior density having support on the parameter space, denoted $\pi(\theta)$, θ_0 is actually the mean of the prior. O'Quigley, Pepe and Fisher [1] initially choose an exponential prior centered on 1, $\pi(\theta) = \exp(-\theta); 0 < \theta < \infty$.

For instance, let us consider the following setting. Suppose we wish to estimate the 30th percentile of the dose-toxicity relationship, based on six discrete dose levels. We first assume that toxic probabilities of these six dose levels are given by 0.01, 0.10, 0.30, 0.50, 0.70 and 0.95 respectively. Considering an exponential prior with mean 1 and a one-parameter logistic model, the dose scale is redefined by computing $x_i = \log[p_i/(1 - p_i)] - a_0$. Figure 6.2 displays some initial guesses of the dose-toxicity curve, according to the value of a_0.

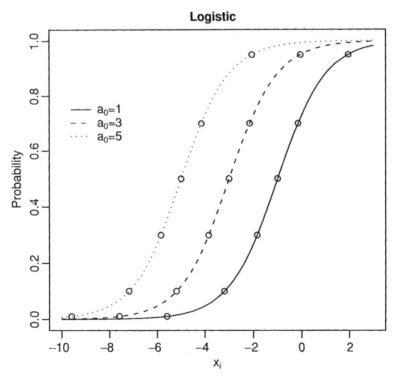

Figure 6.2   Examples of logistic dose-toxicity curves, with $\theta_0 = 1$ and $a_0 = 1, 3, 5$.

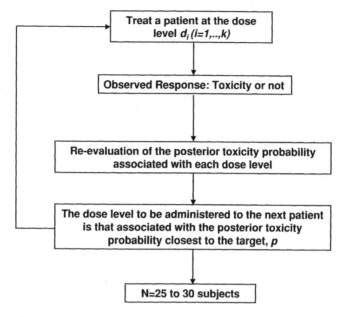

Figure 6.3   Schematic representation of the CRM design.

6.2.2   Design and inference

The CRM is made up of two components: an allocation rule and a statistical procedure. O'Quigley, Pepe and Fisher initially recommended experimentation to start at the lth dose level, where l is the largest integer smaller than $k/2$ [1], or at the level d_s $(1 < s < k)$, whose prior guess of toxic probability is judged closest to the target, p [1]. In other words, the starting dose of the CRM was first selected to be the prior estimate of the MTD.

The main idea of the initial CRM was sequentially to assign incoming patients to one of k possible dose levels, and then, when toxicity outcomes are known for successive patients, to update the information on the probabilities of toxicity in the light of results obtained for the patients already observed. Using the Bayes formula, the results would be further used to determine the dose at which to treat the next patient up to a predetermined number of patients, n. In other words, it mixes the design and estimation procedures of the phase I trial. This is summarized in Figure 6.3.

6.2.3   Inference

Let $x(i)$ be the dose level administered to the ith subject and y_i, his(her) observed response. Let $x = \{(x(1), y_1) \cdots (x(j), y_j)\}$ be the accumulated data after j inclusions. After j observations, the posterior distribution of θ is modified through the use of the

Bayes theorem, as follow

$$\pi(\theta|x) = \frac{f(x|\theta)\pi(\theta)}{\int_\Theta f(x|\theta)\pi(\theta)\,d\theta}, \tag{6.3}$$

where $\pi(\theta)$ is the prior density of θ that reflects our knowledge of the dose-toxicity relationship before experimentation begins and $f(x|\theta)$ is the likelihood function

$$f(x|\theta) = \prod_{r=1}^{j}[\psi(x(r);\theta)]^{y_r}[1 - \psi(x(r);\theta)]^{1-y_r}. \tag{6.4}$$

We then compute the posterior mean of θ as

$$\tilde{\theta}_j = E(\theta|x) = \int_\Theta \theta\pi(\theta|x)d\theta. \tag{6.5}$$

The actualized values of toxic probabilities at each dose level d_i are then computed from

$$\tilde{p}_{ij} = \int_\Omega \psi(x_i;\theta)\pi(\theta|x)d\theta \approx \psi(x_i;\tilde{\theta}_j), \quad i = 1,\dots,k. \tag{6.6}$$

The attribution of doses is iteratively performed after each observation, to minimize, over the $i = 1,\dots,k$ dose levels, some criterion, $L_h(\tilde{\theta}_j)$:

$$X(j+1) = d_h : \min_{h\in(1,\dots,k)} L_h(\tilde{\theta}_j). \tag{6.7}$$

This criterion could be measured on the probability scale, between the target probability of toxicity, p, and the actualized estimates of toxic probabilities, $\tilde{p}_{ij}$, that is minimizing

$$L_h(\tilde{\theta}_j) = [\psi(x_h;\tilde{\theta}_j) - p]^2 \tag{6.8}$$

or on the dose scale

$$L_h(\tilde{\theta}_j) = [x_h - \psi^{-1}(x_h;\tilde{\theta}_j)]^2. \tag{6.9}$$

In other words, rather than minimizing the expectation of a loss function, $E(L_i(\theta|x))$, for computional simplicity, the dose attribution process minimizes the value of a loss function at the expectation of θ, $L_i(E(\theta|x)) = L_i(\tilde{\theta}_j)$.

This inference-design process is continued until the prespecified sample size, n, is reached. Of note, O'Quigley, Pepe and Fisher [1] also proposed a criterion for terminating the CRM, based on the width for a confidence interval of the MTD.

Let $d_R = X(n+1)$ be the recommended dose level at the end of the trial; this is the dose d_i such that, for instance, $[\psi(x_i;\tilde{\theta}_n) - p]^2$ is minimized. In other words, d_R defines the estimated MTD, with an associated mean posterior probability of toxicity

$$\tilde{P}_{R|n} = \psi(x_R, \tilde{\theta}_n). \tag{6.10}$$

The small sample performances of the CRM were assessed on the basis of the simulation results [3].

Of note, the median posterior estimate and the mode posterior estimate were also proposed for providing point estimates less sensitive to asymmetry in the likelihood [5].

6.2.4 Practical considerations

A number of interesting issues emerge from this method. Firstly, as a special case of Bayesian decision procedures [8], the original CRM requires elicitation of a prior and formulation of the design setting. Actually, beyond the likelihood function, $f(x|\theta)$, Bayesian analysis is markedly recognized by a sibling subjective probability belief, which stands out as quantitative *a priori* feelings of θ by $\pi(\theta)$. Berger [9] gave a comprehensive review of univariate prior elicitation, notably with regards to noninformative priors for which inferences should be unaffected by information external to the current data. Actually, for the CRM, one would not like the CRM to depend very strongly on the choice of the prior [1]. The prior subjective distribution of θ was first chosen to be exponential, parameter 1, although priors from truncated-normal or log-normal families were also proposed [1]. Reparametrization of the working model whereby θ is replaced by $\exp(\theta)$ allows the use of normal distribution, with mean 0 and variance sufficiently large to represent vague knowledge [6]. Several approaches of prior elicitation, such as the moment approach or the histogram approach, can be used to specify the prior among the parametric family. Most of the time, the performance of the design relies on simulation results, and the effect of selection of the prior (as well as the intercept parameter of the logistic function) upon operating characteristics of the CRM is investigated through simulation studies. Cheung and Chappell [10] proposed supplement techniques to simulation when planning the trial.

However, this appears as a computational device ignoring potential information available before the trial. Moreover, in situations where a low percentile is targeted, vague priors can lead to undesirable rigidity when given certain trial outcomes that can occur with a nonnegligible probability. Improvement could be achieved by using more informative priors [8, 11]. Notably, a class of informative priors was proposed, using historical data from previous studies [12]. In a Bayesian framework, the $100 \times (1 - \alpha)\%$ Bayesian or credibility interval for the toxicity probability P_R at the dose level d_R can be computed from the posterior density of θ :

$$\{\psi\{x_R, \tilde{\theta}_{\min}\}, \psi\{x_R, \tilde{\theta}_{\max}\}\}, \tag{6.11}$$

where $\{\tilde{\theta}_{\min}, \tilde{\theta}_{\max}\}$ is the 95 % credibility interval of θ, i.e. $\{\tilde{\theta}_{\min}, \tilde{\theta}_{\max}\}$: $\int_{\tilde{\theta}_{\min}}^{\tilde{\theta}_{\max}} f(\theta|\Omega_m)d\theta = 1 - \alpha$. This allows some estimate to be given of the precision around our estimate of P_R.

Finally, the implementation of the CRM requires numerical integrations, in relation to the updating of the prior and to the construction of Bayes intervals. However, the computation of such integrals could become rapidly unwieldy. Algorithms have been proposed to simplify these computations [13]. Nevertheless, the methods used for integrations are still poorly reported.

6.2.5 CRM for phase II dose-finding studies

Though designed for phase I cancer clinical trials, the CRM can easily apply to phase II dose-finding trials with efficacy outcomes. In this setting, we are interested in estimating the minimum effective dose (MED), which can be defined as any targeted percentile of the dose-efficacy relationship. To apply directly, the model should describe the occurrence of failure rather than that of success at each dose level. Actually, it only requires dose levels to be ordered by decreasing instead of increasing levels, so that the first dose level d_1 becames the highest dose level to be tested while d_k denotes the lowest dose level.

6.2.6 Example

A phase II dose-finding trial was previously conducted to assess the MED of nitroglycerin for tocolysis during preterm labor [14]. The MED was defined as the dose of nitroglycerin required to achieve a positive response in 90 % of pregnant women (i.e. 10 % of failure). The trial was designed according to the original CRM design described above, with a prespecified sample size of 25 women. Six dose levels of nitroglycerin were chosen, namely 0.2, 0.4, 0.6, 0.8, 1.0 and 1.2 mg/h. The corresponding initial guesses of failure probability were 0.5, 0.25, 0.2, 0.1, 0.05 and 0.02 respectively. The intercept parameter of the logistic model was fixed at 3 and a unit exponential prior for the model parameter θ was chosen. The first patient was admistered the dose level d_3, our initial guess of the MED.

Table 6.2 represents the dose allocation and the sequential estimation of the response probabilities associated to each dose level. The last dose level, $d_6 = 1.2$ mg/h, which was administered consecutively from the seventh to the last patient, was estimated to be the MED and had an estimated posterior failure probability of 45 % (95 % credibility interval: 24–64 %).

6.3 Likelihood CRM (CRML)

The original CRM was carried out in a Bayesian framework. It was changed thereafter to a more classical framework leaning upon likelihood theory, in which the maximum likelihood estimate is used rather than the posterior mean, resulting in the so-called CRML [5, 6]. A similar approach for the logistic regression model was also proposed by Murphy and Hall [15].

Obviously, the conduct of maximum likelihood estimation requires the observation of heterogeneity in the toxic responses to apply. A requirement for the CRML is thus to first use either original CRM or any standard up-and-down schemes before applying the sequential CRML procedure.

Table 6.2   Sequential dose allocation rule and inference of the nitroglycerin trial. Recommended dose levels (with estimated failure probability closest to 0.1) are in bold.

Patient rank j	Dose (mg/h)	Response	\multicolumn{6}{c}{Dose (mg/h)}

			\multicolumn{6}{c}{Dose (mg/h)}
			d_6 1.2	d_5 1.0	d_4 0.8	d_3 0.6	d_2 0.4	d_1 0.2
			\multicolumn{6}{c}{Initial guesses of failure probabilities}
			p_6 0.02	p_5 0.05	p_4 0.1	p_3 0.2	p_2 0.25	p_1 0.5
Patient rank j	Dose (mg/h)	Response	\multicolumn{6}{c}{Posterior estimated failure probabilities}
			$\tilde{P}_{6j}$	$\tilde{P}_{5j}$	$\tilde{P}_{4j}$	$\tilde{P}_{3j}$	$\tilde{P}_{2j}$	$\tilde{P}_{1j}$
1	0.8	Success	0.00	0.00	0.01	0.03	**0.04**	0.19
2	0.4	Success	0.00	0.00	0.00	0.01	0.01	**0.09**
3	0.2	Success	0.00	0.00	0.00	0.00	0.00	**0.04**
4	0.2	Failure	0.01	0.02	0.05	**0.11**	0.15	0.38
5	0.6	Failure	0.06	**0.12**	0.21	0.34	0.39	0.62
6	1.0	Failure	**0.24**	0.36	0.47	0.59	0.63	0.77
7	1.2	Success	**0.17**	0.27	0.38	0.52	0.56	0.73
8	1.2	Success	**0.13**	0.23	0.33	0.47	0.52	0.70
9	1.2	Failure	**0.27**	0.39	0.50	0.61	0.65	0.78
10	1.2	Success	**0.23**	0.34	0.45	0.58	0.62	0.76
11	1.2	Success	**0.20**	0.31	0.42	0.55	0.59	0.75
12	1.2	Failure	**0.29**	0.41	0.51	0.63	0.66	0.79
13	1.2	Failure	**0.37**	0.49	0.58	0.68	0.71	0.81
14	1.2	Success	**0.33**	0.45	0.55	0.66	0.69	0.80
15	1.2	Success	**0.30**	0.42	0.52	0.63	0.67	0.79
16	1.2	Failure	**0.36**	0.48	0.57	0.67	0.71	0.81
17	1.2	Success	**0.33**	0.45	0.55	0.66	0.69	0.80
18	1.2	Failure	**0.38**	0.50	0.59	0.69	0.72	0.81
19	1.2	Failure	**0.42**	0.54	0.62	0.71	0.74	0.83
20	1.2	Failure	**0.46**	0.57	0.65	0.73	0.75	0.84
21	1.2	Success	**0.43**	0.54	0.63	0.71	0.74	0.83
22	1.2	Failure	**0.47**	0.57	0.65	0.73	0.76	0.84
23	1.2	Failure	**0.49**	0.60	0.67	0.75	0.77	0.84
24	1.2	Success	**0.47**	0.58	0.66	0.73	0.76	0.84
25	1.2	Success	**0.45**	0.56	0.64	0.72	0.75	0.83

The maximum likelihood estimator of θ after j observations, $\widehat{\theta}_j$, is sequentially computed, with approximate variance $\upsilon(\widehat{\theta}_j)$ using

$$\upsilon^{-1}(\widehat{\theta}_j) = \sum_{l=1}^{j-1} (1 - y_l)\psi(x_l;\widehat{\theta}_j)\log\psi(x_l;1)^2/[1 - \psi(x_l - \widehat{\theta}_j)]^2,$$

from which is derived the probability of toxicity at each dose level, $\psi(x_i;\widehat{\theta}_j)$, with approximate $100(1 - \alpha)\%$ confidence intervals [5]:

$$\psi(x_i;\widehat{\theta}_j \pm z_{1-\alpha/2}\upsilon(\widehat{\theta}_j)^{1/2}), \tag{6.12}$$

where z_α is the αth percentile of the standard normal distribution.

The recommended dose will be the dose d_i such that some distance between $\psi(x_i;\widehat{\theta}_j)$ and the target probability of response, p, will be minimized, similarly to the CRM. However, it is not necessary to carry out any integration as in the original CRM, since one works directly with the maximum likelihood estimates of θ. The recommended dose was shown to converge to the target toxicity rate as the sample size increases, with demonstrated consistency and asymptotic normality for the maximum likelihood estimate on large samples [16]. Coverage of the confidence intervals of the probability of toxicity at the MTD for small samples (as small as 12 or 16), close to nominal levels, was assessed through a wide range of simulations [17].

Finally, a stopping rule for the CRML was proposed, based on a binary tree of future responses, suggesting that accrual should stop whenever the probability of the administered dose remaining unchanged along the trial is 1 [18].

6.4   Modified continual reassessment method (MCRM)

Although the original CRM outperforms the traditional $3 + 3$ and up-and-down designs with increased efficiency and precision together with a lower bias, it has some difficulties to be implemented in real practice. Issues raised by some statisticians and clinicians involve the required duration of time for study completion, the possibility of increased toxicity compared to standard designs and sensitivity to the statistical model. Notably, it has been criticised for being too aggressive in recommending escalation and for treating too many patients above the target. To countermeasure these issues, research on the CRM has been quite active in the past decade, including some reviews [19, 20].

6.4.1   Modifications in design

Table 6.3 reports the main proposals for modifying the CRM in its original design. To make clinicians more confortable, a first restriction on the CRM was proposed,

Table 6.3 Summarized proposals of the modified CRM.

CRM (authors)	Design				
	First dose	Cohort size	Skipping	Stopping rule	Model
Original[1]	MTD	1	No	No	Tangent hyperbolic
Modified					
Faries[21]	d_1	1	No	Yes	Logistic
Korn *et al.*[22]	d_1	1	No	Yes	Logistic
Goodman, Zahurak and Piantadosi[23]	d_1	$1 \leq c \leq 3$	No	Yes	Logistic

avoiding skipping dose levels between patients [21, 22]. Although this would tend to make the CRM take longer to reach the MTD, this would also tend to make it more conservative. Similarly, the first lowest dose level was proposed to be the starting dose, as in the traditional designs, by several authors [21, 23]. Two additional conservative adaptations were proposed, incorporating a secondary level of toxicity and assigning three patients to the initial dose level [21]. To accelerate the conduct of the trial, Goodman, Zahurak and Piantadosi [23] proposed to assign more than one patient at a time to each dose level. Actually, the CRM can account for different numbers of patients per dose. Some modified CRM designs proposed to use fixed sample sizes as minimums, continuing until the recommended MTD had $K = 5, 6$ or 7 patients assigned to it [21, 23, 22]. Finally, combined methods were proposed, splitting design into two phases: a first phase with an up-and-down design until the first toxicity is observed and then a second phase with the CRM using all information obtained at that point [24].

6.4.2 Modifications in modelling the dose-response relationship

The original and modified CRM uses an explicit dose-response model, which ought to be realistic, parsimonious and flexible, leaving usually one parameter (θ) to be determined by actual data. Some authors have attempted to reformulate the prior and statistical model by modeling the probabilities of response directly as the unknown parameters of interest, subject only to monotonicity constraints [11, 25]. The curve-free method of Gasparini and Eisele [25] is based on a parametrization of ordinal data, using $\theta_i = (1 - \pi_i)/(1 - \pi_{i-1})$, where $\pi_i = P(Y = 1|d_i)$. Of note, it appears to coincide with the usual model-based CRM, at least in terms of operational performances [26].

The original CRM also requires that each response to treatment is available sufficiently quickly to be used in determining the dose for the next patient. Time-to-event methods such as Tite-CRM [27] will be considered further in the book.

Heterogeneity in phase I clinical trial populations may lead to distinct dose-response relationships along covariate values. When modeling probability of responses, Piantadosi and Lui [28] first proposed to use, in addition to dose, meaningful pharmacokinetic information such as the area under the time–concentration curve (AUC). To account for such differences, an augmented dose-response model with covariates was proposed [12].

Otherwise, Bayesian approaches enable computations to be made of probabilities of future observations, from which several stopping rules can be derived, allowing an easy and reproducible decision either to continue or to stop patient accrual [29, 30]. This will be discussed in Chapter 10.

Table 6.4 reports the main proposals for extending the CRM. Some of them will be detailed elsewhere in this book.

Table 6.4 Summarized proposals of the extended CRM.

CRM (authors)	Proposals
Modeling heterogenity	
Piantadosi and Coworkers[28, 31]	Pharmacokinetic data
O'Quigley, Shen and Gamst[32]	Two-samples CRM
O'Quigley and Paoletti[33]	CRM for ordered groups
Outcomes	
Thall *et al.*[34]	Delayed patient outcome
Thall, Estey and Sung [35]	Bivariate outcomes
Braun[36]	Bivariate CRM
Kramar, Lebecq and Candalh[37]	CRML for 2 drugs
Cheung and Chappell[27]	Time-to-event (Tite-CRM)
Legedza and Ibrahim [38]	Longitudinal dose-response model
Storer[39]	CRML with continuous dose-response curve
Stopping rules	
O'Quigley and Reiner[18]	Stopping rule for the CRML
Zohar and Chevret[29]	Bayes stopping rules
Dose-response model	
Gasparini and Eisele [25]	Curve-free CRM
Ishizuka and Ohashi[20]	Bayes mean posterior of parameter
Leung and Wang[40]	Decision theory
Two-stages CRM(L)	
Zohar and Chevret[41]	Two-stage CRM
O'Quigley, Paoletti and Maccario[42]	Two-stage CRML

Table 6.5   Sequential allocation scheme of the homoharringtonine trial.
Recommended dose levels (with estimated tonic probability closest to the target,
$p = 0.33$) are bolded. Underlined figures correspond to the actual dose given to the
next cohort of patients.

				Dose (mg/m^2/d)				
				d_1	d_2	d_3	d_4	d_5
				0.5	1.0	3.0	5.0	6.0
				Initial guesses of toxicity probabilities				
				p_1	p_2	p_3	p_4	p_5
				0.05	0.100	0.150	0.333	0.500
		Dose		Posterior estimated toxicity probabilities				
Cohort	Patients	(mg/m^2/d)	DLT	$\tilde{p}_{1j}$	$\tilde{p}_{2j}$	$\tilde{p}_{3j}$	$\tilde{p}_{4j}$	$\tilde{p}_{5j}$
1*	3	0.5	0	0.001	0.003	<u>0.006</u>	0.035	**0.108**
2	3	3	1	0.073	0.136	0.195	**<u>0.387</u>**	0.550
3	3	5	1	0.069	0.131	0.189	**<u>0.380</u>**	0.544
4	3	5	0	0.032	0.069	0.109	**<u>0.270</u>**	0.446
5	3	5	1	0.037	0.078	0.121	**<u>0.288</u>**	0.460
6	3	5	2	0.062	0.119	0.174	**<u>0.361</u>**	0.528

The first cohort was administered the lowest dose level, d_1. Next cohort did not receive the recommended
fifth dose level, but the third level, due to physicians fear of toxicity.

6.4.3   Example

A phase I dose-finding trial that aimed to assess the MTD of semi-synthetic homoharringtonine in the treatment of patients with advanced leukemia was conducted. It
used a modified CRM design in the sense that cohorts of three patients were enrolled
at each dose level. The target toxicity probability was fixed at 33 % with a sample
size of 18 patients. Five different dose levels of homoharringtonine were studied
(namely 0.5, 1, 3, 5 and 6 mg/m^2/d), with initial guesses of toxicity probabilities of
0.05, 0.10, 0.15, 0.33 and 0.50 respectively. The CRM used a unit exponential prior
for the logistic model parameter and $a_0 = 3$ for the model intercept. At the end of the
trial, the recommended dose was 5 mg/m^2/d, estimating the MTD, with a posterior
toxicity probability of 36.1 % (95 % credibility interval: 15.8–58.6 %). Table 6.5 represents the dose allocation and the sequential estimation of the toxicity probabilities
associated with each dose level along the trial.

6.5   Concluding remarks

The CRM has been proposed as an alternative method of the traditional "3 + 3" or
up-and-down designs in phase I cancer clinical trials. Its essential features are the
sequential (continual) adaptive design for dose-finding of a dose level for the next

patients based on the dose-toxicity relationship and the updating of the relationship based on patients' response data.

Since the appearance of the original paper [1], the CRM has been the focus of much interest and debate. Several restrictions/extensions of the original design have been proposed and have been widely implemented. Of note, most of the criticisms against the CRM are in fact not criticisms that are specific to the CRM, but are applicable to most dose-finding studies; they are best overcome by close collaboration between clinical pharmacologists, clinicians and statisticians.

Some promising developments will be presented in future chapters of this book, notably to base dose-finding procedure on both toxicity and efficacy [35, 36, 43, 47].

References

1. J. O'Quigley and M. Pepe and L. Fisher (1990) Continual reassessment method: a practical design for phase I clinical trials in cancer. *Biometrics*, **46**, 33–48.
2. H. Robbins and S. Monro (1951) A stochastic approximation method. *Ann. Math. Statistics*, **29**, 400–7.
3. J. O'Quigley and S. Chevret (1991) Methods for dose finding studies in cancer clinical trials: a review and results of a Monte Carlo study. *Statistics in Medicine*, **10**, 1647–64.
4. P.F. Thall and S.J. Lee (1999) Practical model-based dose-finding in phase I clinical trials: methods based on toxicity. *Int. J. Gynecological Cancer*, **13**, 251–61.
5. J. O'Quigley (1992) Estimating the probability of toxicity at the recommended dose following a Phase I clinical trial in Cancer. *Biometrics*, **48**, 853–62.
6. J. O'Quigley and L.Z. Shen (1996) Continual reassessment method: a likelihood approach. *Biometrics*, **52**, 673–84.
7. W.F. Rosenberger (1996) New directions in adaptive designs. *Statistical Sci.*, **11**(2), 137–49.
8. J. Whitehead and H. Brunier (1995) Bayesian decision procedures for dose determining experiments. *Statistics in Medicine*, **14**, 885–93.
9. J.O. Berger (ed.) (1985) *Statistical Decision Theory and Bayesian Analysis*, Springer, New York.
10. Y.K. Cheung and R. Chappell (2002) A simple technique to evaluate model sensitivity in the continual reassessment method. *Biometrics*, **58**, 671–4.
11. Y.K. Cheung (2002) On the use of nonparametric curves in phase I trials with low toxicity tolerance. *Biometrics*, **58**(1), 237–40.
12. A.T.R. Legedza and J.G. Ibrahim (2001) Heterogeneity in phase I clinical trials: prior elicitation and computation using the continual reassessment method. *Statistics in Medicine*, **20**, 867–82.
13. M. Bensadon and J. O'Quigley (1994) Integral evaluation for continual reassessment method. *Computational Methods, Programs in Biomedicine*, **42**(4), 271–3.
14. M. de Spirlet, J. M. Treluyer, S. Chevret, E. Rey, M. Tournaire, D. Cabrol and G. Pons (2004) Tocolytic effects of intravenous nitroglycerin. *Fundamentals Clin. Pharmacology*, **18**(2), 207–13.
15. J.R. Murphy and D.L. Hall (1997) A logistic dose-ranging method for phase I clinical investigations trials. *J. Biopharmaceutical Statistics*, **7**(4), 635–47.

16. L. Shen and J. O'Quigley (1996) Consistency of continual reassessment method under model misspecification. *Biometrika*, **83**(2), 395–405.
17. L. Natarajan and J. O'Quigley (2003) Interval estimates of the probability of toxicity at the maximum tolerated dose for small samples. *Statistics in Medicine*, **22**(11), 1829–36.
18. J. O'Quigley and E. Reiner (1998) A stopping rule for the continual reassessment method. *Biometrika*, **85**, 741–8.
19. C. Ahn (1998) An evaluation of phase I cancer clinical trial designs. *Statistics in Medicine*, **17**(14), 1537–49.
20. N. Ishizuka and Y. Ohashi (2001) The continual reassessment method and its applications: a Bayesian methodology for phase I cancer clinical trials. *Statistics in Medicine*, **20**(17–18), 2661–81.
21. D. Faries (1994) Practical modifications of the continual reassessment method for phase I cancer clinical trials. *J. Biopharmaceutical Statistics*, **4**, 147–64.
22. E.L. Korn, D. Midthune, T.T. Chen, L.V. Rubinstein, M.C. Christian and R.M. Simon (1994) A comparison of two phase I trial designs. *Statistics in Medicine*, **13**, 1799–806.
23. S.N. Goodman, M.L. Zahurak and S. Piantadosi (1995) Some practical improvements in the continual reassessment method for phase I studies. *Statistics in Medicine*, **14**, 1149–61.
24. S. Moller (1995) An extension of the continual reassessment methods using a preliminary up-and-down design in a dose finding study in cancer patients, in order to investigate a greater range of doses. *Statistics in Medicine*, **14**(9–10), 911–22.
25. M. Gasparini and J. Eisele (2000) A curve-free method for phase I clinical trials. *Biometrics*, **56**, 609–15.
26. J. O'Quigley (2002) Curve-free and model-based continual reassessment method designs. *Biometrics*, **58**(1), 245–9.
27. Y.K. Cheung and R. Chappell (2000) Sequential designs for phase I clinical trials with late-onset toxicities, *Biometrics*, **56**, 1177–82.
28. S. Piantadosi and G. Liu (1996) Improved designs for dose escalation studies using pharmacokinetic measurements. *Statistics in Medicine*, **15**, 1605–18.
29. S. Zohar and S. Chevret (2001) The continual reassessment method: comparison of Bayesian stopping rules for dose-ranging studies. *Statistics in Medicine*, **20**(19), 2827–43.
30. S. Zohar, A. Latouche, M. Taconnet and S. Chevret (2003) Software to compute and conduct sequential Bayesian phase I or II dose-ranging clinical trials with stopping rules. *Computational Methods, Programs in Biomedicine*, **72**(2), 117–25.
31. S. Piantadosi, J.D. Fisher and S. Grossman (1998) Practical implementation of a modified continual reassessment method for dose-finding trials. *Cancer Chemotherapy and Pharmacology*, **41**, 429–36.
32. J. O'Quigley, L. Z. Shen and A. Gamst (1999) Two-sample continual reassessment method. *J Biopharmaceutical Statistics*, **9**(1), 17–44.
33. J. O'Quigley and X. Paoletti (2003) Continual reassessment method for ordered groups. *Biometrics*, **59**(2), 430–40.
34. P.F. Thall, J.J. Lee, C.H. Tseng and E.H. Estey (1999) Accrual strategies for phase I trials with delayed patient outcome. *Statistics in Medicine*, **18**, 1155–69.
35. P.F. Thall, E.H. Estey and H.-G. Sung (1999) A new statistical method for dose-finding based on efficacy and toxicity in early phase clinical trials. *Investigational New Drugs*, **17**, 155–67.
36. T. Braun (2002) The bivariate continual reassessment method: extending the crm to phase I trials of two competing outcomes. *Controlled Clin. Trials*, **23**, 240–56.

37. A. Kramar, A. Lebecq and E. Candalh (1999) Continual reassessment methods in phase I trials of the combination of two drugs in oncology. *Statistics in Medicine*, **18**(14), 1849–64.
38. A.T.R. Legedza and J.G. Ibrahim (2000) Longitudinal design for phase I clinical trials using the continual reassessment method. *Controlled Clin. Trials*, **21**, 574–88.
39. B.E. Storer (2001) Phase I trials, in *Biostatistics in Clinical Trials* (eds C. Redmond and T. Colton), John Wiley & Sons, Ltd, Chichester, pp. 337–42.
40. D.H. Leung and Y.G. Wang (2002) An extension of the continual reassessment method using decision theory. *Statistics in Medicine*, **21**(1), 51–63.
41. S. Zohar and S. Chevret (2003) Phase I (or phase II) dose-ranging clinical trials: proposal of a two-stage Bayesian design. *J. Biopharmaceutical Statistics*, **13**(1), 87–101.
42. J. O'Quigley, X. Paoletti and J. Maccario (2002) Non-parametric optimal design in dose finding studies. *Biostatistics*, **3**(1), 51–6.
43. B.N. Bekele and Y. Shen (2004) A Bayesian approach to jointly modeling toxicity and biomarker expression in a phase I/II dose-finding trial. Technical report, The University of Texas, M. D. Anderson Cancer Center.
44. B.N. Bekele and Y. Shen. A Bayesian approach to jointly modeling toxicity and biomarker expression in a phase I/II dose-finding trial. *Biometrics* (to appear).
45. P.F. Thall and K.E. Russell (1998) A strategy for dose-finding and safety monitoring based on efficacy and adverse outcomes in phase I/II clinical trials. *Biometrics*, **54**, 251–64.
46. P.F. Thall and J.D. Cook (2003) Dose-Finding Based On efficacy–toxicity trade-offs. Technical report #006-03, M.D. Anderson Cancer Center, Department of Biostatistics, University of Texas, Nouston, Texas.
47. J. Whitehead, Y. Zhou, J. Stevens and G. Blakey (2004) An evaluation of a Bayesian method of dose escalation based on bivariate binary responses. *J Biopharmaceutical Statistics*, **14**(4), 969–83.

7

Using Bayesian decision theory in dose-escalation studies

John Whitehead

Medical and Pharmaceutical Statistics Research Unit,
The University of Reading, UK

7.1 Introduction

In this chapter, an approach to dose-escalation based on Bayesian decision methodology will be presented. There are similarities between this approach and the continual reassessment method presented elsewhere in this volume. Both are in fact special cases of a wider class of procedures, and although presented 'as a package' readers are encouraged to be aware of the possibility of varying the ingredients chosen here. The essential features of any Bayesian decision procedure are (a) a model for the data, (b) a prior distribution for the unknown parameters, (c) a set of possible actions and (d) a gain function.

In this chapter, a logistic regression model will be used to model the relationship between the probability of some binary event (usually undesirable) and a prespecified transformation of dose. Two parameters will be used to govern the model, in contrast to the CRM, where one of the slopes and the intercept are taken to be fixed. Using two parameters allows the fitted model to have more relevance at doses other than that eventually chosen for further investigation, at no apparent cost in accuracy or safety.

Statistical Methods for Dose-Finding Experiments   Edited by S. Chevret
© 2006 John Wiley & Sons, Ltd

A conjugate prior for the slope and intercept of the model will be used that is equivalent to the observation of extra data, referred to here as 'pseudo-data', available before the study begins. Such a representation allows investigators to understand readily the nature of the prior assumptions as well as allowing straightforward analysis using frequentist software. Of course, investigators usually believe that the dose sought will be one of the higher doses to be tried, and yet they still begin at the lowest dose and move upwards carefully. In order to ensure that the Bayesian procedure mimics this behaviour, the prior will usually be chosen to reflect cautious opinion, representing what is feared rather than what is believed.

The actions from which to choose are those available when a new set of subjects is available for dosing, and consist of all possible combinations of doses that could be applied. No individual subject covariates will be used in making this choice, and so the chosen combination of doses can be administered to the subjects at random; they are not intended for particular people. The decisions begin with the dosing of the first group of subjects and need to repeated for every new group. A further decision concerns when to stop the study.

A gain function can be constructed to reflect what is best for the next group of subjects. This is appropriate when the subjects are themselves patients who could benefit from the study medication. They will be best served by a dose that is high enough to have therapeutic action while low enough to avoid undesirable side-effects. As therapeutic benefit will not be observed during the course of the trial, this requirement becomes a vaguer desire to administer the highest dose considered to be safe. Using such a criterion, every patient in a group being dosed simultaneously will receive the same dose. An alternative gain function can be based on the desire to maximise the information about the relationship between dose and effect, and this can lead to recommendations that subjects in the same group receive varying doses. Such a criterion should usually be operated within the limits of a safety criterion, ensuring that doses believed to be too risky are avoided.

Studies of the form described in this chapter are commonly encountered in oncology, and most statistical approaches to dose-escalation have been motivated by trials in that therapeutic area. A good review of this context is given by Edler [1]. More generally, the methods are applicable to clinical research in life-threatening or otherwise serious conditions in which some level of toxicity is acceptable provided that treatment also brings benefit. The trial described by Dougherty, Porche and Thall [2], and used as an illustration throughout this chapter, is an example of an application outside oncology.

The continual reassessment method (CRM) of O'Quigley, Pepe and Fisher [3] was motivated by cancer studies. Various modifications to that method were proposed, including those by Faries [4], Korn et al. [5] and Goodman, Zahurak and Piantadosi [6], which sought to ensure that the lowest doses are tried first and that escalation is not too quick. Piantadosi and Liu [7] made a different sort of suggestion in which pharmacokinetic observations were taken into account when interpreting treatment effects and setting new doses, while Legedza and Ibrahim [8] make use of pre-study covariates to individualise doses. O'Quigley and Shen [9] responded with their own modification of the CRM in which a more conventional form of dose-escalation preceded a switch to the formal procedure. A more up-to-date review of the CRM has been given by O'Quigley [10] while Rosenberger and Haines [11] give a more general review of the field. Two alternative approaches of interest for the same situation are "escalation with overdose control" described by Babb, Rogatko and Zacks [12] and the curve-free method of Gasparini and Eisele [13].

The methodology described in this chapter was introduced by Whitehead and Brunier [14] and Whitehead and Williamson [15], although it is related to the earlier work of Gatsonis and Greenhouse [16] in which posterior distributions are computed and displayed, but not formally linked to gain functions. Accounts aimed at clinical pharmacologists are given by Whitehead *et al.* [17] and by Zhou [18] and a simulation study of its properties is presented by Zhou and Whitehead [19].

7.2   Example of a dose-escalation study

Dougherty, Porche and Thall [2] describe a dose-escalation study in postoperative analgesia. The novel treatment was nalmefene hydrochloride, an intravenous, long-acting, pure opioid antagonist. Subjects in the study were patients recovering after a surgical operation, prior to which an indwelling epidural catheter had been inserted for the control of postoperative pain. This was used to administer fentanyl towards the end of the operation, and if necessary afterwards, in the postanesthesia care unit. The purpose of administering nalmefene to these patients is to reverse the adverse effects of epidural fentanyl, such as pruritus, nausea, vomiting and somnolence.

Unfortunately, while nalmefene might be effective in reducing adverse effects, it also has the potential to reduce the effectiveness of epidural fentanyl in controlling pain. In this account, the effectiveness of nalmefene in reducing adverse effects induced by epidural fentanyl will be referred to as its efficacy. The degree to which it reduces the effectiveness of epidural fentanyl in controlling pain will be referred to as its peccancy. It was assumed that as the dose of nalmefene was increased, both its efficacy and its peccancy would increase. The dose-escalation study was seen as a precursor to a large double-blind placebo-controlled trial to determine the efficacy of nalmefene. The objective of the dose-escalation study was to find the maximum dose having an acceptable peccancy; efficacy was not formally assessed.

During recovery, patients' experience of pain was monitored using a visual analogue score (VAS) ranging from 0 (no pain) to 10 (worst pain imaginable). Once the VAS had been reduced to 3 or less, a baseline VAS was recorded and a single intravenous injection of nalmefene was administered. Those patients whose scores could not be reduced to 3 or less without the aid of intravenous opioids were not eligible for the study. Once nalmefene had been administered, study patients were infused with epidural fentanyl at a rate intended to maintain their VAS score at 3 or less, and their pain was assessed at least hourly for 4 hours and again at the end of the 8 hour observation period. Reversal of analgesia was defined as an increase in the VAS score of two or more integers above the baseline value at any time during the 8 hour observation period. Here we will refer to reversal of analgesia as a dose-limiting event

Table 7.1   Doses and outcomes for patients in the postoperative analgesia study.

Patient	Dose	DLE	Patient	Dose	DLE	Patient	Dose	DLE
1	0.25	No	10	0.50	No	19	0.50	No
2	0.50	No	11	0.50	No	20	0.50	Yes
3	0.75	Yes	12	0.50	No	21	0.50	No
4	0.25	No	13	0.50	No	22	0.50	No
5	0.50	No	14	0.50	No	23	0.50	Yes
6	0.50	Yes	15	0.50	No	24	0.50	No
7	0.25	No	16	0.50	No	25	0.50	No
8	0.25	No	17	0.75	No			
9	0.50	No	18	0.75	Yes			

(DLE), which in general is a binary response indicating that too high a dose has been administered.

The formal objective of the dose-escalation study was to identify the dose at which the probability of a DLE was equal to 0.20. This will be referred to as the target dose, and denoted by d^*; it will be the dose recommended for comparison with placebo in the subsequent comparative efficacy trial. Setting the probability of a DLE to 0.20 constitutes a compromise between the desire to recommend a dose high enough to have the potential for efficacy and the need to control the risk of peccancy.

Four dose levels of nalmefene were available: 0.25, 0.50, 0.75 and 1.00 µg/kg. Twenty-five patients were treated in the trial, one at a time. The first patient was administered the lowest dose, and subsequently the results from all previous patients were used to select the dose for the next. The doses administered to each patient and the corresponding outcomes are given in Table 7.1 and displayed graphically in Figure 7.1. Dose-escalation was conducted using a modified form of the continual reassessment method, which is described in Section 7.8. The data from this example will be used throughout the chapter to illustrate various dose-escalation procedures.

7.3   A statistical model for the study

The example of section 7.2 illustrates a general form of dose-escalation study. Its essential features are as follows. A set of discrete doses $d_1 < \cdots < d_k$ are available for study. Suitable subjects enter the study in small groups of size c, known as cohorts (in the example $c = 1$). All subjects in a cohort are treated simultaneously, and the results from one cohort are available before the doses are chosen for the next. After a short period of observation, it can be determined whether a subject has experienced a dose-limiting event (DLE). In the example this was reversal of analgesia; in many cancer trials it will be occurrence of a toxicity exceeding a certain grade.

The study will focus on the peccancy of the treatment, with efficacy being the subject of a subsequent, larger trial. It is assumed that both peccancy and efficacy

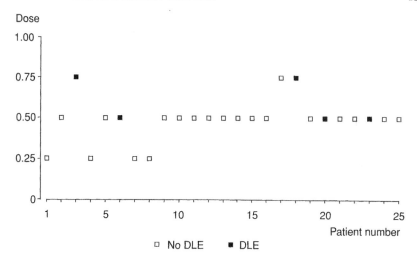

Figure 7.1 Graphical display of the dose-escalation in the postoperative analgesia study.

increase as the dose increases. The objective of the study is to find the maximum dose associated with acceptable peccancy. This will be defined as the dose d^* at which the probability of a DLE is equal to π, where π takes a small value such as 0.20. In some contexts it is appropriate to refer to d^* as the 'toxic dose 100π' (TD100π). Introducing the notation $p(d)$ for the probability of a DLE after administration of a dose d, d^* will be the solution of the equation $p(d^*) = \pi$.

Statistical approaches to the design and conduct of dose-escalation studies require the assumption of a model for the form of $p(d)$. This can be as minimal as merely assuming that $p(d)$ is increasing in d. Here, a parametric model will be assumed of the form

$$p(d) = \frac{\exp[\theta_1 + \theta_2 g(d)]}{1 + \exp[\theta_1 + \theta_2 g(d)]}, \tag{7.1}$$

where $g(d)$ represents some transformation of dose. The most usual forms for g are identity ($g(d) = d$) and the natural logarithm ($g(d) = \log(d)$). This is a logistic regression model [20], which can also be written as

$$\log\left[\frac{p(d)}{1 - p(d)}\right] = \theta_1 + \theta_2 g(d). \tag{7.2}$$

The relationship between the transformed dose $g(d)$ and $p(d)$ implicit in this model is illustrated in Figure 7.2.

At first sight it appears that the imposition of the model shown in Figure 7.2 will be a major assumption. The inverse symmetry about $p(d) = 0.5$ means that the shape of the upper part of the curve will be constrained by what is discovered about the lower part. However, in practice there should be little or no data relating to the upper part of

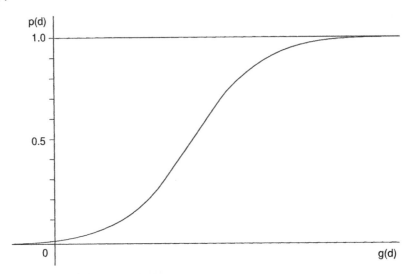

Figure 7.2   Assumed relationship between dose *d* and the probability of a DLE.

the curve as this relates to doses that are clearly undesirable. The necessary inferences concern the lower part of the curve in the restricted region shown in Figure 7.3. Thus it can be seen that all that is being assumed is an increasing and accelerating relationship between $p(d)$ and $g(d)$ that should not be too restrictive.

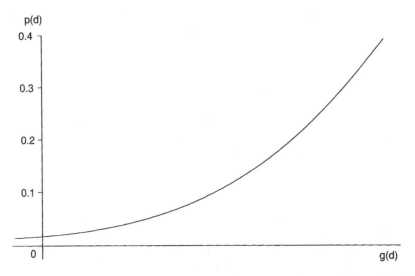

Figure 7.3   Detail of the region of the relationship between dose *d* and the probability of a DLE that is of interest.

Table 7.2 Data summary for a
dose-escalation study.

Dose	Number of administrations	Number of DLEs
d_1	n_1	t_1
d_2	n_2	t_2
$\vdots$	$\vdots$	$\vdots$
d_k	n_k	t_k

The data relating to the relationship shown in Figure 7.3 collected during the study can be summarised as shown in Table 7.2. The likelihood of (θ_1, θ_2) based on these data (denoted by x) is

$$L(\theta_1, \theta_2 | x) = \prod_{i=1}^{k} \{p(d_i)\}^{t_i} \{1 - p(d_i)\}^{n_i - t_i}, \qquad (7.3)$$

where $p(d)$ is defined by equation (7.1). The likelihood depends on (θ_1, θ_2) as each of the $p(d_i)$ can be expressed in terms of those parameters. Standard logistic regression software (such as PROC LOGISTIC in SAS) can be used to find the maximum likelihood estimates of (θ_1, θ_2) that maximise equation (7.3).

The data in Table 7.1 can be summarised in the style of Table 7.2, to give Table 7.3. Fitting the model of equation (7.1) with $g(d)$ set as the identity ($g(d) = d$) gives maximum likelihood estimates of $\widehat{\theta}_1 = -6.568$ (with standard error 2.881) and $\widehat{\theta}_2 = 9.812$ (with standard error 5.168). This gives respective fitted probabilities of a DLE of 0.016, 0.160, 0.688 and 0.962 at the doses 0.25, 0.50, 0.75 and 1.00. The first three of these can be compared with the observed proportions of 0, 0.167 and 0.667, suggesting a satisfactory fit. The estimated TD20 is 0.528, with a 95 % confidence interval (0.413, 0.643).

If instead, the model of equation (7.1) is fitted with $g(d) = \log(d)$, then the maximum likelihood estimates are $\widehat{\theta}_1 = 2.400$ (with standard error 2.073) and $\widehat{\theta}_2 = 5.806$ (with standard error 3.263). This gives respective fitted probabilities of a DLE of

Table 7.3 Data summary for the
postoperative analgesia study.

Dose	Number of administrations	Number of DLEs
0.25	4	0
0.50	18	3
0.75	3	2
1.00	0	0

0.004, 0.165, 0.675 and 0.917 at the doses 0.25, 0.50, 0.75 and 1.00. The estimated TD20 is 0.521, with a 95 % confidence interval (0.428, 0.633). The results are very similar to those obtained from setting $g(d)$ to be identity, which is not surprising as there are two unknown parameters in each model and only two doses providing appreciable information. The fitted probabilities in this latter model for doses 0.25, 0.50 and 0.75 are even closer to the observed proportions than for the identity model, while the extrapolation to dose 1.00, which was never used, suggests a lower risk of a DLE.

7.4   Prior information

Dose-escalation designs based on Bayesian decision theory make use of subjective opinions about the form of the curve $p(d)$ expressed before the study begins. A model for $p(d)$, such as that displayed in equation (7.1), is assumed to be true. Thus, everything is known about the relationship between the dose and the probability of a DLE except for the values of the pair of parameters (θ_1, θ_2). In the Bayesian paradigm, uncertainty about parameters is allowed for by treating them as random variables with a statistical distribution. Such a distribution characterises opinion about them even before any study data are collected. This is known as prior opinion, and in this case it is expressed in the form of a statistical distribution for (θ_1, θ_2). Prior opinion reflects subjective intuitive beliefs about the values of unknown parameters that might be formed from expert scientific judgement or from the analysis of previously collected relevant data or from a mixture of the two. In some applications, such as that considered here, the prior opinion expressed might be deliberately pessimistic. This forces the data to work against and overcome the prior and ensures that the procedure and inferences drawn from it err on the safe side. Once a prior distribution has been determined, new data are observed and prior opinion is transformed to posterior opinion (expressed through a posterior distribution) using Bayes theorem.

One possible way of expressing prior opinion is through consideration of pseudo-data, which by their nature and amount express both the position of the parameters (θ_1, θ_2) and the strength of that opinion. In essence, we imagine that we already have some data of the form shown in Table 7.2. Notation describing the pseudo-data is displayed in Table 7.4. This opinion is that, at some dose d_{-1} chosen by the expert, the probability of a DLE is equal to t_{-1}/n_{-1} and that the strength of that opinion is

Table 7.4   Pseudo-data expressing prior opinion.

Dose	Number of administrations	Number of DLEs
d_{-1}	n_{-1}	t_{-1}
d_0	n_0	t_0

Table 7.5 Default setting for pseudo-data.

Dose	Number of administrations	Number of DLEs
d_1	3	3π
d_k	3	1.5

as if n_{-1} real subjects had been observed. Similarly, the expert is of the opinion that, at some other dose d_0, the probability of a DLE is equal to t_0/n_0 and that the strength of that opinion is as if n_0 real subjects had been observed. In principle, the expert has a free choice in constructing a table like Table 7.4. In practice, this is not easy to do, and experience of the consequences of the choice made will be needed before it can be done sensibly.

In Section 7.7, the evaluation of Bayesian designs through simulation will be described. This allows the exploration of proposed designs, and their modification and reassessment. When the TD100π is sought with $\pi < 0.5$, the pseudo-data shown in Table 7.5 can be explored as they often gives a sensible design. These pseudo-data express the belief that the lowest dose in the dose schedule is the target dose achieving $p(d^*) = \pi$. The values of t_{-1} and t_0 can, as in this example, be noninteger, emphasising the imaginary nature of the pseudo-data. In principle n_{-1} and n_0 can be noninteger as well, but such a choice is more difficult to implement in software. The highest dose is believed (according to this prior) to have a fifty–fifty chance of leading to a DLE. Both opinions are equivalent to the observation of three subjects.

This is a pessimistic opinion, perhaps expressing what is feared rather than what is believed. It suggests that only the lowest dose is safe; the data have to work against this prior pessimism and prove that other doses are safe too. It will have the effect of forcing investigators to begin the trial with the administration of the lowest dose, which accords with traditional practice. It is also a weak opinion; the real data will soon overcome and dominate the imaginary findings from six subjects. The assumption that the highest dose corresponds to a risk of a DLE equal to one-half is the most arbitrary part of this setting. If π is not close to 0.2, then the risk set at d_k may be raised or lowered accordingly.

Mathematically, the opinion expressed in Table 7.4 can be characterised by taking $p_{-1} = p(d_{-1})$ to follow the beta distribution parameters t_{-1} and $(n_{-1} - t_{-1})$ and $p_0 = p(d_0)$ independently to follow the beta distribution parameters t_0 and $(n_0 - t_0)$. This can be transformed to a prior $h_0(\theta_1, \theta_2)$ density for (θ_1, θ_2) which takes the form

$$h_0(\theta_1, \theta_2) = |g(d_{-1}) - g(d_0)| \prod_{i=-1}^{0} \frac{p(d_i)^{t_i} \{1 - p(d_i)\}^{n_i - t_i}}{B(t_i, n_i - t_i)},$$

where B denotes the beta function and $||$ denotes absolute value. This form of prior is due to Tsutakawa [21]. The essential feature of this prior is

$$h_0(\theta_1, \theta_2) \propto \prod_{i=-1}^{0} p(d_i)^{t_i} \{1 - p(d_i)\}^{n_i - t_i}, \tag{7.4}$$

where $\propto$ denotes proportionality.

Application of the Bayes theorem, using the likelihood expressed by equation (7.3), shows that the posterior density $h(\theta_1, \theta_2 | x)$, following observation of the data shown in Table 7.2, satisfies

$$h_0(\theta_1, \theta_2 | x) \propto \prod_{i=-1}^{k} p(d_i)^{t_i} \{1 - p(d_i)\}^{n_i - t_i}. \tag{7.5}$$

Thus, the Tsutakawa prior is a conjugate prior, in that it leads to a posterior density of similar form to the prior. By comparing equation (7.5) with equation (7.3), it can be seen that the posterior is exactly the same as the likelihood would be if the pseudo-data were real. The values of (θ_1, θ_2) that maximise $h(\theta_1, \theta_2 | x)$, known as posterior modal estimates of (θ_1, θ_2), are the same as maximum likelihood estimates of the combined (pseudo- and real) datasets. This makes it possible to fit the Bayesian model using frequentist logistic regression software such as PROC LOGISTIC of SAS. It is also straightforward to fit the Bayesian model using Bayesian software such as WinBUGS, but this gives the expectation and median of the posterior distribution of (θ_1, θ_2) rather than the mode of the density. Wang and Faries [22] use 'seed data' in a similar manner to the use of pseudo-data here. Like the approach here, their seed data are chosen to reflect prior belief about the properties of the test drug, but crucially their method is non-Bayesian, the seed data being used as if it were real in a conventional likelihood approach.

In the example of Section 7.2, four dose levels of nalmefene were available: 0.25, 0.50, 0.75 and 1.00 µg/kg. Using prior opinion of the form displayed in Table 7.5, with $g(d) = \log d$ in equation (7.1) and with $\pi = 0.2$ as it is the TD20 that is required, gives the prior density for (θ_1, θ_2) displayed in Figure 7.4. By coincidence, this choice of prior has modal estimates of $\widetilde{\theta}_1 = 0$ and $\widetilde{\theta}_2 = 1$, and these can be seen to correspond to the highest point of h_0. Combining the prior opinion with the complete data shown in Table 7.4 leads to the posterior density $h(\theta_1, \theta_2 | x)$ shown in Figure 7.5. This demonstrates the considerable reduction in uncertainty due to observation of the data.

Fitting a logistic regression model (on PROC LOGISTIC) to both the pseudo-data and the real data yields the posterior modal estimates of $\widetilde{\theta}_1 = 0.288$ (with standard deviation 0.889) and $\widetilde{\theta}_2 = 2.314$ (with standard deviation 1.327). These can be compared with the maximum likelihood estimates computed in Section 7.3, which were $\widehat{\theta}_1 = 2.400$ (with standard error 2.073) and $\widehat{\theta}_2 = 5.806$ (with standard error 3.263). The Bayes estimates are shifted towards the prior values, but the maximum likelihood estimates do appear to be on the ridge shown in Figure 7.5, albeit below the summit.

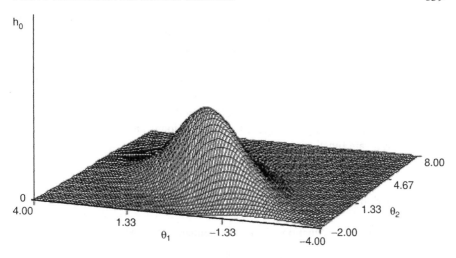

Figure 7.4   Prior density for (θ_1, θ_2) for the postoperative analgesia study.

7.5   Gain functions

So far, a model for the data has been suggested, and frequentist and Bayesian analyses have been described and illustrated by application to the complete postoperative analgesia study. In a Bayesian dose-escalation procedure, the model is fitted using the Bayesian approach prior to observing any data and then after every cohort of subjects. Thus, every time the decision is to be made concerning the doses to administer to the

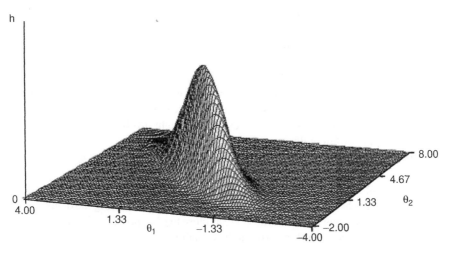

Figure 7.5   Posterior density for (θ_1, θ_2) on completion of the postoperative analgesia study.

next cohort, an expression of opinion about the values of θ_1 and θ_2 will be available, and in particular their modal estimates $\tilde{\theta}_1$ and $\tilde{\theta}_2$ will be known.

Substituting $\tilde{\theta}_1$ and $\tilde{\theta}_2$ for θ_1 and θ_2 in equation (7.1) will provide estimated values of $p(d_i)$ for each available dose. A subject in the study will typically be a patient who would like to benefit from the efficacy of the drug without suffering from its peccancy. Usually, this will mean that the ideal dose is the target dose d^* satisfying $p(d^*) = \pi$. Thus the best dose for each subject in the next cohort will be d_i, where $p(d_i)$ is closest to π among $i = 1, \ldots, k$. This criterion is known as the patient gain. Technically, a gain function G_p can be defined as

$$G_p(d_i; \theta_1, \theta_2) = \{p(d_i) - \pi\}^{-2} \tag{7.6}$$

and the criterion for choosing the dose can be regarded as choosing d_i to maximise $G_p(d_i; \tilde{\theta}_1, \tilde{\theta}_2)$.

An alternative gain function, G_v, can be defined as follows:

$$G_v(\theta_1, \theta_2) = \theta_2^2 \frac{\left[\sum n_i p_i(1 - p_i)\right]\left[\sum n_i p_i(1 - p_i)(g_i - \bar{g})^2\right]}{\sum n_i p_i(1 - p_i)(g_i - g^*)^2}, \tag{7.7}$$

where $p_i = p(d_i)$ and $g_i = g(d_i)$, $i = 1, \ldots, k$, $g^* = g(d^*)$, and

$$\bar{g} = \frac{\sum n_i p_i(1 - p_i)g_i}{\sum n_i p_i(1 - p_i)}, \tag{7.8}$$

so that $\bar{g}$ is a weighted average of the g_i. The doses for the next cohort will be chosen to maximise $G_v(d_i; \tilde{\theta}_1, \tilde{\theta}_2)$, where $\tilde{\theta}_1$ and $\tilde{\theta}_2$ are computed from the data observed so far, and the $p_i = p(d_i)$ used in equation (7.7) are evaluated from equation (7.1) using these values $\tilde{\theta}_1$ and $\tilde{\theta}_2$. The sums in equations (7.7) and (7.8) are over $i = -1, \ldots, k$ and include all pseudo-subjects featuring in the pseudo-data, all subjects who have actually been treated and observed, plus all subjects in the next cohort about to be treated. The responses to treatment do not appear in equation (7.7) for once the current posterior modal parameter estimates have been supplied, only the doses administered are needed. Therefore $G_v(d_i; \tilde{\theta}_1, \tilde{\theta}_2)$ is evaluated for all of the doses featuring in the pseudo- and real data and all possible combinations of doses that could be applied to the next cohort. All possible combinations are searched over in order to find that which maximises equation (7.7). The best choice might involve subjects in the same cohort receiving different doses.

Maximisation of G_v is an attempt to reconcile two competing considerations. Maximising the numerator is achieved by maximising the spread of the doses used in the sense of making the weighted sum of squared deviations of the g_i from their weighted mean $\bar{g}$ as large as possible. On the other hand, minimising the denominator is achieved by ensuring that all of the g_i are as close to g^* as possible. The transformed target dose g^* depends on θ_1 and θ_2 via the equation

$$g^* = \frac{\log\left[\pi/(1 - \pi)\right] - \theta_1}{\theta_2}$$

and its prior and posterior distributions can be derived from the joint prior and posterior distributions of θ_1 and θ_2. The expression for G_v is the inverse of the asymptotic posterior variance of g^*, and for this reason it is known as the variance gain. Although samples will be small, especially during the early part of the study, it turns out that use of G_v leads to attractive dose-escalation schemes, as can be demonstrated through simulation (see Section 7.7).

Consider the example of postoperative analgesia introduced in Section 7.2, modelled using equation (7.1) with $g(d) = \log(d)$. Suppose that prior opinion corresponds to three pseudo-subjects treated at dose 0.25 giving a total of 0.6 DLEs and three treated at dose 1.00 giving 1.5 DLEs. In Section 7.4, it was pointed out that this choice of prior has modal estimates of $\tilde{\theta}_1 = 0$ and $\tilde{\theta}_2 = 1$. Substituting these values in equation (7.1) gives prior predictions of $p(0.25) = 0.200$, $p(0.50) = 0.333$, $p(0.75) = 0.429$ and $p(0.50) = 0.500$. The first and last of these values are intentionally fixed; the prior was set to accord with the pseudo-data in Table 7.5 – i.e. make the prior estimate of the target dose equal to the lowest dose available and to associate the top dose with a fifty–fifty chance of a DLE. The patient gain takes the values $G_p = \infty$, 56.53, 19.07 and 11.11 respectively at the available doses, and so the lowest dose, 0.25, will be administered to the first cohort of subjects. The prior and the patient gain have been constructed specifically to guarantee this outcome in every case.

Table 7.6 shows the progress of dose-escalation for the postoperative analgesia trial based on the logistic regression model against log dose, the cautious prior described above, the patient gain and for eight cohorts of size 3. The scheme is illustrated in Figure 7.6. The real data shown in Table 7.1 are used, but in the order required by the Bayesian procedure. Where necessary, subjects are used twice, going back to the earliest recruits. The subject numbers according to the original data are shown in Table 7.6. Also shown are the estimates $\tilde{d}^*$ of the target dose, calculated after inclusion of each cohort. The initial value of $\tilde{d}^*$ is its prior estimate, 0.25.

Table 7.6 Progress of dose-escalation for the postoperative analgesia study based on the patient gain and eight cohorts of size 3.

Cohort	Doses	Subject numbers	DLE	$\tilde{d}^*$
1	0.25, 0.25, 0.25	1, 4, 7	0, 0, 0	0.417
2	0.50, 0.50, 0.50	2, 5, 6	0, 0, 1	0.382
3	0.50, 0.50, 0.50	9, 10, 11	0, 0, 0	0.481
4	0.50, 0.50, 0.50	12, 13, 14	0, 0, 0	0.560
5	0.50, 0.50, 0.50	15, 16, 19	0, 0, 0	0.621
6	0.50, 0.50, 0.50	20, 21, 22	1, 0, 0	0.562
7	0.50, 0.50, 0.50	23, 24, 25	1, 0, 0	0.521
8	0.50, 0.50, 0.50	2, 5, 6	0, 0, 1	0.491

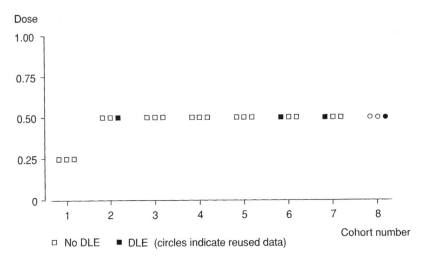

Figure 7.6   Graphical display of the dose-escalation in the postoperative analgesia study based on the patient gain and eight cohorts of size 3.

After all eight cohorts have responded, the posterior modal estimates are $\tilde{\theta}_1 = -0.201$ (with standard deviation 0.989) and $\tilde{\theta}_2 = 1.668$ (with standard deviation 1.354). The corresponding estimate of d^* is 0.491, so that the recommended dose would probably be 0.50. The 95 % credibility interval for d^* is (0.281, 0.860), which excludes 0.25 but not 0.75. These estimates can be compared with maximum likelihood estimates, computed ignoring the prior pseudo-data, which are $\widehat{\theta}_1 = 9.309$, $\widehat{\theta}_2 = 15.518$ and $\widehat{d}^* = 0.502$. Because only two doses have been used there are no degrees of freedom from which to estimate the standard errors of the maximum likelihood estimates, which are effectively infinite. Although the Bayesian and frequentist estimates for the slope and intercept are quite different, the resulting estimates for d^* are very similar. From the Bayesian model, fitted probabilities of a DLE at doses 0.25, 0.50, 0.75 and 1.00 are 0.075, 0.205, 0.336 and 0.500 respectively. The data used in Table 7.6 give the corresponding proportions 0 and 0.190 for the first two of these, whereas the actual data listed in Table 7.1 give proportions 0, 0.167 and 0.667 for the first three. The Bayesian model fits well at the doses actually administered, but the prior continues to dominate at those doses never tried.

The dose-escalation scheme shown in Table 7.6 avoids the higher doses 0.75 and 1.00 altogether, and with the hindsight offered by the real data this policy was wise. Having found a dose, 0.50, for which the estimated probability of a DLE was running consistently close to 0.20, there was no reason to offer any patient anything else. Regardless of how the relationship between dose and risk of DLE develops for doses higher than 0.50, the data from Table 7.6 suggest that dose 0.50 is associated with the target peccancy and thus should be used in subsequent studies. There is no need to risk exposure to higher doses to confirm this.

Table 7.7   Progress of dose-escalation for the postoperative analgesia study based on the variance gain and eight cohorts of size 3.

Cohort	Doses	Subject numbers	DLE	$\widetilde{d}^*$
1	0.25, 0.25, 0.25	1, 4, 7	0, 0, 0	0.417
2	0.50, 0.50, 0.25	2, 5, 8	0, 0, 0	0.533
3	0.75, 0.50, 0.50	3, 6, 9	1, 1, 0	0.395
4	0.25, 0.25, 0.25	1, 4, 7	0, 0, 0	0.428
5	0.50, 0.50, 0.50	10, 11, 12	0, 0, 0	0.488
6	0.50, 0.50, 0.50	13, 14, 15	0, 0, 0	0.535
7	0.75, 0.75, 0.50	17, 18, 16	0, 1, 0	0.533
8	0.50, 0.50, 0.50	19, 20, 21	0, 1, 0	0.506

Running the same scheme, but with cohorts of size 1, gives precisely the same pattern of results. The escalation to dose 0.50 occurs after the third subject, and dose 0.75 is never tried. A run with cohorts of size 3 in which no DLEs were ever observed would escalate to 0.75 after one cohort on 0.25 and two cohorts on 0.50, and to 1.00 after a further two cohorts on 0.75.

Table 7.7 and Figure 7.7 show the progress of dose-escalation for a similar design, but based on the variance gain. At the end of the study the posterior modal estimates are $\widetilde{\theta}_1 = 0.347$ (with standard deviation 0.888) and $\widetilde{\theta}_2 = 2.546$ (with standard deviation 1.311). The corresponding estimate of d^* is 0.506, so the recommended dose would once more be 0.50. The 95 % credibility interval for d^* is $(0.339, 0.757)$. These results

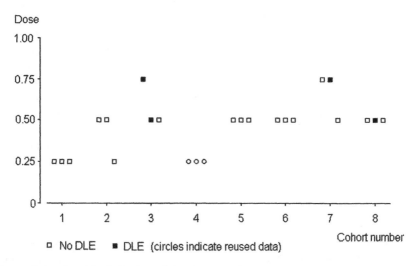

Figure 7.7   Graphical display of the dose-escalation in the postoperative analgesia study based on the variance gain and eight cohorts of size 3.

are closer to the Bayesian results from the full data reported in Section 7.4 than to those obtained from the patient gain, because in this run the dose 0.75 has been explored. The estimate of d^* is nevertheless very similar to that obtained using the patient gain and the credibility interval around it is tighter, as would be expected, given the objective of the variance gain. Maximum likelihood estimates based on these data are $\widehat{\theta}_1 = 2.537$ (with standard error 2.082), $\widehat{\theta}_2 = 6.279$ (with standard error 3.385) and $\widehat{d}^* = 0.535$ (with standard error 0.057). From the Bayesian model, fitted probabilities of a DLE at doses 0.25, 0.50, 0.75 and 1.00 are 0.040, 0.195, 0.405 and 0.586 respectively.

The variance gain has led to a dose-escalation scheme similar to that actually used. The method allows 'split cohorts', i.e. cohorts such as numbers 2, 3 and 7 above in which different subjects receive different doses. High doses are likely to be tried in an effort to improve estimation of d^*, although it is interesting to note that dose 1.00 was never tried, partly because the pseudo-data already provide supposed information about its risk. The procedure also tends occasionally to go back to lower doses (as in cohort 4) in order to estimate the slope of the model better.

7.6   Safety constraints and stopping rules

In cohort 3 of the dose-escalation scheme presented in Table 7.7 and Figure 7.7, the first subject receives dose 0.75 and suffers a DLE. It could be argued that dose-escalation proceeded too quickly and that this subject was placed at too great a risk (even though the actual dose-escalation scheme reached this point for the third subject in the study).

Every dose-escalation study is likely to result in some subjects suffering a DLE; indeed if they do not then a further study of higher doses might be initiated in order to identify the 'danger zone'. However, there are genuine reasons for avoiding DLEs among the early subjects. This is because, although the mathematical model of the process recognises only the outcomes 'DLE' and 'no DLE', in reality there are finer gradations of outcome. In particular, there could be severe DLEs and even lethal DLEs, and these are to be avoided at all costs. Modelling the risks of more severe grades of DLE is not feasible; as there will be so few of them, or better none at all, any model will be supported almost entirely by prior opinion. Here it will be assumed only that, as the probability of any sort of DLE increases, so do the probabilities of severe DLEs. Thus, doses d for which $p(d)$ is large are to be avoided. For some chosen value g, doses for which the current estimate of $p(d) \geq \gamma$ will not be used, the current estimate of $p(d)$ being found from equation (7.1) with θ_1 and θ_2 replaced by their posterior modal estimates. If the TD100π is being sought, then γ will be chosen to be a little larger than π; e.g. if the target dose is the TD20, then $\gamma = 0.25$ or 0.30 might be used.

Figures 7.8 and 7.9 present graphical displays of dose-escalation in the postoperative analgesia study using the variance gain and with the safety constraint γ set at 0.25 and 0.30 respectively. In Figure 7.8, the dose 0.75 is avoided altogether, whereas the more lenient setting of $\gamma = 0.30$ shown in Figure 7.9 only delays its eventual administration.

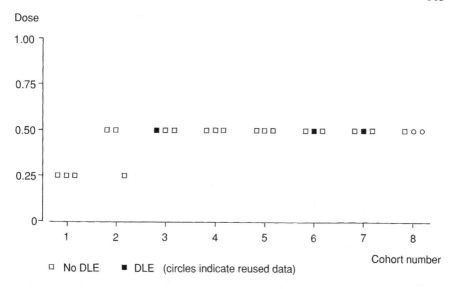

Figure 7.8   Graphical display of the dose-escalation in the postoperative analgesia study, with variance gain and safety constraint γ set at 0.25.

For any dose-escalation study a maximum number of cohorts will be set in advance. If a safety constraint is set, then this will imply a safety stopping rule: stop when none of the doses available satisfy the safety constraint. An additional accuracy stopping rule can also be imposed in order to save unnecessary investigation. Zhou

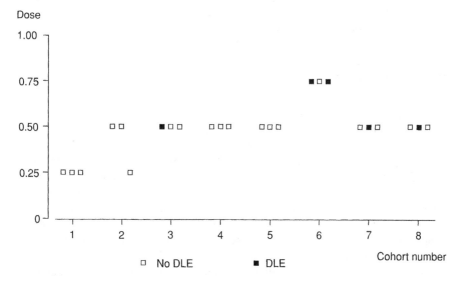

Figure 7.9   Graphical display of the dose-escalation in the postoperative analgesia study, with variance gain and safety constraint γ set at 0.30.

Table 7.8 Credibility intervals following each cohort of subjects for the postoperative analgesia study based on the variance gain with a safety constraint.

	Safety constraint $\gamma = 0.25$				Safety constraint $\gamma = 0.30$			
Cohort	$\tilde{d}^*$	$\tilde{d}_L^*$	$\tilde{d}_U^*$	$\tilde{d}_U^*/\tilde{d}_L^*$	$\tilde{d}^*$	$\tilde{d}_L^*$	$\tilde{d}_U^*$	$\tilde{d}_U^*/\tilde{d}_L^*$
0	0.250	0.015	4.232	286.53	0.250	0.015	4.232	286.53
1	0.417	0.127	1.364	10.70	0.417	0.127	1.364	10.70
2	0.533	0.213	1.334	6.27	0.533	0.213	1.334	6.27
3	0.466	0.207	1.049	5.06	0.466	0.207	1.049	5.06
4	0.545	0.268	0.109	4.15	0.545	0.268	0.109	4.15
5	0.607	0.314	1.173	3.73	0.607	0.314	1.173	3.73
6	0.550	0.301	1.007	3.35	0.522	0.330	0.827	2.51
7	0.512	0.291	0.900	3.09	0.494	0.315	0.775	2.46
8	0.553	0.323	0.947	2.93	0.474	0.305	0.736	2.41

and Whitehead [19] suggest stopping when the ratio of the upper to the lower limits of the 95 % posterior credibility interval for the target dose d^* falls below some critical value, R. This interval is taken to be $(\exp(\tilde{g}^* - 1.96/\sqrt{G_v}), \exp(\tilde{g}^* + 1.96/\sqrt{G_v}))$, where $\tilde{g}^*$ is the estimate of $\log(d^*)$ based on the posterior modal estimates of θ_1 and θ_2, and G_v is the inverse of its asymptotic variance as given by equation (7.7). In this setting G_v is computed from the pseudo- and observed data, and not from potential data from future cohorts.

Table 7.8 shows the emerging credibility intervals for the simulated runs shown in Figures 7.8 and 7.9. Until the sixth cohort, the two sequences are the same. When $\gamma = 0.30$, dose 0.75 is used for the sixth cohort, and although two DLEs are observed the gain in information is clearly reflected in a greater narrowing of the credibility interval than when $\gamma = 0.25$ and dose 0.75 is avoided. Applying the accuracy rule with $R = 3$ would lead to stopping after the eighth cohort for $\gamma = 0.25$ (i.e. no early stopping) and after the sixth cohort for $\gamma = 0.30$.

7.7 Evaluation of the Bayesian approach

Having designed a Bayesian dose-escalation procedure, it is sensible to evaluate its properties before using it in practice. This is best achieved through simulation. Consider a trial assessing doses 0.25, 0.50, 0.75 and 1.00 mg, conducted in cohorts of size 3 using the variance gain, which is one of the designs explored in Section 7.6. An upper limit of eight cohorts is used, the TD20 is sought and a safety constraint with $\gamma = 0.25$ is set. A stopping rule based on a 95 % credibility limit ratio of $R = 3$ is applied. The prior is equivalent to observing three subjects at dose 0.25 resulting in 0.6 DLEs and three at 1.00 with 1.5 DLEs.

The properties of the design will be assessed under each of six scenarios, described in Table 7.9. Also shown in Table 7.9 is the prior model. This is a deliberately

Table 7.9 The prior model and six simulation scenarios for the relationship between the probability of a DLE and dose.

Scenario	Intercept, θ_1	Slope, θ_2	TD20	TD25	TD50
Prior	0	1	0.25	0.333	1.00
1. Standard	1.342	4.283	0.529	0.566	0.731
2. Toxic	2.887	5.505	0.460	0.485	0.592
3. Safe	0.562	5.505	0.702	0.740	0.903
4. Steep	2.850	9.098	0.628	0.648	0.731
5. Very toxic	0.599	1.913	0.354	0.412	0.731
6. Very safe	−1.411	2.407	1.011	1.139	1.797

pessimistic prior, constructed to force a start at the lowest available dose. It is not used as a simulation scenario. Some results from 10 000-fold simulations are shown in Table 7.10.

The efficiency of each procedure is assessed in terms of the number of subjects needed to achieve the required accuracy of estimation. The maximum number allowed

Table 7.10 Results of the simulation investigation, with 10 000 runs of each scenario. Italic entries indicate the administration of doses exceeding the TD25 and bold entries the administration of doses exceeding the TD50.

Scenario	1	2	3	4	5	6
numbers of subjects per run	19.50	18.48	19.84	17.60	15.14	21.63
numbers of safety stops	285	269	31	1	3614	284
numbers of accuracy stops	8722	9250	8329	9385	3753	4752
numbers of DLEs per run	2.47	2.70	1.79	1.99	2.74	1.39
Intercept	0.121	0.423	−0.337	0.019	0.234	−0.835
Slope	2.230	2.204	2.488	2.668	1.456	1.965
Target dose (PME)	0.509	0.439	0.665	0.598	0.300	0.755
Standard deviation	*0.107*	*0.078*	*0.099*	*0.068*	*0.145*	*0.208*
Target dose (MLE)	0.527	0.467	0.712	0.669	0.299	0.742
Standard error	*0.126*	*0.094*	*0.119*	*0.075*	*0.175*	*0.213*
Precision error	0.140	0.140	0.143	0.222	0.132	0.103
MLE failures	26	6	209	9	542	1668
Administration of doses (average number per run)						
0.25	7.48	9.77	4.55	4.43	10.47	4.79
0.50	10.94	8.45	10.63	10.15	*4.56*	10.16
0.75	*1.07*	**0.26**	*4.22*	**3.01**	**0.11**	4.74
1.00	**0.01**	**0.00**	**0.44**	**0.02**	**0.00**	1.93

is 24, while the average number required varies according to a scenario between 15 and 22. For all scenarios, the majority of runs stop before reaching 24 subjects, although it is a very small majority in the case of scenario 6. Most stopping is due to achieving the required accuracy, although stopping because no dose appears to be safe is also common. The average number of DLEs per run is maintained below three in all cases.

The accuracy of estimation can be assessed in various ways. Firstly, the posterior modal estimates (PMEs) of the intercept, slope and target dose (TD20) are presented, together with the standard deviation of the last quantity. In all cases, the intercept and slope are poorly estimated. This is because only four doses are available. The top dose of 1.00 mg was rarely used under any of the scenarios because it would have seldom appeared to be safe, and for most scenarios this was appropriate because of the high risk of a DLE at this dose. The bottom dose was not often used, so that the majority of observations were at just two doses. This led to poor estimation of these parameters, with a strong influence of the prior. In general, both the slope and the intercept are underestimated (bear in mind that all doses are ≤ 1 so that all log doses are ≤ 0). However, the predicted DLE probabilities are quite accurate around the target dose, which is itself well estimated. Also given are maximum likelihood estimates (MLE), ignoring the prior. Sometimes this method leads to infinite, zero or negative slopes, and in each case these are recorded as 'MLE failures'. When they exist, these frequentist estimates are similar to their Bayesian counterparts. Finally, the precision error is listed and is defined as

$$\text{Precision error} = \sqrt{\text{average}\left[p(\widehat{d}^*) - \pi\right]^2},$$

where $\widehat{d}^*$ is the final maximum likelihood estimate of the TD100π that is being sought ($\pi = 0.20$ in this case). The value of $p(\widehat{d}^*)$ is found from equation (7.1) using the true intercept and slope underlying the simulation model. Thus, the precision error assesses the discrepancy between the DLE probability that will be obtained if the estimated target dose is actually used and the target probability.

The majority of subjects received doses that lie below the TD25, indicating the success of the safety constraint. The greatest number exceeding the TD25 occurs for scenario 2 in which dose 0.50 lies just above the TD25 of 0.485. Few subjects receive doses exceeding the TD50, the worst case being scenario 4, which has the steepest slope. The dose recommended for use in subsequent trials could be the dose closest to the estimated TD20, the highest dose below the estimated TD20 or derived from some other consideration.

Following an evaluation of this nature, the design can be modified and then re-evaluated. In this case, it would be interesting to try including more dose levels (especially as with this design some of them can be skipped), relaxing the safety constraint and trying an alternative, less pessimistic, prior.

7.8   Discussion

In this chapter, a Bayesian decision procedure has been applied to the problem of dose-escalation, based on a two-parameter logistic regression model for the relationship between the probability of a DLE and some prespecified transformation of the dose. Since 1990, a wide variety of rival procedures has been developed for dose-escalation studies in which each subject receives a single dose once, and exhibits some form of DLE or does not. Prominent among these is the continual reassessment method (CRM), introduced by O'Quigley, Pepe and Fisher [3], and discussed elsewhere in this book (chapter 6). Dougherty, Porche and Thall [2] used a modified form of the CRM to conduct the postoperative analgesia study used as an example throughout this chapter.

In the real trial, subjects were treated in cohorts of size 1. A logistic regression model was assumed between the probability of a DLE and the coded doses d(0.25), d(0.50), d(0.75) and d(1.00), with the intercept fixed to be 3. Coded doses are often used when implementing the CRM, and here their values were taken to be d(0.25) $= -5.197$, d(0.50) $= -4.386$, d(0.75) $= -3.405$ and d(1.00) $= -1.614$. A unit exponential distribution was used as a prior for the slope. Thus the prior mean of the slope was 1, and the corresponding prior estimates of the DLE probabilities at the four doses were 0.1, 0.2, 0.4 and 0.8 respectively. The coded doses were found from the latter values, which were chosen to provide a study design with good properties as judged by simulation results. No untried doses could be skipped as doses were increased, but otherwise every subject was assigned to the dose with a prior or posterior estimate of the DLE probability closest to 0.2. Estimation was based on expectation over the prior or posterior distribution of the TD20. A total of 25 subjects were used in the study and 5 DLEs were observed. The dose 0.50 was identified as the 'maximum tolerated dose'.

In order to determine whether the Bayesian decision procedure described in this chapter was more suitable for this trial than the modified CRM actually used would require comparing a simulation evaluation of the latter to that presented in Section 7.7 for the former. No such comparison is presented here. There are many variations of both the Bayesian decision theory approach and the CRM. In an application it would be wise to identify approaches from more than one camp and to evaluate them carefully. Once a design has been found to behave suitably for two or three similar studies, then it might be adopted as standard, until dose-escalation is required for a drug likely to exhibit qualitatively different behaviour.

One consideration in developing the methods described in this chapter has been a desire to devise a procedure that can be modified for use in other types of dose-escalation study. The same principles have been applied by Patterson et al. [23] and Whitehead et al. [24] (see also Zhou in this volume, chapter 9) to trials in healthy volunteers where each subject receives more than one dose and is assessed in terms of some continuously distributed pharmacokinetic response. They have also been extended to trials in which desirable outcomes may be observed as well as DLEs [25,26].

The computations and simulations presented in this chapter have all been prepared using the software 'Bayesian ADEPT' [27]. Thus, the methodology and the associated software are in place. It is hoped that this and similar articles will encourage phase I statisticians and clinical pharmacologists to assess the methodology further, perhaps retrospectively applying it to their own datasets, and then to go further and apply it prospectively in future trials. It must be stressed that the whole procedure is intended to operate in an advisory role. Its recommendations for dosing are only recommendations, to be confirmed or overruled by the clinical investigators or their designated safety committee. Additional constraints can be operated and alternative doses can be substituted at any stage. The responses to those doses can be entered into the procedure and used to advise the next dose allocation. The procedure is made to be operated flexibly, and with experience users should be able to learn how to choose a design that will seldom require being overruled.

References

1. L. Edler (2001) Overview of phase I trials, in *Statistics in Clinical Oncology* (ed. J. Crowley), Marcel Dekker, New York, pp. 1–34.
2. T. B. Dougherty, V. H. Porche and P. F. Thall (2000) Maximum tolerated dose of nalmefene in patients receiving epidural fentanyl and dilute bupivacaine for postoperative analgesia. *Anesthesiology*, **92**, 1010–16.
3. J. O'Quigley, M. Pepe and L. Fisher (1990) Continual reassessment method: a practical design for phase I clinical trials in cancer. *Biometrics*, **46**, 33–48.
4. D. Faries (1994) Practical modifications of the continual reassessment method for phase I cancer clinical trials. *J. Biopharmaceutical Statistics*, **4**, 147–64.
5. E.L. Korn, D. Midthune, T.T. Chen, L.V. Rubinstein, M.C. Christian and R.M. Simon (1994) A comparison of two phase I designs. *Statistics in Medicine*, **13**, 1799–806.
6. S.N. Goodman, M.L. Zahurak and S. Piantadosi (1995) Some practical improvements in the continual reassessment method for phase I studies. *Statistics in Medicine*, **14**, 1149–61.
7. S. Piantadosi and G. Liu (1996) Improved designs for dose escalation studies using pharmacokinetic measurements. *Statistics in Medicine*, **15**, 1605–18.
8. A. Legedza and J.G. Ibrahim (2001) Heterogeneity in phase I clinical trials: prior elicitation and computation using the continual reassessment method. *Statistics in Medicine*, **20**, 867–82.
9. J. O'Quigley and L.Z. Shen (1996) Continual reassessment method: a likelihood approach. *Biometrics*, **52**, 673–84.
10. J. O'Quigley (2001) Dose-finding designs using continual reassessment method, in *Statistics in Clinical Oncology* (ed. J. Crowley), Dekker, New York, pp. 35–72.
11. W. F. Rosenberger and L. M. Haines (2002) Competing designs for phase I clinical trials: a review. *Statistics in Medicine*, **21**, 2757–70.
12. J. Babb, A. Rogatko and S. Zacks (1998) Cancer phase I clinical trials: efficient dose escalation with overdose control. *Statistics in Medicine*, **17**, 1103–20.
13. M. Gasparini and J. Eisele (2000) A curve-free method for phase I clinical trials. *Biometrics*, **56**, 609–15.
14. J. Whitehead and H. Brunier (1995) Bayesian decision procedures for dose determining experiments. *Statistics in Medicine*, **14**, 885–93.
15. J. Whitehead and D. Williamson (1998) An evaluation of Bayesian decision procedures for dose-finding studies. *J. Biopharmaceutical Medicine*, **8**, 445–67.
16. C. Gatsonis and J.B. Greenhouse (1992) Bayesian methods for phase I clinical trials. *Statistics in Medicine*, **11**, 1377–89.
17. J. Whitehead, Y. Zhou, S. Patterson, N.D. Webber and S. Francis (2001) Easy-to-implement Bayesian methods for dose-escalation studies in healthy volunteers. *Biostatistics*, **2**, 47–61.

18. Y. Zhou (2004) Choice of designs and doses for early phase trial. *Fundamental Clin. Pharmacology*, **18**, 1–7.
19. Y. Zhou and J. Whitehead (2003) Practical implementation of Bayesian dose escalation procedure. *Drug Information J.*, **37**, 45–59.
20. D. Collett (ed.) (2003) *Modelling Binary Data*, 2nd edn, Chapman and Hall/CRC, Florida.
21. R.K. Tsutakawa (1975) Technical Report 52, Mathematical Sciences, University of Missouri, Columbia, Missouri.
22. O. Wang and D.E. Faries (2000) A two-stage dose selection strategy in phase I trials with wide dose ranges. *J. Biopharmaceutical Statistics*, **10**, 319–33.
23. S. Patterson, S. Francis, M. Ireson, D. Webber and J. Whitehead (1999) A novel Bayesian decision procedure for early-phase dose finding studies. *J. Biopharmaceutical Statistics*, **9**, 583–97.
24. J. Whitehead, Y. Zhou, S. Stallard, S. Todd and A. Whitehead (2001) Learning from previous responses in phase I dose-escalation studies. *Br. J. Clin. Pharmacology*, **52**, 1–7.
25. J. Whitehead, Y. Zhou, J. Stevens, G. Blakey, J. Price and J. Leadbetter (2006) Bayesian decision procedures for dose-escalation based on evidence of undesirable events and therapeutic benefit. *Statistics in Medicine*, **25**, 37–53.
26. J. Whitehead, Y. Zhou, J. Stevens and G. Blakey (2006) An evaluation of a Bayesian method of dose-escalation based on bivariate binary responses, *Statistics in Medicine*, **25**, 433–445.
27. Y. Zhou and J. Whitehead (2002) *Bayesian Adept: Operating Manual*. The University of Reading, Reading, UK.

8

Dose-escalation with overdose control

Mourad Tighiouart and André Rogatko

Department of Biostatistics and Winship Cancer Institute,
Emory University, Atlanta, Georgia, USA

8.1 Introduction

The primary goal of a cancer phase I clinical trial is to determine the dose of a new drug or combination of drugs for subsequent use in phase II trials to evaluate its efficacy. The dose sought is typically referred to as the maximum tolerated dose (MTD) and its definition depends on the treatment under investigation, the severity and reversibility of its side-effects, and on clinical attributes of the target patient population. Since it is generally assumed that toxicity is a prerequisite for optimal antitumor activity (see Wooley and Schein [1]) the MTD of a cytotoxic agent typically corresponds to the highest dose associated with a tolerable level of toxicity. More precisely, the MTD is defined as the dose expected to produce some degree of medically unacceptable, dose-limiting toxicity (DLT) in a specified proportion θ of patients (see Gatsonis and Greenhouse [2]). Hence, we have

$$\text{Prob}\{\text{DLT}|\text{dose} = \gamma\} = \theta.$$

Due to the sequential nature of these trials, the small number of patients involved and the severity of dose-toxicity, designs with the following desirable properties are sought:

Statistical Methods for Dose-Finding Experiments   Edited by S. Chevret
© 2006 John Wiley & Sons, Ltd

1. *A priori* information about the drug from animal studies or similar trials should be easily implemented in the entertained model.

2. The design should be adaptive [3], in the sense that uncertainty about the toxicity associated with the dose level to be given to the next patient (or cohort of patients) should be reduced when data collected thus far are taken into account.

3. The design should control the probability of overdosing patients at each stage.

4. The design should produce a sequence of doses that approaches the MTD as rapidly as possible.

5. The design should take into account the heterogeneity nature of cancer phase I clinical trial patients.

A number of statistical designs have been proposed and extensively studied in the past three decades. Nonparametric approaches to this problem have been developed by Durham and Flournoy [4] and Gasparini and Eisele [5]. Within a parametric framework, a model for the dose-toxicity relationship is typically specified and the unknown parameters are estimated sequentially. Bayesian approaches to estimating these parameters are natural candidates for designs that satisfy properties (1) and (2) above. Among such designs, we mention the pioneering work of Tsutakawa [6,7], Grieve [8] and Racine *et al.* [9]. More recent Bayesian models include the continual reassessment method (CRM) of O'Quigley, Pepe and Fisher [10], escalation with overdose control (EWOC) described by Babb, Rogatko and Zacks [11], the decision-theoretic approach of Whitehead and Brunier [12] and the constrained Bayesian C- and D-optimal designs proposed by Haines, Perevozskaya and Rosenberger [13]. The CRM and EWOC schemes both produce consistent sequences of doses but the latter takes into account the ethical constraint of overdosing patients. The last two designs are optimal in the sense of maximizing the efficiency of the estimate of the MTD. A discussion on the performance of these designs can be found in Rosenberger and Haines [14].

In this chapter, we describe EWOC in detail and present two real-life applications. EWOC is the first statistical method to incorporate formal safety constraints directly into the design of cancer phase I trials. In Section 8.2, we show how the method controls the frequency of overdosing by selecting dose levels for use in the trial so that the predicted proportion of patients administered a dose exceeding the MTD is equal to a specified upper bound. This approach allows more patients to be treated with potentially therapeutic doses of a promising new agent and fewer patients to suffer the deleterious effects of a toxic dose. EWOC has been used to design over a dozen phase I studies approved by the Research Review Committee and the Institute Review Board of the Fox Chase Cancer Center, Philadelphia, USA. Also, EWOC was adopted by the University of Miami (UM) for its NCI/CTEP-approved study of Cytochlor, a new radio-sensitizing agent synthesized at UM. Additionally, EWOC has been used in trials sponsored by pharmaceutical companies such as Pharmacia-Upjohn, Jensen and Bristol-Myers-Squibb.

In Section 8.3, we show how EWOC permits the utilization of information concerning individual patient differences in susceptibility to treatment. The extension of EWOC to covariate utilization made it the first method described to design cancer clinical trials that not only guides dose escalation but also permits personalization of the dose level for each specific patient (see Babb and Rogatko [15] and Cheng et al. [16]). The method adjusts doses according to patient-specific characteristics and allows the dose to be escalated as quickly as possible while safeguarding against overdosing. The extension of EWOC to covariate utilization was implemented in four Food and Drug Administration (FDA)-approved phase I studies. Section 8.4 addresses the issue of the choice of prior distributions by exploring a wide range of vague and informative priors. In Section 8.5, we give some final remarks and discussion of current and future work.

Based on the research work we describe in Sections 8.1, 8.2 and 8.3, the EWOC methodology satisfies the above five desirable properties and, to our knowledge, no other design has been shown to be flexible enough to accommodate those properties simultaneously.

8.2 Escalation with overdose control design

The main attribute underlying EWOC is that it is designed to approach the MTD as fast as possible subject to the ethical constraint that the predicted proportion of patients who receive an overdose does not exceed a specified value. The design has many advantages over some competing schemes such as up-and-down designs and the continual reassessment method. In this section, we describe the methodology in detail and give a real-life example illustrating this technique.

8.2.1 EWOC design

Let $X_{\min}$ and $X_{\max}$ denote the minimum and maximum dose levels available for use in the trial. One chooses these levels in the belief that $X_{\min}$ is safe when administered to humans and $\gamma \in [X_{\min}, X_{\max}]$ with prior (and hence posterior) probability 1. Denote by Y the indicator of toxicity. The dose-toxicity relationship is modeled parametrically as

$$P(Y = 1|\text{dose} = x) = F(\beta_0 + \beta_1 x), \qquad (8.1)$$

where F is a specified cumulative distribution function (CDF). We assume that $\beta_1 > 0$ so that the probability of a DLT is a monotonic increasing function of the dose. The model is reparameterized in terms of the MTD and the probability of DLT at the starting dose ρ_0, parameters that clinicians can easily interpret. This might be advantageous since γ is the parameter of interest and one often conducts preliminary studies at or near the starting dose so that a meaningful informative prior for ρ_0 can be selected. Assuming a logistic distribution for F, model (8.1) becomes

$$P(Y = 1|\text{dose} = x) = \frac{\exp\left\{\ln\left(\dfrac{\rho_0}{1 - \rho_0}\right) + \ln\left[\dfrac{\theta(1 - \rho_0)}{\rho_0(1 - \theta)}\right]\dfrac{x}{\gamma}\right\}}{1 + \exp\left\{\ln\left(\dfrac{\rho_0}{1 - \rho_0}\right) + \ln\left[\dfrac{\theta(1 - \rho_0)}{\rho_0(1 - \theta)}\right]\dfrac{x}{\gamma}\right\}}. \tag{8.2}$$

Denote by y_i the response of the ith patient where $y_i = 1$ if the patient exhibits DLT and $y_i = 0$ otherwise. Let x_i be the dose administered to the ith patient and $D_k = \{(x_i, y_i), i = 1, \ldots, k\}$ be the data after observing k patients. After specifying a prior distribution $h(\rho_0, \gamma)$ for (ρ_0, γ), denote by $\Pi_k(x)$ the marginal posterior cdf of γ given D_k.

EWOC can be described as follows. The first patient receives the dose $x_1 = X_{\min}$ and, conditional on the event $\{y_1 = 0\}$, the kth patient receives the dose $x_k = \Pi_k^{-1}(\alpha)$ so that the posterior probability of exceeding the MTD is equal to the feasibility bound α. Such a procedure is called Bayesian-feasible of level $1 - \alpha$ (see Eichhorn and Zacks [17]). The corresponding sequence of doses generated by this design converges to the unknown MTD while minimizing the amount by which patients are underdosed. Calculation of the marginal posterior distribution of γ was performed using numerical integration. In practice, phase I clinical trials are typically based on a small number of prespecified dose levels $d_1, d_2, \ldots, d_r$. In this case, the kth patient receives the dose

$$D_k = \max\{d_1, \ldots, d_r : d_i - x_k \leq T_1 \text{ and } \Pi_k(x_k) - \alpha \leq T_2\},$$

where T_1, T_2 are nonnegative numbers we refer to as tolerances. The resulting dose sequence is Bayesian-feasible of level $1 - \alpha$ if and only if T_1 or T_2 is zero. We note that this design scheme does not require that we know all patient responses before we can treat a newly accrued patient. Instead, we can select the dose for the new patient on the basis of the data currently available.

At the conclusion of the trial, the MTD is estimated by minimizing the posterior expected loss with respect to some suitable loss function l. One should consider asymmetric loss functions since underestimation and overestimation have very different consequences. Indeed, the dose x_k selected by EWOC for the kth patient corresponds to the estimate of γ having minimal risk with respect to the asymmetric loss function:

$$l_\alpha(x, \gamma) = \begin{cases} \alpha(\gamma - x) \text{ if } x \leq \gamma, & \text{i.e. if } x \text{ is an underdose;} \\ (1 - \alpha)(x - \gamma) \text{ if } x > \gamma, & \text{i.e. if } x \text{ is an overdose.} \end{cases}$$

Note that the loss function l_α implies that for any $\delta > 0$, the loss incurred by treating a patient at δ units above the MTD is $(1 - \alpha)/\alpha$ times greater than the loss associated with treating the patient at δ units below the MTD. This interpretation might provide a meaningful basis for the selection of the feasibility bound.

The above methodology can be implemented using the user-friendly software of Rogatko *et al.* [18].

8.2.2 Example

EWOC was used to design a phase I clinical trial that involved the R115777 drug at Fox Chase Cancer Center in Philadelphia, USA, in 1999. R115777 is a selective nonpeptidomimetic inhibitor of farnesyltransferase (FTase), one of several enzymes responsible for post-translational modification that is required for the function of p21(ras) and other proteins. This was a repeated-dose, single-center trial designed to determine the MTD of R115777 in patients with advanced incurable cancer.

The dose-escalation scheme was designed to determine the MTD of R115777 when the drug is administered orally for 12 hours during 21 days followed by a 7 day rest. Toxicity was assessed by the NCIC Expanded Common Toxicity Criteria. Dose limiting toxicity (DLT) was determined by week 3 of cycle 1, as defined by grade 3 nonhematological toxicity (with the exception of alopecia or nausea/vomiting) or hematological grade 4 toxicity with a possible, probable or likely casual relationship to administration of R115777. Dosing continued until there was evidence of tumor progression or DLT leading to permanent discontinuation. The initial dose for this study was 60 mg/m^2 for 12 hours. The drug was supplied in 50 mg and 100 mg capsules; therefore the patient's dose was averaged to the closest 50 mg. In a previous pilot study, five patients received doses ranging from 100 to 300 mg/m^2 and no toxicity was noted. An accelerated dose-escalation scheme was then used whereby the dose of R115777 was increased by increments of approximately 50 % in successive patients treated at 21 day intervals because no dose-limiting toxicity was encountered in any of the preceding patients. The first patient received 240 mg, and doses for subsequent patients were selected from the set 360, 510, 750 mg/m^2. The dose of R115777 at which the first DLT occurred during cycle 1 of the treatment was denoted by Dl. Once a DLT occurred in any treated patient, all subsequent patients were assigned a dose based on the EWOC algorithm using Dl as the dose upon which subsequent dose levels were derived. Figure 8.1 shows the posterior distributions of the MTD as the trial progressed.

The prior probability density function of (ρ_0, γ) was taken as

$$h(\rho_0, \gamma) = \begin{cases} \dfrac{1}{180} & \text{if } (\rho_0, \gamma) \in [0, 0.333] \times [60, 600]; \\ h(\rho_0, \gamma) = 0 & \text{otherwise.} \end{cases}$$

Thus, ρ_0 and γ are independent *a priori*, uniformly distributed over their corresponding interval. The EWOC scheme assumed (a) that the dose of R115777 below which the DLT was first observed is the safe starting dose, (b) that the maximum dose achieved will not exceed four times the value of D1, (c) that $\theta = 0.333$ and (d) that $\alpha = 0.3$. This modification of the EWOC scheme allowed rapid dose-escalation at nontoxic doses of the drug, which resulted in a more efficient yet safe determination of the MTD.

Figure 8.2 shows the posterior density of the MTD after 10 patients have been treated. The posterior mode is 372 which corresponds to the 40th percentile of the distribution. However, by design, since $\alpha = 0.3$, patient 11 was given the dose 340.

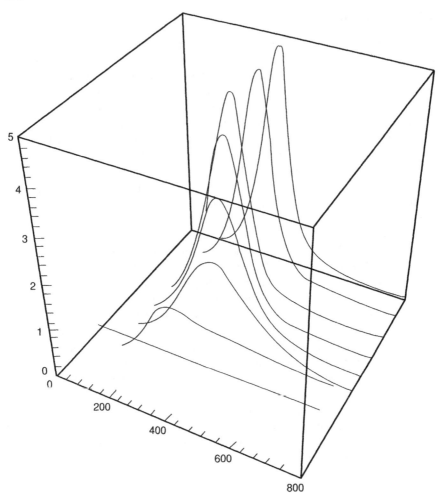

Figure 8.1   Posterior density of the MTD when the number of treated patients (from bottom to top) is 1, 5, 10, 15, 20, 25, 30 and 33.

8.3   Adjusting for covariates

8.3.1   Model

In the previous section, the MTD was assumed to be the same for every member of the patient population; no allowance is made for individual patient differences in susceptibility to treatment. Recent developments in our understanding of the genetics of drug-metabolizing enzymes and the importance of individual patient differences in pharmacokinetic and relevant clinical parameters is leading to the development of

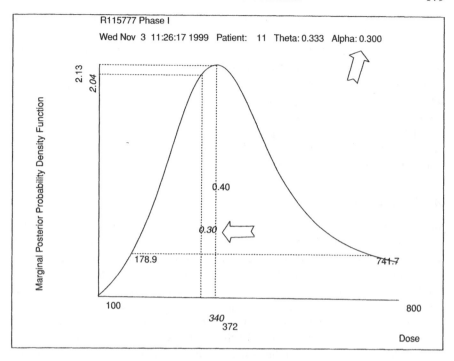

Figure 8.2   Posterior density of the MTD after 10 patients have been treated.

new treatment paradigms (see, for example, Decoster, Stein and Holdener [19] and Ratain *et al.* [20].

In cancer clinical trials, the target patient population can often be partitioned according to some categorical assessment of susceptibility to treatment. A phase I investigation can then be conducted to determine the appropriate dose for each patient subpopulation. As an example, the NCI currently accounts for the contribution of prior therapy by establishing separate MTDs for heavily pretreated and minimally pretreated patients. In such contexts, independent phase I trials can be designed for each patient group according to the methods outlined above. Alternatively, a single trial might be conducted with relevant patient information directly incorporated into the trial design. Thus, the dose-toxicity relationship is modeled as a function of patient attributes represented by the vector c of covariate measurements. For simplicity of presentation, we consider the case where a single covariate observation c_i is obtained for the ith patient and the relationship between dose and response is characterized as

$$P(Y = 1|\text{dose} = x, \text{covariate} = c) = \frac{\exp(\beta_0 + \beta_1 x + \beta_2 c)}{1 + \exp(\beta_0 + \beta_1 x + \beta_2 c)}. \tag{8.3}$$

Assuming that the covariate assessment is made before the initial course of treatment, the dose recommended for phase II testing can be tailored to individual patient needs.

Specifically, the MTD for patients with covariate c is defined as the dose $\gamma(c)$ such that $P(Y = 1|\text{dose} = \gamma(c), \text{covariate} = c) = \theta$. In other words, $\gamma(c)$ is the dose that is expected to induce DLT in a proportion θ of patients with pretreatment covariate observation c. Since estimation of the MTD is the primary aim of cancer phase I clinical trials and in order to accommodate prior information about the toxicity of the agent for selected groups of patients (if available), it is convenient to reparameterize model (8.3) in terms of $\gamma(c_0)$, $\rho_{x_1}(c_1)$ and $\rho_{x_2}(c_2)$, where $\gamma(c_0)$ is the maximum tolerated dose associated with a patient with covariate value c_0, and $\rho_{x_1}(c_1)$, $\rho_{x_2}(c_2)$ are the probabilities of DLT associated with patients with covariate values c_1 and c_2 when treated with dose levels x_1 and x_2 respectively.

8.3.2   Example

In this example, we describe the use of EWOC using the above reparameterization in a phase I study of PNU-214565 (PNU) involving patients with advanced adenocarcinomas of gastrointestinal origin. Preclinical studies demonstrated that the action of PNU is moderated by the neutralizing capacity of anti-SEA antibodies. Based on this, the MTD was defined as a function of, and dose levels were adjusted according to, each patient's plasma concentration of anti-SEA antibodies. Specifically, the MTD for patients with pretreatment anti-SEA concentration c was defined as the dose $\gamma(c)$ that results in a probability equal to $\theta = 0.1$ that a DLT will be manifest within 28 days. The small value chosen for θ reflects the severity of treatment-attributable toxicities (e.g. myelosuppression) observed in previous studies.

We assume that $\beta_1 > 0$ and $\beta_2 < 0$ in model (8.3) so that the probability of DLT is (a) an increasing function of dose for fixed anti-SEA and (b) a decreasing function of anti-SEA for fixed dose since anti-SEA has a neutralizing effect on PNU. A previous clinical trial showed that patients could be safely treated at 0.5 ng/kg dose of PNU irrespective of their anti-SEA concentration. Furthermore, it was observed that patients with anti-SEA concentration equal to c (pmol/ml) could receive PNU doses up to the minimum of 3.5 and $c/30$ ng/kg without the induction of significant toxicity. Consequently, dose levels for patients with pretreatment anti-SEA concentration c will be selected above

$$X_{\min}(c) = 0.5I_{(0,15]}(c) + (c/30)I_{[15,105]}(c) + 3.5I_{[105,\infty)}(c).$$

Owing to the nature of the agent and as a precaution, it was also decided that no patient with anti-SEA titer greater than 5 pmol/ml should be administered a dose level greater than his(her) pretreatment anti-SEA concentration. Since the FDA mandated that no patient in the trial be treated at a dose in excess of 1000 ng/kg, each patient received a dose below

$$X_{\max}(c) = 0.5I_{(0,5]}(c) + cI_{[5,1000]}(c) + 1000I_{[1000,\infty)}(c).$$

Model (8.3) is re-expressed in terms of $\gamma_{\max} = \rho(c_2)$, $\gamma_1 = \rho0.5(c_1)$ and $\rho = \rho0.5(c_2)$ for values $c_1 = 0.01$ and $c_2 = 1800$ selected to span the range of anti-SEA concentrations expected in the trial. Since the probability of DLT at a given dose is a decreasing function of anti-SEA concentration, we have $\rho_2 < \rho_1$. Furthermore, since the MTD was assumed to be greater than 0.5 ng/kg for all values of anti-SEA concentrations, we have $\rho_1 < \theta$. The prior distribution of $(\gamma_{max}, \rho_1, \rho_2)$ was then specified by assuming that γ_{max} and (ρ_1, ρ_2) are independent *a priori*, with (ρ_1, ρ_2) uniformly distributed on $\Gamma = \{(x, y) : 0 \leq y \leq x \leq \theta\}$ and $\ln(\gamma_{max})$ uniformly distributed on the interval $[\ln(3.5), \ln(1000)]$.

The PNU trial was designed according to the scheme described in Section 8.2. Accordingly, each patient was administered the dose level corresponding to the frac-tile of the marginal posterior cumulative distribution function (CDF) of the MTD. Specifically, after $k - 1$ patients had been observed, the dose for the next patient accrued to the trial became the marginal posterior CDF of the MTD given the data from the previous $k - 1$ patients. Prior to the onset of this trial, 76 patients with a known pretreatment anti-SEA concentration were treated with PNU. These data were used during the phase I trial in order to maximize statistical efficiency (see Babb and Rogatko [15] for more details).

A total of 56 patients were treated in the phase I trial of which three (5.4 %) experienced DLT. The data from patients with anti-SEA concentrations less than 100 pmol/ml, treated either during or prior to the phase I trial, are depicted in Figure 8.3. Patients were observed to tolerate doses of PNU as high as 44 % of

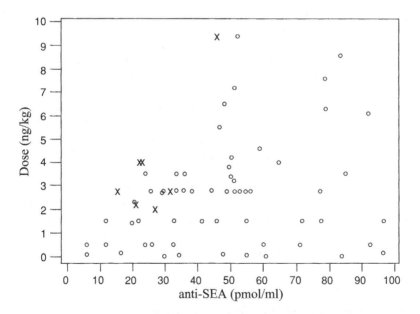

Figure 8.3 The dose level and anti-SEA of each phase I patient with anti-SEA con-centration less than 100 pmol/ml. Patients experiencing treatment-attributable dose-limiting toxicity (DLT) are indicated by a cross, those without DLT by an open circle.

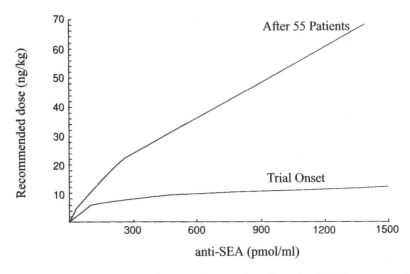

Figure 8.4   The recommended dose of PNU as a function of anti-SEA concentration at both the onset and the conclusion of the phase I trial.

their anti-SEA concentration without significant toxicity. None of the 96 patients treated at a dose less than 7 % of their anti-SEA concentration exhibited DLT. Of the 63 patients treated with a dose greater than their anti-SEA/30 (the lowest permissible dose during the phase I trial) seven patients (11.1 %) manifest DLT, a rate of toxicity not far above the targeted proportion.

Figure 8.4 shows the recommended dose level as a function of anti-SEA at both the start and the conclusion of the trial. The latter (uppermost) curve corresponds to the dose levels recommended for phase II evaluation. At trial onset the recommended dose curve was nearly horizontal beyond an anti-SEA concentration of 100 pmol/ml. In other words, nearly the same dose was recommended for all patients with sufficiently high anti-SEA concentration. Essentially, this was a reflection of the fact that data from only 36 patients with anti-SEA concentrations greater than 100 were available at the start of the trial. Since all of these patients received a dose less than 2.6 % of their anti-SEA concentration (no dose exceeded 4 ng/kg) and none experienced DLT, little was initially known about the effect of high anti-SEA concentrations on treatment response. The amount of information gained during the trial is demonstrated in Figure 8.5, which shows the change in the marginal posterior distribution of the MTD for patients with anti-SEA concentration equal to 5, from the start to the end of the phase I trial.

8.4   Choice of prior distributions

In this section, we address the issue of the choice of prior distributions. Specifically, we extend the class of restrictive priors used in Sections 8.2 and 8.3 by relaxing some

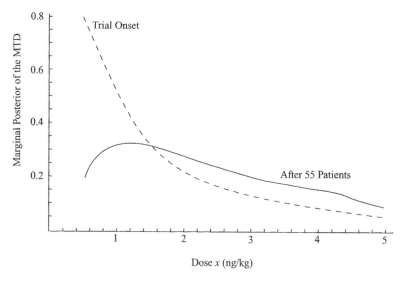

Figure 8.5 The marginal posterior distribution of the MTD for patients with anti-SEA concentration equal to 5 pmol/ml, at both the onset and the conclusion of the phase I trial.

of the constraints placed on (ρ_0, γ). We show through simulations that a candidate joint prior distribution for (ρ_0, γ) with negative *a priori* correlation between these two components results in a safer trial than the one that assumes independent priors for these two parameters while keeping the efficiency of the estimate of the MTD essentially unchanged.

8.4.1 Independent priors

In Sections 8.2 and 8.3, we assumed that the support of the MTD was contained in $[X_{\min}, X_{\max}]$; i.e. it was assumed that dose levels $X_{\min}$ and $X_{\max}$ could be identified *a priori* such that $\gamma \in [X_{\min}, X_{\max}]$ with prior (and hence posterior) probability 1. Although simulation studies showed that the logistic-based model (8.2) works well in practice, the assumption that the support of γ is bounded from above is too restrictive. In the absence of toxicity, this assumption causes the dose-escalation rate to slow down and, in general, the target MTD will never be achieved if it lies outside the support of γ. Furthermore, since the support of the probability of DLT at the initial dose ρ_0 is $[0, \theta]$ and γ is a function of θ, the assumption of prior independence between ρ_0 and γ may not be realistic. Intuitively, the closer ρ_0 is to θ, the closer the MTD is to $X_{\min}$. We also note that when independent priors are specified for (β_0, β_1) as in Tsutakawa [7] and Racine *et al.* [9], then a negative correlation between ρ_0 and γ will result in the induced prior for these two parameters. Such observations are useful if a researcher plans to compare the EWOC methodology we described with the designs used by Tsutakawa [7] and Racine *et al.* [9]. In the next section, we examine a class of prior distributions for (ρ_0, γ) defined on $[0, \theta] \times [X_{\min}, \infty)$ and study their properties through simulations.

8.4.2   Correlated priors

For simplicity of notation, ρ_0, γ and v will denote both random variables and arguments of the corresponding densities. Let ρ_0 be a random variable defined on $(0, \theta)$ and $v \sim N(b, \sigma_1^2)$ truncated to the interval (b, ∞). Given ρ_0 and v, let $\gamma \sim N(\mu(\rho_0, v), \sigma_2^2)$ truncated to the interval (a, v) with $a < \mu(\rho_0, v) < v$ and $a < b$. Denote by $g_{\mu(.)}(\gamma)$ the marginal distribution of γ. This density depends on the functional form of $\mu(\rho_0, v)$ specified below.

Model M_1

ρ_0 and γ are independent with $\rho_0 \sim U(0, \theta)$ and $\gamma \sim U(a, b)$. This is the prior used in the 5F-U trial.

Model M_2

ρ_0 and γ are independent with $\rho_0 \sim U(0, \theta)$ and γ has density $g_{\mu(.)}(\gamma)$ with $\mu(\rho_0, v) = (a + v)/2$. This prior allows the support of the MTD to extend beyond b (which corresponds to the maximum allowable dose in the 5-FU trial) and keeps a vague prior for ρ_0 on $(0, \theta)$.

Model M_3

ρ_0 and γ are independent with $\rho_0/\theta \sim \text{beta}(\alpha_1, \alpha_2)$ and γ has density $g_{\mu(.)}(\gamma)$ with $\mu(\rho_0, v) = (a + v)/2$. Again, the support of the MTD is extended to $[a, \infty)$ but the prior distribution for ρ_0 puts more mass near 0 for suitable choices of the hyperparameters α_1 and α_2 as in Gatsonis and Greenhouse [2].

Model M_4

$\rho_0 \sim U(0, \theta)$ and γ has density $g_{\mu(.)}(\gamma)$ with $\mu(\rho_0, v) = (\rho_0/\theta)a + (1 - \rho_0/\theta)v$. Here, we introduced an *a priori* correlation structure between the MTD, γ and ρ_0 by forcing the distribution of the MTD to concentrate towards its upper tail whenever the probability of DLT at the initial dose is close to 0.

Model M_5

$\rho_0/\theta \sim \text{beta}(\alpha_1, \alpha_2)$ and γ has density $g_{\mu(.)}(\gamma)$ with $\mu(\rho_0, v) = (\rho_0/\theta)a + (1 - \rho_0/\theta)v$. The prior structure is similar to that of model M_4 except that the prior distribution for ρ_0 puts more mass near 0 as in model M_3.

Since γ is the parameter of interest, ρ_0 and ν will be treated as nuisance parameters. Under M_2 and M_3, the marginal prior density of the MTD is given by

$$\frac{1}{\pi \sigma_1 \sigma_2} \int_{\max(\gamma, b)}^{\infty} C_1^{-1} \exp\left[-(2\gamma - a - \nu)^2/(8\sigma_1^2)\right] \exp\left[-(\nu - b)^2/(2\sigma_2^2)\right] d\nu, \quad (8.4)$$

where

$$C_1(\nu) = 2\Phi[(\nu - a)/(2\sigma_1)] - 1$$

and $\Phi(z)$ is the CDF of the standard normal.

The marginal prior density of the MTD under M_4 is given by

$$\frac{1}{\pi \theta \sigma_1 \sigma_2} \int_{\max(\gamma, b)}^{\infty} \exp\left[-(\nu - b)^2/(2\sigma_2^2)\right]$$

$$\times \int_0^{\theta} C_2^{-1}(\nu, \rho_0) \exp\left\{ -[\gamma - \mu(\rho_0, \nu)]^2/(2\sigma_1^2)\right\} \partial\rho_0 \, \partial\nu, \quad (8.5)$$

where

$$C_2(\nu, \rho_0) = 2\Phi\{[\nu - \mu(\rho_0, \nu)]/\sigma_1\} - 1$$

and

$$\mu(\rho_0, \nu) = \frac{\rho_0}{\theta} a + \left(1 - \frac{\rho_0}{\theta}\right)\nu.$$

A similar expression for this prior is obtained under model M_5 by replacing $1/\theta$ by the density of $\theta \times \beta(\alpha_1, \alpha_2)$. These priors are clearly intractable and Markov Chain Monte Carlo (MCMC) methods will be used to extract features of the marginal posterior distribution of the MTD.

The marginal density of g under models M_2, M_3 and M_4 contains four hyperparameters a, b, σ_1 and σ_2. Under model M_5, two extra hyperparameters α_1 and α_2 are inherited from the prior of ρ_0. The parameter is usually set to be the dose administered to the first patient. Parameter b can be selected by the clinicians on the basis of previous trials and prior information about the agent as in the 5-FU trial. Parameters σ_1 and σ_2 control the spread of the marginal distribution of g. As $\sigma_1 \to 0$ and $\sigma_2 \to \infty$, these models become essentially the same as model M_1. After experimenting with several choices of these parameters, we recommend the following strategy for choosing them. Fix σ_2 according to the desired level of flatness of the density of g in (a, b); typically, values of σ_2 greater than or equal to $b - a$ tend to flatten this density. Next, we ask the clinicians to provide their best guess of the prior probability that the MTD exceeds b. These are then solved using either equations (8.4) or (8.5).

The Bayesian statistical software WinBUGS [21] can be used to fit the above five models and the codes can be found in Tighiouart, Rogatko and Babb [22].

8.4.3 Simulations

We compared the performance of models M_2 with M_3 and M_4 with M_5 by simulating a large number of trials from each model. An MCMC sampler based on the Metropolis–Hastings algorithm [23,24] was devised to estimate features of the marginal posterior distribution of γ. For each of the above four models, we simulated 5000 trials, each consisting of $n = 30$ patients. Comparisons of these models were based on the proportion of patients that were assigned dose levels higher than the MTD, the proportion of patients exhibiting DLT, the average bias and the estimated mean square error (MSE). We found that, on the average, fewer patients were overdosed under M_4 compared to M_2 whereas the proportions of patients exhibiting dose-limiting toxicity were about the same under these two models. The efficiency of the estimated MTD as measured by the root mean square error was about the same on the average. Based on the above remarks, we recommend the use of model M_4 with our proposed *a priori* correlation structure between ρ_0 and γ; while the efficiency of the estimated MTD is about the same under the two models, fewer patients are overdosed under model M_4. Under models M_3 and M_5, the prior distribution of the probability of dose-limiting toxicity at the initial dose is more concentrated towards 0. Since ρ_0 and γ are negatively correlated *a priori* under model M_5, this resulted in more patients being overdosed and exhibiting DLT under this model compared to model M_3. In other words, model M_5 uses a more aggressive scheme in search of the MTD. On the other hand, model M_5 performs much better in terms of the efficiency of the estimated MTD. Details on the above simulations can be found in Tighiouart, Rogatko and Babb [22].

8.5 Concluding remarks

We described a dose-escalation scheme (EWOC) for cancer phase I clinical trials that addresses the ethical demands that underlie cancer phase I trials by selecting doses while controlling for the probability of overdosing patients. Simulation results presented in Babb, Rogatko and Zacks [11] showed that (a) relative to CRM, EWOC overdosed a smaller proportion of patients, exhibited fewer dose-limiting toxicities and estimated the MTD with slightly lower average bias and marginally higher mean squared error and (b) relative to the nonparametric dose-escalation schemes, EWOC treated fewer patients at dose levels that were either subtherapeutic or severely toxic, treated a higher proportion of patients at doses near the MTD and estimated the MTD with lower average bias and mean squared error.

We also showed through a phase I clinical trial how EWOC permits the utilization of information concerning individual patient differences in susceptibility to treatment. This extension to a continuous covariate utilization made it the first method described to design cancer clinical trials that not only guides dose-escalation but also permits personalization of the dose level for each specific patient. *A priori* information and uncertainty about the agent under consideration can easily be implemented into the methodology and the corresponding computations of dose allocations can be easily carried out using WinBUGS. We are currently working on extensions of this methodology to accommodate more than one continuous covariates utilization of categorical covariates and ordered groups with respect to their susceptibility to treatment.

References

1. P.V. Wooley and P.S. Schein (1979) Clinical pharmacology and phase I trial design, in *Methods of Cancer Research* (eds V. de Vita and H. Busch), Academic Press, New York, pp. 177–98.
2. C. Gatsonis and J.B. Greenhouse (1992) Bayesian methods for phase I clinical trials. *Statistics in Medicine*, **11**(10), 1377–89.
3. B.E. Storer (1989) Design and analysis of phase I clinical trial. *Biometrics*, **45**(3), 925–37.
4. S.D. Durham and N. Flournoy (1994) Random walks for quantile estimation, in *Statistical Design Theory and Related Topics V* (eds S.S. Gupta and J.O. Berger), Springer, New York, pp. 467–76.
5. M. Gasparini and J. Eisele (2000) A curve-free method for phase I clinical trials. *Biometrics*, **56**(2), 609–15.
6. R.K. Tsutakawa (1972) Design of experiment for bioassay. *J. Am. Statistical Assoc.*, **67**, 584–90, 2183–96.
7. R.K. Tsutakawa (1980) Selection of dose levels for estimating a percentage point on a logistic quantal response curve. *Appl. Statistics*, **29**, 25–33.
8. A.P. Grieve (1987) A Bayesian approach to the analysis of LD50 experiments. Technical report 8708, CIBA-GEIGY AG.
9. A. Racine, A.P. Grieve, H. Fluehler and A.F.M. Smith (1986) Bayesian methods in practice: experiences in the pharmaceutical industry. *Appl. Statistics*, **35**, 93–150.
10. J. O'Quigley, M. Pepe and L. Fisher (1990) Continual reassessment method: a practical design for phase I clinical trials in cancer, *Biometrics*, **46**(1), 33–48.
11. J. Babb, A. Rogatko and S. Zacks (1998) Cancer phase I clinical trials: efficient dose escalation with overdose control. *Statistics in Medicine*, **17**(10), 1103–20.
12. J. Whitehead and H. Brunier (1995) Bayesian decision procedures for dose determining experiments. *Statistics in Medicine*, **14**(9), 885–93.
13. L.M. Haines, I. Perevozskaya and W.F. Rosenberger (2003) Bayesian optimal designs for phase I clinical trials. *Biometrics*, **59**(3), 591–600.
14. W.F. Rosenberger and L.M. Haines (2002) Competing designs for phase I clinical trials: a review. *Statistics in Medicine*, **21**(18), 2757–70.
15. J. Babb and A. Rogatko (2001) Patient specific dosing in a cancer phase I clinical trial. *Statistics in Medicine*, **20**(14), 2079–90.
16. J. Cheng, J.S. Babb, C. Langer, S. Aamdal, F. Robert, L.R. Engelhardt, O. Fernberg, J. Schiller, G. Forsberg, R.K. Alpaugh, L.M. Weiner and A. Rogatko (2004) Individualized patient dosing in phase I clinical trials: the role of escalation with overdose control in PNU-214936. *J. Clin. Oncology*, **22**(4), 602–9.
17. B.H. Eichhorn and S. Zacks (1973) Sequential search of an optimal dosage, I. *J. Am. Statistical Assoc.*, **68**, 594–8.
18. A. Rogatko, M., Tighiouart and X. Zhiheng (2005) *EWOC 2.0 application software.* Winship Cancer Institute, Emory University. Atlanta, Georgia. http://sisyphus.emory.edu/ewoc.html.

19. G. Decoster, G. Stein and E.E. Holdener (1989) Responses and toxic deaths in phase I clinical trials, in Sixth NCI-EORTC Symposium on *New Drugs in Cancer Therapy*, Amsterdam, 1989, pp. 175–81.
20. M.J. Ratain, R. Mick, R.L. Schilsky and M. Siegler (1993) Statistical and ethical issues in the design and conduct of phase I and II clinical trials of new anticancer agents. *J. Natl Cancer Inst.*, **85**(20), 1637–43.
21. D.J. Spiegelhalter, A. Thomas and N.G. Best (1999) *WinBUGS Version 1.2 User Manual*, MRC Biostatistics Unit.
22. M. Tighiouart, A. Rogatko and J.S. Babb (2005) Flexible Bayesian methods for cancer phase I clinical trials: dose escalation with overdose control. *Statistics in Medicine*, **24**, 2183–2196.
23. N. Metropolis, A.W. Rosenbluth, M.N. Rosenbluth, A.H. Teller and E. Teller (1953) Equation of state calculations by fast computing machines. *J. Chem. Physics*, **21**, 1087–92.
24. W.K. Hastings (1970) Monte Carlo sampling methods using Markov chains and their applications. *Biometrika*, **57**, 97–109.

9

Dose-escalation methods for phase I healthy volunteer studies

Y. Zhou
Medical and Pharmaceutical Statistics Research Unit,
The University of Reading, Reading, UK

9.1 Introduction

After laboratory and animal data have been obtained from preclinical studies, any new therapeutic compound has to be experimented on human subjects for the first time. Apart from those concerning cytotoxic drugs for cancer patients, the majority of first-into-man studies is done on healthy volunteers in order to establish safety and to explore the absorption, distribution, metabolism and elimination of the drug. These volunteers are carefully examined, monitored and treated throughout their participation in the study. Many outcomes are measured. Here, we focus on a single pharmacokinetic variable derived from the curve relating the concentration of the drug in plasma to the time since administration [1]. Commonly used summaries such as the area under the curve (AUC) and the maximum concentration (C_{max}) are often modelled by the normal distribution, after a logarithmic transformation [2]. It is desirable to avoid excessive drug concentrations, as reflected by large values of AUC or C_{max}, although knowledge of suitable upper limits is often vague. Figure 9.1 shows a typical concentration–time curve for a single dose.

Statistical Methods for Dose-Finding Experiments   Edited by S. Chevret
© 2006 John Wiley & Sons, Ltd

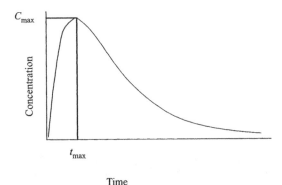

Figure 9.1   A typical concentration–time curve.

Primary objectives of dose-escalation studies are usually to evaluate the safety and tolerability of the new compound. A 'maximum safe dose' is to be identified. Secondary objectives can be to evaluate the relationship between pharmacokinetic responses and dose. A series of ascending dosing levels are identified in advance, with the lowest apparently very safe as far as extrapolation from animal data can determine. A group of subjects (known as a cohort) is treated concurrently, and each member may receive just one dose, or else a dose in each of a series of consecutive treatment periods. A placebo might be administered so that any adverse effects following administration of the active drug can be put into context, and to introduce an element of blindness. Data from each cohort, or from each period within a cohort, are collected and assessed prior to choosing the next set of doses for administration. This is a statistical sequential procedure: we collect data, perform analyses and then draw conclusions to make decisions about whether to continue the study, and if so which doses to administer next. However, in many cases the nature of this statistical procedure is not formalized: no equations are used and no probabilistic models are fitted. Instead, 'clinical judgement' is used to make sense of what has been observed and to determine what will happen next. Regardless of how it is described, this process of 'data in–decision out' should be subjected to evaluation and assessment according to statistical criteria.

A design commonly used for first-into-man healthy volunteer studies is described by Patterson *et al.* [3]. This is a placebo-controlled, dose-rising, four-period crossover study of two to six cohorts of four healthy volunteers. In the first cohort, each volunteer receives three active doses in an ascending order and a placebo dose, inserted in a random position in the sequence, as illustrated in Table 9.1. The doses are denoted by $d_1, d_2, \ldots, d_k$, where $d_1 < d_2 < \cdots < d_k$. Administration of the doses is separated by a washout period.

The pharmacokinetic data for each volunteer are expressed in terms of the concentrations of active drug substance in the plasma against time after administration. The study may be terminated or the dosing regimen altered if volunteers exceed some predefined exposure level or if an unacceptable adverse event profile is seen. The

Table 9.1 The dosing schedule for the first cohort in a conventional dose-escalation study.

Period	Subject 1	Subject 2	Subject 3	Subject 4
1	d_1	d_1	d_1	Placebo
2	d_2	d_2	Placebo	d_1
3	d_3	Placebo	d_2	d_2
4	Placebo	d_3	d_3	d_3

maximum exposure level is defined prior to the start of the study based on the toxicity profile for the compound observed in the most sensitive animal species.

If it is deemed safe to continue with the dose-escalation, then the next cohort of volunteers will receive three active doses (d_3, d_4, d_5) with the placebo arranged in a similar pattern to the first cohort. The lowest dose used in the second cohort is the highest dose used in the previous one. This procedure continues until all planned doses have been administered, or the study is terminated due to an unacceptable adverse event profile or to values of AUC or C_{max} in excess of the set limits. The starting and top doses in first-into-man studies are usually fixed based on preclinical and toxicology data for that drug [4].

These studies can take a long time to complete. Each cohort usually takes a month to complete the dosing schedule, and there may be up to six cohorts of volunteers. Furthermore, information is not always gathered at the most appropriate doses. Often, the majority of the information is gathered at very low doses, with few volunteers receiving the higher doses likely to be used when developing the drug further. There are no formal guidelines for determining dose-escalation, which proceeds by informal evaluation of the data observed so far. The results are generally summarized descriptively and graphically and are not analysed formally.

9.2 Frequentist analysis

Although formal analysis of dose-escalation data is not usually performed, straightforward and appropriate methods exist. To illustrate these, a recent dose-escalation study conducted by GlaxoSmithKline (GSK) involving 25 healthy volunteers will be considered. The principal pharmacokinetic measure was C_{max}, the maximum recorded concentration in plasma and the dataset is presented in Table 9.2. When a subject has a nonquantifiable C_{max} corresponding to low doses, the response is treated as missing and is ignored in the analysis. Seven doses were used according to the schedule: 2.5, 5, 10, 25, 50, 100, 150 µg. An appropriate safety cut-off for this response was 200 mcg/ml.

We use a power model to fit the data: $C_{max} = e^{\theta_1}(\text{dose})^{\theta_2}$. Here $\theta' = (\theta_1, \theta_2)$ is a vector representing two unknown parameters. Consider the natural logarithm of C_{max}, which will be denoted by y. Taking logarithms on both sides of the power model,

Table 9.2   Real data from the C_{max} trial.

	Period							
	1		2		3		4	
Subject	Dose	C_{max}	Dose	C_{max}	Dose	C_{max}	Dose	C_{max}
1	2.5	.	5	.	10	11.0		
2	2.5	.	5	14.5			10	20.4
3	2.5	.			5	10.0	10	19.7
4	10	24.1			25	33.3	50	74.6
5			2.5	.	5	10.2	10	29.7
6			2.5	10.4	5	20.6		
7	2.5	.	5	13.5	10	28.5		
8	2.5	.	5	.			10	14.6
9	2.5	.			5	.	10	27.0
10			10	14.6	25	19.4	50	47.7
11	10	29.0	25	34.1	50	71.6		
12	10	.			25	37.1	50	59.2
13	10	15.0	25	34.9			50	76.1
14	10	21.8	25	70.6			50	166.6
15	10	23.0	25	40.7	50	73.4		
16			10	16.6	25	53.0	50	87.1
17			2.5	.	5	14.4	10	17.8
18	50	54.7	100	125.6				
19			50	79.4	100	108.1		
20	50	161.5						
21	50	101.4	100	131.3				
22	50	194.1	100	232.5				
23	50	61.6			100	104.5		
24	50	81.7	100	84.2	150	217.6		
25			50	113.8	100	178.9		

we obtain the following equation: $y = \log(C_{max}) = \theta_1 + \theta_2 \log(\text{dose})$. The power model is familiar to pharmacologists, while its log transformation yields a regression equation more familiar to statisticians. So far the model described is deterministic. To model variability, a random error term ε, is introduced. Thus, denoting by l_{ij} the logarithm of the jth active dose received by the ith subject, the response y_{ij} for the jth observation on the ith subject is

$$y_{ij} = \theta_1 + \theta_2 l_{ij} + \varepsilon_{ij}.$$

Placebo administrations are ignored in this analysis, as there will be no drug detected in plasma.

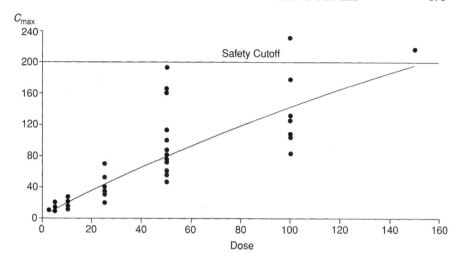

Figure 9.2 Dose-response relationship. Data are from Table 9.2. The model is $C_{\max} = e^{\theta_1}(\text{dose})^{\theta_2}$.

The model is not yet complete. Since each volunteer reacts to the drug differently, a subject effect should be added in the above model, with a common value for all observations on the same subject:

$$y_{ij} = \theta_1 + \theta_2 l_{ij} + s_i + \varepsilon_{ij}. \qquad (9.1)$$

The term s_i is a random effect relating to the ith subject. The s_i and ε_{ij} are modelled as mutually independent, normally distributed random variables with mean zero, and variances τ^2 and σ^2 respectively. The correlation, ρ, between two responses on the same subject can be shown to be equal to $\tau^2/(\sigma^2 + \tau^2)$. The linear mixed model (9.1) is described in reference [5].

Figures 9.2 and 9.3 show dose-response data of Table 9.2 on a direct scale and on a log scale respectively. Figure 9.2 also shows the fitted power curve and Figure 9.3 the fitted regression line. The bulk of the information is gathered at lower doses.

In this chapter, the maximum safe dose, d_f^*, for a new untested subject is defined as a dose at which the probability of $C_{\max}$ exceeding some safety cut-off, denoted by L, is equal to some small value, π_0. For the illustration, L will be taken to have the value 200 and π_0 to be 0.05. Thus, if Y_f denotes the $\log(C_{\max})$ of a new untested subject, then d_f^* can be calculated from the equation: $P(Y_f > \log(200)|d_f^*) = 0.05$. To find the value of d_f^*, the distribution $Y_f \sim N(\theta_1 + \theta_2 \log(d_f^*), \sigma^2 + \tau^2)$ is used.

Model (9.1) is an approximate representation of the dose-response relationship. Our approach is to fit a model that claims validity only for doses between d_1 and d_k (2.5 and 150 mcg in the example) and to avoid extrapolation. If the nonobservable $C_{\max}$ values in Table 9.2 are replaced by fixed values, then these imputed values prove to be very influential and lead to very small estimates of the between-subject variance

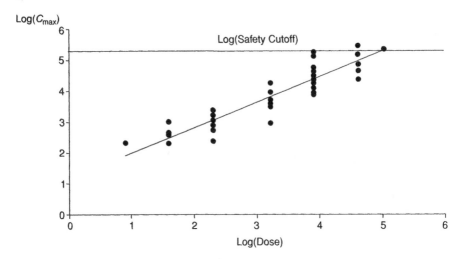

Figure 9.3   Dose-response relationship on a log scale. Data are from Table 9.2. The model is $\log(C_{\max}) = \theta_1 + \theta_2 \log(\text{dose})$.

τ^2. Multiple imputation methods may provide an alternative form of analysis, but we have not investigated such an approach. Instead, the nonobservable values have been ignored.

From a SAS PROC MIXED [6] analysis, maximum likelihood estimates of the parameters in equation (9.1) are $\widehat{\theta}_1 = 1.167, \widehat{\theta}_2 = 0.822, \widehat{\sigma}^2 = 0.053$ and $\widehat{\tau}^2 = 0.073$, from which it follows that $\widehat{\rho} = 0.579$. According to this fitted model, for dose 10 µg and dose 100 µg, the expected values for $C_{\max}$ are 21.3 µg/ml and 141.5 µg/ml respectively. For a typical subject with zero subject effect, i.e. $s_i = 0$, there is a 95 % chance that $C_{\max}$ lies within (13.6, 33.5) at dose 10 µg and within (90.1, 222.1) at dose 100 µg. However, the subject effect itself is random, with a 95 % chance of lying within ($-0.530, 0.530$). Thus, for a new untested subject, the total variance of $\log(C_{\max})$ is $\sigma^2 + \tau^2$ and there is a 95 % chance that $C_{\max}$ lies within the wider interval (10.6, 42.8) at dose 10 µg and between (70.5, 283.7) at dose 100 µg. For a new untested subject, the maximum safe dose, d_f^*, is estimated as 65.3 µg (by maximum likelihood).

9.3   A Bayesian analysis

Bayesian decision theory supplies a general framework for making decisions under uncertainty which can be applied in many scientific and business fields [7–9]. In this chapter, a Bayesian decision procedure for dose-escalation is developed, but in order to use the approach, a model for the data to be observed must first be specified and prior opinion concerning unknown parameters of the model must be expressed. Bayesian decision–theoretic methods for dose-escalation studies on healthy volunteers have been described by Patterson et al. [3] and Whitehead et al. [10], and in this section the Bayesian model underlying them will be described. The Bayesian analysis of the complete dataset provides an alternative interpretation to the frequentist analysis described in Section 9.2, as well as playing a vital role in the decision–theoretic approach to the collection of the data.

Bayes' theorem involves conditional probabilities. Suppose θ is some quantity that is currently unknown. Some information or expert opinion will be available about the unknown parameter θ before the dose-escalation study begins. This information can be formulated as a probability density function for θ, denoted by $h_0(\theta)$ and known as the 'prior density'. Let x denote the data collected in the dose-escalation study, and $f(x|\theta)$ be its likelihood function of the data. Then, the posterior density function of the unknown parameter θ, $h(\theta|x)$, can be derived using Bayes' theorem:

$$h(\theta|x) = \frac{h_0(\theta)f(x|\theta)}{\int h_0(\varphi)f(x|\varphi)\partial\varphi}.$$

This posterior represents the opinion about θ formed by combining the prior opinion with the data. See reference [11] for introductory descriptions of the Bayesian approach.

Equation (9.1) in Section 9.2, $y_{ij} = \theta_1 + \theta_2 l_{ij} + s_i + \varepsilon_{ij}$, will be adopted as the model. Parameters θ and v will be treated as random, where θ is the vector $\theta' = (\theta_1, \theta_2)$ and v is the within-subject precision, $v = \sigma^{-2}$. In order to avoid complications, the correlation ρ will be treated as fixed and known. In Bayesian terms, this amounts to the imposition of a point prior for ρ with zero variance. As $\rho = \tau^2/(\sigma^2 + \tau^2)$, this strategy avoids the need for a separate prior for τ^2. A normal–gamma prior distribution is used to express prior information on θ and v, as this is easy to fit and is also conjugate. We take

$$\theta|v \sim N\left(\mu_0, (v\mathbf{Q}_0)^{-1}\right)$$

and

$$v \sim Ga(\alpha_0, \beta_0), \tag{9.2}$$

where N denotes a normal distribution, Ga a gamma distribution and the values of μ_0, $\mathbf{Q}_0$, α_0 and β_0 are chosen to represent prior knowledge. The expressions in (9.2) define the prior conditional density of θ, given v, and the unconditional density of v. Their product is the joint density of θ and v.

The likelihood function of the data, $f(y|\theta, v)$, follows from the normal distribution: $Y|\theta, v \sim N\left(m, (v\mathbf{M})^{-1}\right)$, where m and $\mathbf{M}$ are functions of the unknown parameter θ. Bayes theorem gives a posterior distribution of the same form:

$$\theta|v \sim N\left(\mu, (v\mathbf{Q})^{-1}\right)$$

and

$$v \sim Ga(\alpha, \beta), \tag{9.3}$$

where α, β, μ and $\mathbf{Q}$ depend on the prior values α_0, β_0, μ_0 and $\mathbf{Q}_0$ and the data, in a way described in reference [10].

To set the prior, the responses y_{01} and y_{02} to two log dose levels l_{01} and l_{02} are predicted (such data are called 'pseudo-data'). The components μ_{01} and μ_{02} of μ_0 are taken to be the intercept and slope of the line joining these two points. The matrix Q_0 satisfies $(\nu Q_0)^{-1} = \text{Var}(\mu_0)$, and its values and those of α_0 and β_0 are generally more difficult to set: this point will be revisited in Section 9.4. An advantage of the use of pseudo-data to define prior distributions is that posterior distributions of a relatively simple form are obtained. First consider how studying data on the ith subject changes our belief about that person's subject effect s_i (conditional on θ and ν). Suppose that n_i observations have already been made on this subject.

Here we present two Bayesian analyses with two different priors. We return to the example introduced in Section 9.2. We fix the value for ρ to be 0.6. The two priors differ in their settings for μ_0. The first is a realistic, best guess of the relationship between C_{max} and the dose, predicting C_{max} to be equal to 6.8 and 197.5 at dose 2.5 μg and dose 150 μg respectively. We impose the value $\alpha_0 = 1$ and choose β_0 so that $\pi_0 = P(C_{max} > L|d_1) = 0.05$ for the first subject when receiving the lowest dose d_1. This reflects the investigators' prior opinion that it is safe to start with dose d_1. It follows that $\beta_0 = 0.268$. We can deduce that

$$Q_0 = \begin{pmatrix} 0.817 & -0.095 \\ -0.095 & 0.032 \end{pmatrix}.$$

This prior is referred as 'pseudo-data', as it is equivalent to two observations made on the pseudo subject 0. Under this prior, Bayesian prior modal estimates for the parameters of model (9.1) are $\widetilde{\theta}_1 = 1.163$, $\widetilde{\theta}_2 = 0.822$, $\widetilde{\sigma}^2 = 0.267$ and $\widetilde{\tau}^2 = 0.402$. After observing the data in Table 9.2, the Bayesian posterior modal estimates are $\widetilde{\theta}_1 = 1.166$, $\widetilde{\theta}_2 = 0.822$, $\widetilde{\sigma}^2 = 0.050$ and $\widetilde{\tau}^2 = 0.075$. The estimates of θ have changed very little, indicating that the prior opinion was very good, while the variance estimates are smaller, indicating that the linear model will be considerably more accurate and the first dose is considerably safer than first thought. In this illustration, in the absence of true opinion prior to data collection, maximum likelihood estimates of θ and ρ have been used to form the prior opinion, which is an option not available in practice as the prior must be formed before the data are collected.

The second prior is intentionally cautious, imagining a potentially hazardous drug. We predict that doses 12.5 and 25 would give high C_{max} values of 26.6 and 53.2 respectively. Again we impose the values $\alpha_0 = 1$ and $\pi_0 = 0.05$, and this time deduce that $\beta_0 = 0.076$ and

$$Q_0 = \begin{pmatrix} 2.745 & -0.903 \\ -0.903 & 0.314 \end{pmatrix}.$$

Under this prior, Bayesian prior modal estimates are $\widetilde{\theta}_1 = 0.755$, $\widetilde{\theta}_2 = 1.000$, $\widetilde{\sigma}^2 = 0.076$ and $\widetilde{\tau}^2 = 0.113$. After observing the data, the posterior modal estimates are $\widetilde{\theta}_1 = 1.163$, $\widetilde{\theta}_2 = 0.824$, $\widetilde{\sigma}^2 = 0.050$ and $\widetilde{\tau}^2 = 0.075$. Although the two priors are very different, the Bayesian posterior modal estimates are similar. In particular, the cautious choices made in the second prior have been overcome by the more encouraging data.

9.4 Conducting dose-escalation using a Bayesian decision–theoretic approach

The decision to which Bayesian theory is to be applied is the choice of which dose to administer to each subject in each successive cohort. Bayesian decision theory demands that this is done in a way that uses a predefined criterion.

At any stage of the dose-escalation procedure, the posterior predictive probability $P(y_{if} > \log L | d_f, y)$ can be computed, where y_{if} is a future response on subject i, and conditioning is on y, all the data so far observed, and d_f, the future dose administered. A safety constraint can be imposed, such that only doses d_f for which the posterior predictive probability is $\leq \pi_0$ will be administered. This can be used to find the 'maximum safe dose', d_{if}^*, for the ith subject, the dose for which the posterior predictive probability above is equal to π_0. This dose is not to be exceeded for subject i. If some responses are already available from subject i, d_{if}^* might differ from the maximum safe dose for another subject or for a new subject, being lower if subject i absorbed more drug than expected and higher if absorption was less.

In Whitehead $et\ al.$ [10], two criteria for dose-escalation are used. One administers the maximum safe dose d_{if}^* to the ith subject. This is referred to as 'maxsafe', simply treating each subject at the highest dose permitted by the safety constraint. This will have the effect of gathering information efficiently about both the maximum dose that can be safely administered and about the response to that dose. The other criterion aims for D-optimality, the optimal choice of doses is one that maximizes the determinant of the variance–covariance matrix of their joint posterior distribution based on pseudo- and real data. This determinant is a linear combination of two components: a weighted between-subject sum of squares of log doses and a within-subject sum of squares of log doses. Thus, it is desirable to have both contrasting patterns of doses between subjects and a wide spread of doses within each individual subject. If D-optimality is used without a safety constraint, then one or more subjects will typically be allocated very high doses in order to achieve the latter contrast, even at relatively early stages of a trial. This is unlikely to be acceptable in practice, where dose-escalation has usually proceeded in a gradual manner, but it can be avoided by operating the sequential D-optimal design within the confines of a safety constraint. Whitehead $et\ al.$ [12] proposed another selection criterion, i.e. to minimize $\mathrm{Var}(\eta | y^+, \nu)$, where $\eta = \theta_1 + \theta_2 \log d_f^*$ and y^+ denotes the data that will be available after the next treatment period. This will be referred to as the variance criterion. According to the normal approximation used here for the distribution of η, the required variance depends on the doses already administered and on those about to be used in the current cohort, but not on the pharmacokinetic responses of the latter.

The parameters α_0 and β_0 of the gamma prior for ν are more difficult to choose. However, values for α_0 and β_0 can be determined from considerations of the safety constraint. The prior will be set so that the prior probability $P_0(y > \log L | d_1)$ is equal to π_0 when the lowest available dose d_1 is administered, as was done in the example of Section 9.3. This will make the lowest dose, d_1, be the only dose allowed by the safety constraint for the first period of treatment of the first cohort, consistent with usual clinical practice. The values of α_0 and π_0 are fixed, and the value of β_0 can then

Table 9.3   A simulated dose-escalation study based on the maxsafe criterion and fixed $\rho = 0.6$.

		Dose/$C_{\max}$					
Cohort	Period	Subject 1	Subject 2	Subject 3	Subject 4	d_f^*	Ratio R
1	1	Placebo	2.5, 4.3	2.5, 6.6	2.5, 6.1	36.39	7.27×10^8
	2	25,54.2	Placebo	25, 44.9	25, 49.7	63.44	4.36
	3	50, 72.6	50, 70.0	Placebo	50, 94.8	74.44	3.27
	4	50, 92.0	100, 124.1	50, 127.5	Placebo	70.99	2.88
		Subject 5	Subject 6	Subject 7	Subject 8		
2	1	Placebo	50, 76.4	50, 56.0	50, 79.1	79.50	2.32
	2	50, 80.4	Placebo	100, 145.1	50, 69.8	81.82	2.13
	3	50, 83.9	50, 91.0	Placebo	100, 179.3	80.80	2.05
	4	50, 119.1	50, 107.3	100, 140.5	Placebo	76.38	1.99
		Subject 9	Subject 10	Subject 11	Subject 12		
3	1	Placebo	50, 47.9	50, 58.8	50, 32.7	79.49	1.78
	2	50, 67.0	Placebo	100, 105.0	150, 209.4	77.20	1.66
	3	50, 56.6	100, 115.4	Placebo	100, 130.9	78.18	1.62
	4	100, 119.6	100, 160.9	100, 118.6	Placebo	77.67	1.59

be deduced. The value of α_0 is chosen to represent the relative weighting of the prior information to the observed data. A single-point prior is used for ρ, fixing its value. Alternatively, ρ can be treated as unknown in the same way as all of the other model parameters, e.g. a discrete prior can be used [12], taking the value ρ_r with probability $a_{0r}, r = 1, \ldots, R$: $a_{01} + \cdots + a_{0R} = 1$.

Since the Bayesian decision procedure is sequential, stopping rules may be used to terminate a trial when enough information is gathered. Of course a maximum number of cohorts will be set, and stopping will have to occur if none of the doses satisfy the safety constraint. Additionally, an accuracy rule can be set, for example stopping when the ratio, R, of the upper 97.5 % credibility limit for the linear term, $\eta = \theta_1 + \theta_2 \log d_f^*$, to the lower 2.5 % limit becomes small enough.

For an illustrative dose-escalation, we use the second prior described in the previous section based on predictions that doses 12.5 and 25 would give $C_{\max}$ values of 26.6 and 53.2 respectively. The specification of the prior is completed by setting $\pi_0 = 0.05$, $\alpha_0 = 1$ and fixing ρ at 0.6. Data comprising $C_{\max}$ values are simulated from three cohorts of four healthy volunteers, each treated in four consecutive periods and receiving three active doses and one randomly placed placebo. The selection criterion is to give the next subject the maximum safe dose. The maximum sample size is 12 subjects.

Table 9.3 gives the complete simulated dataset with Bayesian predicted values of d_f^*. Figure 9.4 shows the doses administered to each subject and the corresponding

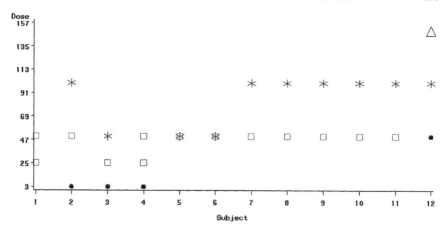

Key: ● $C_{max} \in [0, 0.2L)$; □ $C_{max} \in [0.2L, 0.5L)$; ✳ $C_{max} \in [0.5L, L)$; △ $C_{max} \in [L, \infty)$

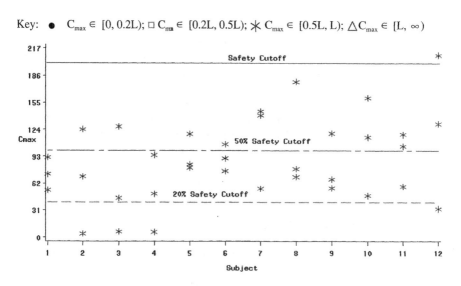

Figure 9.4 An illustration of a single simulation run (data from Table 9.3).

responses. All subjects receive the lowest dose 2.5 in the first period of the active treatment. In the second period, all subjects receive dose 25, the maximum safe dose for each of them. The dose-escalation skips two doses: 5 and 10 μg. In the last period of the first cohort, subject 2 receives dose 100 μg higher than the doses for subjects 1 and 3. This is because subject 2 absorbed less of doses 2.5 and 50. In the first period of the second cohort, all subjects receive dose 50, the predicted d_f^* for a new untested subject being 70.99 μg. Only two doses are used in the second cohort, with subjects 5 and 6 being repeatedly dosed at 50 μg, as their C_{max} values at that dose are quite high. The third cohort begins at dose 50, as the predicted d_f^* has only risen to

Table 9.4   Maximum likelihood estimates (MLE) and Bayesian modal estimates of
the simulated data in Table 9.3 (with standard errors or standard deviations).

	θ_1	θ_2	σ^2	τ^2	ρ	d_f^*
Truth for simulations	1.167	0.822	0.053	0.073	0.579	74.86
(MLE from real data)	(0.158)	(0.046)				
Final MLE	0.754	0.913	0.043	0.027	0.386	90.08
	(0.169)	(0.042)				
Bayesian prior	0.755	1.000	0.076	0.113	0.6	2.5
modal estimates	(1.657)	(0.561)				
Bayesian posterior	0.701	0.932	0.039	0.058	0.6	77.67
modal estimates	(0.171)	(0.041)				

76.38 µg after two cohorts. Subject 12 exceeds the safety limit in the second period
of the third cohort after receiving dose 150. Dose 100 is given to that subject in the
third period. In practice, such a subject may be excluded from the trial after exceeding
the safety limit. The ratio, R, of the upper 97.5 % credibility limit to the lower 2.5 %
limit is reported in Table 9.3. If the accuracy stopping rule was used, say stop when
the current ratio is 2, then the trial would have been stopped after only two cohorts.

Table 9.4 gives the maximum likelihood estimates from the real data in Table 9.2
that were used as the true values in the simulation, together with the maximum
likelihood estimates from the simulated data in Table 9.3. Results show that σ^2 and τ^2
were underestimated from the simulated data. Consequently, the estimated correlation
from the simulated data is smaller than the true value.

9.5   Multiple simulations

Powerful computers make multiple simulation runs possible. Simulations can demonstrate that the Bayesian approach is of potential value for dose-escalation and provide
insight into the design choices required for implementation. Thus, simulations are
highly recommended as an evaluation tool to check and compare designs prior to
running a study.

Tables 9.5 and 9.6 give an example of such simulation results. The prior used is
the same as in the previous section, except that three choices for α_0 are investigated:
0.1, 1 and 5. The scenario used here is also the same as that in the previous section:
the model derived from the maximum likelihood estimates from the real data. The
maxsafe gain function is used in all simulations. Each design is explored with the
maximum sample size set at 12 subjects and without an accuracy stopping rule. For
each of the 1000 runs conducted, the number of subjects for whom an undesirable
C_{max} value exceeding $L = 200$ are counted. No runs were stopped due to there being
no safe doses available. The number of administrations leading to C_{max} in each of the

Table 9.5   Multiple simulation results: distribution of values of C_{max} and of doses administered.

π_0	0.05		
α_0	0.1	1	5
Number of subjects with	1.257	1.028	0.326
$C_{max} \in [L, \infty)$ per run standard deviation	(1.219)	(1.126)	(0.651)
Number of responses per run with $C_{max} \in$			
[0.0.2L)	5.481	6.399	11.257
[0.2L, 0.5L)	19.870	20.211	19.411
[0.5L, L)	9.381	8.353	5.005
[L, \infty)	1.268	1.0137	0.327
Number of administrations per run of dose			
2.5	3	3	3
5.0	0	0	0
10.0	0.070	0.049	3.408
25.0	5.170	7.538	12.660
50.0	22.297	20.918	15.682
100.0	4.677	3.906	1.107
150.0	0.786	0.589	0.143

intervals $[0, 0.2L)$, $[0.2L, 0.5L)$, $[0.5L, L)$ and $[L, \infty)$ are counted, together with the usage of each dose. The value of $E(\log C_{max})$ at dose 150 for a new untested subject is $5.286 = \log(197.6)$, which is close to the limiting value of $\log(200)$. Therefore, dose 150 is on the borderline of safety. The safety of the Bayesian prodecure is reflected

Table 9.6   Multiple simulation results: precision of estimates (RMSE, root mean square error).

π_0	0.05		
α_0	0.1	1	5
True $\log(d_f^*)$	4.317		
Mean $\log(d_f^*)$, Bayes	4.053	4.045	3.886
RMSE $\log(d_f^*)$, Bayes	0.328	0.327	0.462
Mean $\log(d_f^*)$, frequentist	4.338	4.334	4.326
RMSE $\log(d_f^*)$, frequentist	0.174	0.171	0.191
True σ^2	0.053		
Mean σ^2, Bayes	0.082	0.083	0.108
RMSE σ^2, Bayes	0.041	0.039	0.060
Mean σ^2, frequentist	0.078	0.079	0.079
RMSE σ^2, frequentist	0.038	0.037	0.038

in Table 9.5 where less than one administration per simulation run is made on the borderline dose 150.

From the final dataset, the Bayesian posterior modal estimates and the frequentist maximum likelihood estimates are found for $\log d_f^*$ and σ^2. These are summarized over each set of 1000 runs in terms of means and root mean square errors. Results indicate that the bigger α_0 is, the more safe the approach is. Dose 5.0 is not used by any of the designs. There is little difference between designs with $\alpha_0 = 0.1$ and 1 according to accuracy, but setting $\alpha_0 = 5$ gives worse Bayesian estimates. This shows that if a prior is too conservative then Bayesian estimates are inaccurate, which is to be expected. All designs achieve similar maximum likelihood estimates. Here we only explore three designs under one scenario. In practice, many designs should be evaluated under different scenarios, to investigate different numbers of doses, different stopping rules, different gain functions and different prior settings (see reference [12]).

9.6 Conclusions

In practice, the decision as to whether to accept the recommended doses determined by the Bayesian procedure will lie with the investigating clinicians. Recommendations might be overruled because of safety data or other outcomes not modelled by the procedure. Alternatively, the clinicians' experience may indicate that different doses are appropriate. An advantage of the procedure is that it can learn from the results of administering any doses. As users become familiar with the procedure it is expected that it will be overruled less frequently, and that persistent discrepancies between recommendations and practice will lead to a fine tuning of the options used in the procedure.

The principles underlying the procedure are open to flexible interpretation and so various components can easily be varied. The modelling of the responses y_{ij} described in equation (9.1) could be amended in various ways. Instead of the subject effect being expressed as a random intercept, it could be included as a random slope: indeed both random terms could be included. However, we note that in our own fitting of models to pharmacokinetic data, random slopes have not been found to improve the model significantly. Covariates relating to the volunteers can be easily introduced, as could a factor relating to period effects. Complex procedures, perhaps based on multiple imputation or on exact treatment of censored values, could be used to overcome the problem of nonobservable pharmacokinetic responses. However, the desire to allow for the many potential influences on outcome must be tempered by the realization that the data available are very few, especially in the early cohorts. It will seldom be desirable to use models that are much more sophisticated than (9.1).

References to work that has sought to introduce other novel statistical procedures to phase I studies include an application of Bayesian methodology [13], and a detailed account of frequentist design and analysis [14]. The Bayesian decision–theoretic approach as a whole could be applied with other pharmacokinetic endpoints, such as the area under the curve, or to pharmacodynamic responses, such as blood pressure or pulse, serving as the y_{ij}. In the latter case, models more sophisticated than (9.1) may be required.

Acknowledgements

The author would like to thank Tony Sabin from GlaxoSmithKline, Greenford, UK, for permission to use the data and John Whitehead at the MPS Research Unit for advice and helpful comments.

References

1. S.C. Chow and J.P. Liu (eds.) (1999) *Design and Analysis of Bioavailability and Bioequivalence studies*, Marcel Dekker, New York.
2. W.J. Westlake (1988) Bioavailability and bioequivalence of pharmaceutical formulations, in *Biopharmaceutical Statistics for Drug Development* (ed. K.E. Peace), Marcel Dekker, New York, pp. 329–352.
3. S. Patterson, S. Francis, M. Ireson, D. Webber and J. Whitehead (1999) A novel Bayesian decision procedure for early-phase dose finding studies, *J. Biopharmaceutical Statistics*, **9**(4), 583–97.
4. H. Boxenbaum and C. DiLea (1995) First-time-in-human dose selection: allometric thoughts and perspectives. *J. Clin. Pharmacology*, **35**(10), 957–66.
5. M.N. Laird and J.H. Ware (1982) Random effects models for longitudinal data. *Biometrics*, **38**(4), 963–74.
6. R.C. Littell, G.A. Milliken, W.W. Stroup and R.D. Wolfinger (1996) *SAS System for Mixed Models*, SAS Institute Inc., pp. 253–66.
7. J.O. Berger (ed.) (1985) *Statistical Decision Theory and Bayesian Analysis*, Springer, New York.
8. D.V. Lindley (ed.) (1971) *Making Decisions*, John Wiley & Sons Ltd, Chichester.
9. J.Q. Smith (ed.) (1988) *Decision Analysis: A Bayesian Approach*, Chapman and Hall, London.
10. J. Whitehead, Y. Zhou, S. Patterson, N.D. Webber and S. Francis (2001) Easy-to-implement Bayesian methods for dose-escalation studies in healthy volunteers. *Biostatistics*, **2**(1), 47–61.
11. P.M. Lee (ed.) (1989) *Bayesian Statistics: An Introduction*, Oxford University Press, Oxford.
12. J. Whitehead, Y. Zhou, A. Mander, S. Ritchie, A. Sabin and A. Wright (2006) An evaluation of Bayesian designs for dose-escalation studies in healthy volunteers. *Statistics in Medicine*, **25**(3), 433–445.
13. A. Racine-Poon and J.P. Dubois (1989) Predicting the range of plasma carbemazepine concentrations in patients with epilepsy. *Statistics in Medicine*, **8**(11), 1327–37.
14. P.C. Boon and K.C. Roes (1999) Design and analysis issues for crossover designs in phase I clinical studies. *J. Biopharmaceutical Statistics*, **9**(1), 109–28.

Part IV

Future Trends for Past Issues

10

Defining stopping rules

Sarah Zohar

Département de Biostatistique et Informatique Médicale, U717 Inserm
Hôpital Saint-Louis, Paris, France

10.1 Introduction

Formal statistical methods for dose-finding studies have been mainly developed in oncology trials. In this context, there is an ethical conflict between undertreating and overtreating too many patients. If the first dose level is lower than some toxicity target, the dose-escalation of the standard designs may lead to treat too many patients at nontherapeutic levels. On the contrary, if the first dose level is more toxic than warranted, such designs may expose too many patients to levels with higher toxicity than necessary.

In order to address these ethical concerns better and optimize the trial sample size, efficient stopping rules that allow easy and reproducible decision rules, such as either continue or stop patient accrual, have been proposed in the last 30 years. However, most of these stopping rules have been developed for uncontrolled phase II trials or randomized phase III trials [1–6]. By contrast, only few authors in the last 10 years have dealt with the development of stopping rules in the setting of dose-finding studies [7–12]. Besides empirical ones, these stopping rules have been mainly proposed in the setting of Bayesian approaches.

This chapter aims to give an overview of existing statistical stopping rules for dose-finding clinical trials that allow the ethical concerns of these trials to be addressed.

Statistical Methods for Dose-Finding Experiments Edited by S. Chevret
© 2006 John Wiley & Sons, Ltd

10.2   Background

One of the first authors who used the term 'stopping rule' in the context of clinical trials was Peter Armitage, when introducing sequential clinical trial designs [13,14]. This development was the result of ethical considerations, focusing on the conflict of interests between monitoring a clinical trial and randomizing further patients [15]. This conflict of interest was largely discussed, by introducing the concept of 'theoretical or clinical equipoise', i.e. when there is no preference between treatment options to be compared [16–21]. However, even if such equipoise can be assumed at the beginning of the trial, the more the trial progresses and data have been accumulating, the more a discernible trend in the favour of one of the treatments appeared before the inclusion of the planned number of patients. Nevertheless, in classical clinical trials, the sample size is determined and fixed before the beginning of the trial, without any readjustment along the trial that could consider the accumulated data.

In order to optimize sample size and to stop a clinical trial when there is sufficient evidence of either effectiveness or ineffectiveness of a new treatment, sequential designs were proposed. Sequential clinical trials are based on sequential stopping rules in the way that they involve a sequence of decisions to terminate or continue enrolment in the clinical trial. In fixed sample size designs, any choice of stopping rules can lead to a biased estimation of the treatment effect because, if the trial stops early, maximum likelihood can overestimate or underestimate the underlying effect [22]. One of the key features of sequential designs is that they allow the type I error rate to be controlled, despite repeated interim analyses.

From a practical point of view, several grouped sequential frequentist designs were proposed in which the interim analyses are performed after each inclusion of a number of predetermined patients or events [1–6, 13]. Although these procedures can differ from one design to another on particular points, they share several common features: (a) a sequence of statistics is used to test the null hypothesis; (b) the stopping rule is defined as a sequence of constant or increasing nominal significance levels for each test; (c) the sequence is chosen in order to maintain a predefined type I error rate, in which are fixed either the number of analyses or the rate of the overall significance [19, 23]. In this setting, three main sequential stopping approaches with associated test statistics were proposed in order to measure the treatment difference [24, 25]. In the first sequential approaches, traditional test statistics are used, such as the chi-square statistic or the t-statistic, computed after the observed responses of k patients, where k is defined at the beginning of the trial [1–3, 14]. The second sequential designs use a boundaries approach, like the triangular test, based on the cumulative measure of the advantage of the experimental over the standard treatment, Z, and on the amount of information about the treatment difference contained in Z, denoted V [4, 24, 26]. Finally, the third sequential approaches are based on repeated confidence intervals for the treatment difference computed at each interim analysis [5]. In all cases, the stopping of patient's inclusion results from the rejection or not of the null hypothesis.

Otherwise, to address the issue of stopping rules, Bayesian approaches have been proposed [27–34]. By contrast to the frequentist point of view, which relies on significance tests or confidence intervals of a fixed parameter of interest, Bayesian methods assume that the unknown true treatment difference is a random variable for which a prior distribution has to be determined [35]. The collected information during the trial with the prior opinion are combined into a posterior distribution as a basis for the trial conclusions. Such a Bayesian framework allows sequential monitoring of results and also prediction of the consequences of continuing the trial in terms of sample size or precision of estimated treatment difference. In this context, the stopping rules are based on either the posterior and/or the predictive distributions of the treatment difference [36]. Nevertheless, Bayesian approaches with associated stopping rules have been mostly developed and analyzed in noncomparative phase II studies [27–30,37], while proposals in randomized clinical trials have remained rather theoretical [31–34,38].

In this chapter, stopping rules in the context of dose-finding trials will be presented and discussed. Several authors have proposed stopping criteria that are all associated to a specific dose-allocation scheme [7–11,39–41]. The chapter is organized as follows: firstly, dose-finding specificities are presented and, secondly, statistical methods and their mathematical formulations are described. In the fourth section, these stopping rules are applied to three real datasets, one from a dose-finding phase I clinical trial (the Nalmefene trial [42]) and two from dose-finding phase II clinical trials (the Prantal trial and the nitroglycerine trials [43]). Finally, some discussion and concluding remarks for clinical decision making in using these stopping rules are provided in the last section.

10.3 Dose-finding specificities

In dose-finding studies, patient's accrual is performed sequentially. Therefore, the inclusion of new patients in the trial depends on previous observations in terms of dose level and response. Even if accrual is done sequentially, there are still major differences between these trials and other traditional sequential clinical trials (Table 10.1).

Firstly, dose-finding trials are used in the early phases of the development of a new treatment while standard sequential trials are used in phases II or III. Secondly, the number of dose levels to be tested in dose-finding, and therefore the number of potential groups of patients, is at least four and usually around six. By contrast, in standard sequential trials, usually one or two arms are used in phase II or phase III trials respectively. Thirdly, standard sequential trials deal with hypothesis testing, based on the Newman and Pearson test statistics approach, which leads to stop the trial if there is sufficient evidence of the superiority of one treatment over the other. By contrast, the aim of dose-finding trials is to estimate a dose level and the trials are not placed in the context of hypothesis testing; the commonly used stopping rules are design–based, in the context of the standard '3 + 3' approach. More recent dose-finding methods have been developed in order to optimize sample size, as well as minimizing the number of patients treated at ineffective doses and minimizing the number of patients treated at doses that are too toxic [44–46]. In recently developed

Table 10.1 Comparaison of dose-finding and standard sequential clinical trials.

	Dose-finding trials	Sequential trials
Development phase	Phase I or II. Evaluation of the MTD or MED	Phase II or III. Evaluation and comparison of the efficacy
Number of tested dose levels	Several dose levels (at least 4)	Two arms in randomized trials or one in nonrandomized trials
Hypothesis testing	—	
Sample size	Small sample size (15–30 subjects)	Sample size depends on the treatment effect that one wishes to observe, the type I error probability and the type II error probability
Repeated analyses	As much as the number of cohorts in the trial. The dose level to be administered to the next cohort of patients depends on the dose levels and observations of previous cohorts	The number of repeated analyses is determined and fixed before the beginning of the trial in order to control the overall type I error
Stopping rules	Design-based stopping rules in the case of '3+3' design. The trial ending is recommended when the wanted dose level has been found	At each repeated analysis one determines whether to stop or to continue enrolment in the clinical trial

methods, the sample size is usually computed from simulation studies, where the recommended number of patients is the number of patients that allows, on average, the desired maximal tolerated dose with good statistical properties to be reached.

Thus, stopping rules designed for standard sequential trials based on frequentist approaches are not well suited for dose-findings. By contrast, stopping rules based on Bayesian approaches seem more adapted in this context.

In the next sections, stopping rules that are 'design-based' or 'statistically based' for frequentist or Bayesian approaches will be presented. Readers should not forget that the presented stopping rules are often associated with a particular dose-finding allocation scheme, but they can be adapted to schemes other than the 'native' ones.

10.3.1 Algorithm-based stopping rules

Design-based stopping rules rely on patient observations, with recommendation to stop the trial resulting from an arbitrary choice, such as the number of patients who experienced toxicity. Two main design-based stopping rules can be distinguished. First, stopping and ending the trial is recommended when at least a minimum number of patients, noted n_1, were treated at the estimated MTD (usually, $n_1 = 3, 6$) [39,47–50]. Otherwise, stopping rules are based on the minimum number of DLT observed, n_2 ($n_2 = 3, 4$), among a fixed number of patients (9 or 18) [51]. In all cases, no statistical justification is given and the threshold numbers (either n_1 or n_2) are arbitrarily chosen.

10.3.2 Model-based stopping rules: frequentist approaches

Statistically based approaches rely on adjustment of the underlying dose-response model parameters that came from patient observations. Statistically based stopping rules address two separate questions, namely the early detection of either (a) a mischoice in dose range or (b) a suitable estimation of the MTD (or MED). Several stopping rules that specifically address these questions have been proposed for dose-finding studies conducted through frequentist or a Bayesian framework.

10.3.2.1 Stopping criterion (SC) based on the binary outcome tree

The stopping criterion developed by O'Quigley and Renier [8] is based on the probability that the administrated dose level remains unchanged for some additional patients (from j to $j + z$, where j is the number of included patients and z is the number of additional subjects to be recruited) and is represented by a binary tree. Let $P\{X(j + 1) = \ldots X(j + z)|\text{data}\}$ be the true probability of no change in the administrated dose of z additional inclusions, with $X(j + 1), \ldots, X(j + z)$ the dose levels to be administered from the j to the $j + z$ patients. This probability is estimated by (SC1)

$$\tilde{P}\{X(j + 1) = \cdots X(j + z)|\text{data}\} = \sum_{r=0}^{z} A r (1 - \tilde{p})^{z-r} \tilde{p}^r, \tag{10.1}$$

where $\bar{p}$ is the estimated toxicity probability associated with the administered dose level evaluated with the maximum likelihood based CRM and Ar is the number of paths of the binary tree that contains the same number of toxicities (r) from the root to the leaf. If this probability is higher than some threshold (in $[0, 1]$) then the trial is stopped. The use of this stopping criterion was extended to Bayesian approaches, where $\bar{p}$ is estimated by the CRM [10].

10.3.2.2   Stopping criterion based on the sequential ratio test

This stopping criterion was developed in the context of phase I/II clinical trials where the dose-toxicity and the dose-response relationships are jointly modeled [52,53]. The aim is to identify the situation when the experimented dose level, d_i (with $i = 1, \ldots, k$ and k the number of dose levels), has a too low or high efficacy. This stopping criteria is defined by (SC2)

$$X_i(n) \log \frac{p_1}{p_0} + [N_i(n) - X_i(n)] \log \frac{1 - p_1}{1 - p_0}, \tag{10.2}$$

where $X_i(n)$ is the number of responses observed at the dose level d_i, $N_i(n)$ the total number of patients treated at this dose level and p_0 and p_1 are the response rates associated with the null and the alternative hypotheses respectively. If an upper threshold (in $[0, 1]$) is crossed, the trial is stopped and d_i is recommended for further experimentations; conversely, if a lower threshold (in $[0, 1]$) is crossed, then this dose level and lower ones are removed and the target toxicity probability is updated.

10.3.3   Model-based stopping rules: Bayesian approaches

10.3.3.1   Stopping criteria (SC) based on posterior distribution

In the context of phase I/II clinical trials, two stopping criteria based on posterior probabilities being given the accumulated data at any interim point in the trial have been proposed [7,54,55]. The dose level d_i is considered to have an unacceptably high adverse outcome if the following posterior probability is higher than a predetermined threshold (in $[0, 1]$)(SC3):

$$P\{P_{i|j} > \pi_1 | \text{data}\}, \tag{10.3}$$

where $P_{i|j}$ is the estimated probability of toxicity at the dose level i after j inclusions and π_1 is the toxicity target probability.

Moreover, the dose level d_i is considered to have unacceptably low efficacy if the following posterior probability is higher than a prespecified threshold (in $[0, 1]$)(SC4):

$$P\{Q_{i|j} < \pi_2 | \text{data}\}, \tag{10.4}$$

with $Q_{i|j}$ being the estimated probability of response at the dose level i after j inclusions and π_2 the targeted probability of efficacy.

The first stopping criterion was also used in phase I clinical trials [10,41], and extended to evaluate too low efficacy at the dose level d_i in phase II dose-finding clinical trials. The second stopping criterion was extended, in the context of phase I oncology trials, in order to evaluate the probability that the estimated toxicity probability at the last dose level is lower than the toxicity target [10].

10.3.3.2 Stopping criterion (SC) based on credibility intervals

One stopping criterion recommends that the trial should stop when the width of the credibility interval of the estimated parameter of the dose-toxicity relationship reaches some threshold [9,40,50]. Let θ be the random parameter of the dose-toxicity relationship model. The credibility interval of level α for θ is defined by $(\tilde{\theta}_{min}, \tilde{\theta}_{max})$: $\int_{\tilde{\theta}_{min}}^{\tilde{\theta}_{max}} f(\theta|\text{data})d\theta = 1 - \alpha$. The width of this credibility interval is thus (SC5)

$$w = \tilde{\theta}_{max} - \tilde{\theta}_{min}. \tag{10.5}$$

If the width of the credibility interval is less than some threshold ($\in [0, 2]$) then stopping the trial is recommended [9].

This stopping criterion was extended in the setting of the maximum likelihood based CRM in the evaluation of the confidence intervals width [11].

10.3.3.3 Stopping criteria (SC) based on predictive probabilities distribution

Four stopping criteria based on the mean and maximum predictive gain of z additional patients on either the estimated probability of toxicity or the width of its credibility interval have been proposed [10,12]. If three out of the four stopping criteria are lower than some threshold (in $[0, 1]$), then stopping the trial is recommended.

- The predictive mean gain of z additional inclusions on the estimated response probability is defined by (SC6)

$$\sum_{y_1=0}^{1} \cdots \sum_{y_z=0}^{1} |\tilde{P}_{R|j+z} - \tilde{P}_{R|j}| P(Y_{j+1} = y_1, \ldots, Y_{j+z} = y_z|\text{data}), \tag{10.6}$$

where $y_1, \ldots, y_z$ are all the possible responses observed in the $(j + 1)$th, $\ldots, (j + z)$th patients, $\tilde{P}_{R|j}$ is the estimated probability of toxicity at the dose level R (R is the recommended dose level associated with the MTD $R \in d_i, \ldots, d_k$) after the inclusion of j patients and $P(Y_{j+1} = y_1, \ldots, Y_{j+z} = y_z|\text{data})$ is the predictive probability of the z future responses.

- The maximal predictive gain of z additional inclusions on the estimated response probability of the recommended dose level is (SC7)

$$\max_{(y_1, \ldots, y_z)} |\tilde{P}_{R|j+z} - \tilde{P}_{R|j}|. \tag{10.7}$$

- The predictive mean gain of z additional inclusions on the credibility interval width, of the response probability of the recommended dose level (d_R), P_R, is defined by (SC8)

$$\sum_{y_1=0}^{1} \cdots \sum_{y_z=0}^{1} |\{c_{\alpha, j+z}(P_R) - c_{\alpha, j+1}(P_R)\}| P(Y_{j+1} = y_1, \ldots, Y_{j+z} = y_z | \text{data}),$$

(10.8)

where $y_1, \ldots, y_z$ are all the possible responses observed in the $(j+1)$th, $\ldots, (j+z)$th patients, $c_{\alpha,.}(P_R)$ is the credibility interval of the toxicity probability and $P(Y_{j+1} = y_1, \ldots, Y_{j+z} = y_z | \text{data})$ is the predictive probability of the z future responses.

- The maximal predictive gain of z additional inclusions on the credibility interval width is (SC9)

$$\max_{(y_1, \ldots, y_z)} |c_{\alpha, j+z}(P_R) - c_{\alpha, j}(P_R)|.$$

(10.9)

10.4   Examples

In this section, some of the previously presented statistically based stopping rules are applied to two illustrative examples. These two examples deal with dose-finding trials in the setting of either a phase I clinical trial, the Nalmefene trial [42], or a phase II clinical trial, the Prantal trial.

10.4.1   The Nalmefene trial

This is a phase I dose-finding trial that has previously been conducted and published [42]. It aimed at evaluating the MTD of the opioid antagonist, Nalmefene, which does not reverse analgesia in an acceptable number of postoperative patients receiving epidural fentanyl. It used a modified CRM design, in the sense that the dose-allocation scheme started with the lowest dose level and does not allow any dose to be skipped before escalating the dose in the next patients. The target toxicity probability was fixed at 20 % and the fixed sample size at 25. Four dose levels of Nalmefene were studied, namely 0.25, 0.50, 0.75 and 1.00 µg.kg, with initial guesses of toxicity probability of 0.10, 0.20, 0.40 and 0.80 respectively. Published results [42] that used a unit exponential prior for the logistic model parameter and three for the model intercept selected the second dose level (0.50 µg/kg) as the MTD, with posterior toxicity probability of 18 % (95 % credibility interval: 6–36 %). Table 10.2 reports the dose allocation and the sequential estimation of the toxicity probabilities associated with each dose level.

Seven stopping criteria (SC) were retrospectively applied to this dataset (Table 10.3). Of note, stopping criteria SC2 and SC4, which aim to evaluate some efficacy outcome, were not computed in this setting of a phase I trial. Each stopping criterion was associated with a stopping threshold, according to literature values, as

Table 10.2 Sequential allocation scheme of the Nalmefene trial. At each step, the estimated failure probability closest to 0.20 is shown in bold.

			Dose (µg/kg)			
			Prior estimated toxicity probabilities			
			0.25	0.50	0.75	1.0
	Dose		Posterior estimated toxicity probabilities			
Patient	(µg/kg)	Response	0.1	0.2	0.4	0.8
1	0.25	No Toxicity	0.01	0.03	**0.11**	0.65
2	0.50	No Toxicity	0.00	0.01	**0.05**	0.54
3	0.75	Toxicity	**0.15**	0.27	0.472	0.82
4	0.25	No Toxicity	0.10	**0.19**	0.39	0.80
5	0.50	No Toxicity	0.06	**0.14**	0.33	0.78
6	0.50	Toxicity	**0.19**	0.32	0.52	0.83
7	0.25	No Toxicity	**0.15**	0.28	0.48	0.82
8	0.25	No Toxicity	0.13	**0.25**	0.45	0.81
9	0.50	No Toxicity	0.11	**0.21**	0.41	0.80
10	0.50	No Toxicity	0.09	**0.19**	0.39	0.80
11	0.50	No Toxicity	0.08	**0.17**	0.36	0.79
12	0.50	No Toxicity	0.07	**0.15**	0.34	0.78
13	0.50	No Toxicity	0.06	**0.14**	0.32	0.77
14	0.50	No Toxicity	0.05	**0.13**	0.30	0.77
15	0.50	No Toxicity	0.05	**0.12**	0.29	0.76
16	0.50	No Toxicity	0.04	0.11	**0.28**	0.75
17	0.75	No Toxicity	0.04	0.10	**0.25**	0.75
18	0.75	Toxicity	0.06	**0.13**	0.31	0.78
19	0.50	No Toxicity	0.05	**0.12**	0.30	0.76
20	0.50	Toxicity	0.08	**0.17**	0.37	0.79
21	0.50	No Toxicity	0.08	**0.16**	0.35	0.79
22	0.50	No Toxicity	0.07	**0.15**	0.34	0.78
23	0.50	Toxicity	0.10	**0.19**	0.39	0.78
24	0.50	No Toxicity	0.09	**0.19**	0.38	0.79
25	0.50	No Toxicity	0.08	**0.18**	0.37	0.79

follows: SC1 = 1.00, SC3 ≥ 0.90, SC5 ≤ 0.75 and SC6; SC7; SC8 and SC9 (three criteria from four) lower than 0.05.

Results from Table 10.3 show that the trial could have been stopped before the enrolment of the prespecified fixed sample size of 25, after the inclusion of 19–20 patients, with the conclusions that the second dose level is the estimated MTD and that no marked gain in terms of precision in estimates would have been expected

Table 10.3 Sequential computation of the stopping criteria for the Nalmefene trial.

	Stopping criteria						
	SC1	SC3	SC5	SC6	SC7	SC8	SC9
	Stopping threshold						
Patient	≥ 1.00	≥ 0.90	≤ 0.75	< 0.05	< 0.05	< 0.05	< 0.05
1	0.00	0.29	4.03	0.31	0.74	0.39	0.86
2	0.07	0.14	4.00	0.19	0.74	0.18	0.26
3	0.24	0.45	1.41	0.15	0.54	0.30	0.42
4	0.00	0.33	1.31	0.14	0.45	0.10	0.19
5	0.00	0.22	1.27	0.10	0.43	0.15	0.23
6	0.39	0.50	0.88	0.09	0.34	0.18	0.26
7	0.20	0.41	0.84	0.07	0.30	0.12	0.17
8	0.43	0.34	0.82	0.09	0.27	0.04	0.06
9	0.59	0.26	0.81	0.08	0.26	0.06	0.10
10	0.74	0.19	0.80	0.06	0.25	0.06	0.09
11	0.87	0.14	0.79	0.05	0.22	0.06	0.08
12	0.89	0.10	0.79	0.05	0.21	0.05	0.08
13	0.36	0.08	0.78	0.04	0.20	0.05	0.07
14	0.27	0.06	0.78	0.04	0.17	0.05	0.07
15	0.14	0.04	0.77	0.04	0.16	0.05	0.07
16	0.38	0.03	0.77	0.06	0.17	0.10	0.11
17	0.54	0.02	0.78	0.06	0.18	0.04	0.05
18	0.37	0.04	0.76	0.04	0.14	0.14	0.16
19	0.26	0.03	**0.75**	0.03	0.13	0.03	0.06
20	**1.00**	0.07	—	**0.03**	0.12	**0.03**	**0.04**
21	—	0.05	—	—	—	—	—
22	—	0.04	—	—	—	—	—
23	—	0.09	—	—	—	—	—
24	—	0.07	—	—	—	—	—
25	—	0.05	—	—	—	—	—

from further inclusions. Such conclusions relied on the computation of all the stopping criteria but SC3, which, actually remained far below the stopping threshold all along the trial, indicating that a too high toxicity probability at any dose level is unlikely.

10.4.2 The Prantal trial

This phase II dose-finding trial was conducted to assess the MED of Prantal (diphemanil methylsulfate) in the treatment of vagal bradycardia in infants. The MED was defined as the dose of Prantal required to decrease vagal bradycardia in 90 % of infants

Table 10.4 Sequential allocation scheme of the Prantal trial. At each step, the estimated failure probability closest to 0.1 is shown in bold.

			Dose (mg/kg/d)				
			Prior estimated failure probabilities				
			10	8	6	4	2
			Posterior estimated failure probabilities				
Patient	Dose (mg/kg/d)	Response	0.01	0.1	0.3	0.5	0.7
1	8	Success	0.00	0.01	**0.06**	0.19	0.45
2	6	Success	0.00	0.00	0.02	**0.08**	0.29
3	4	Failure	0.01	**0.10**	0.30	0.50	0.70
4	8	Failure	**0.13**	0.42	0.63	0.75	0.83
5	10	Success	**0.08**	0.33	0.56	0.70	0.81
6	10	Success	**0.06**	0.28	0.52	0.67	0.80
7	10	Success	**0.05**	0.26	0.50	0.66	0.79
8	10	Success	**0.04**	0.23	0.48	0.64	0.78
9	10	Failure	**0.15**	0.44	0.65	0.76	0.84
10	10	Failure	**0.27**	0.56	0.72	0.80	0.87
11	10	Failure	**0.36**	0.64	0.77	0.83	0.88
12	10	Failure	**0.44**	0.69	0.79	0.85	0.89
13	10	Success	**0.39**	0.65	0.78	0.84	0.88
14	10	Success	**0.35**	0.63	0.76	0.83	0.88
15	10	Success	**0.32**	0.61	0.75	0.82	0.87
16	10	Failure	**0.38**	0.65	0.77	0.83	0.88
17	10	Success	**0.35**	0.63	0.76	0.83	0.88

(resulting in 10 % of targeted failure). The trial was designed according to the original CRM design. Five dose levels were studied, namely 2, 4, 6, 8 and 10 mg/kg/d, with initial guesses of failure probability of 0.7, 0.5, 0.3, 0.1 and 0.01 respectively. A logistic model was used. Based on model operating characteristics, the intercept was fixed at 3, while an exponential prior with unit mean was retained for the model parameter. The sample size was 17. Table 10.4 summarizes the dose allocation and the sequential estimation of the mean posterior failure probability associated with each dose level throughout the trial. At the end of the trial, the highest dose level (10 mg/kg/d) that was administered consecutively from the 5th to the 17th patient was estimated to be the MED, with an estimated posterior mean failure probability of 35 % (95 % credibility interval: 13–60 %).

Table 10.5 reports the retrospective sequential application of seven stopping criteria, with threshold values fixed at SC1 = 1.00, SC3 ≥ 0.90, SC5 ≤ 0.80 and SC6; SC7; SC8 and SC9 (three criteria from four) lower than 0.05.

Table 10.5   Sequential computation of the stopping criteria for the Prantal trial.

	Stopping criteria						
	SC1	SC3	SC5	SC6	SC7	SC8	SC9
	Stopping threshold						
Patient	≥ 1.00	≥ 0.90	≤ 0.75	<0.05	<0.05	<0.05	<0.05
1	0.00	0.20	4.03	0.27	0.82	0.42	0.61
2	0.00	0.07	4.04	0.24	0.78	0.24	0.44
3	0.61	0.21	1.56	0.16	0.71	0.32	0.42
4	**1.00**	0.58	1.02	0.16	0.62	0.32	0.45
5	—	0.47	0.90	0.09	0.53	0.23	0.30
6	—	0.39	0.84	0.06	0.44	0.16	0.20
7	—	0.34	0.81	0.04	0.37	0.13	0.24
8	—	0.29	0.79	0.03	0.32	0.10	0.25
9	—	0.70	**0.75**	0.07	0.29	0.10	0.14
10	—	**0.91**	—	0.07	0.23	0.09	0.14
11	—	—	—	0.07	0.19	0.08	0.13
12	—	—	—	0.07	0.15	0.07	0.11
13	—	—	—	0.06	0.15	0.07	0.10
14	—	—	—	0.05	0.15	0.05	0.08
15	—	—	—	0.05	0.14	0.05	0.08
16	—	—	—	0.05	0.12	0.05	0.07
17	—	—	—	0.04	0.12	0.05	0.07

As previously, it appears that the trial could have been stopped earlier than with the fixed sample size, though with a somewhat rather different conclusion. Indeed, the application of stopping rules would have allowed the trial to stop patient inclusion after at most 10 patients, for a mis-choice of dose levels. Actually, such a stopping decision only relies on the computed stopping criteria SC1 and SC3, indicating that subsequent patients would receive the same – highest – dose level, and that its associated failure probability was too high as compared to the target of 0.10 respectively. The stopping criterion SC5 also indicated that the width of its 95 % credibility interval was satisfactory.

10.4.3   The nitroglycerin trial

A phase II dose-finding trial was conducted to assess the MED of the nitroglycerin tocolytic effect during preterm labor [43]. The MED was defined as the dose of nitroglycerin required to achieve a positive response in 90 % of pregnant women (i.e. 10 % failure). The trial was designed according to the original CRM design with

Table 10.6 Sequential allocation scheme of the nitroglycerin trial.

			Dose (mg/h)					
			Prior estimated failure probabilities					
			1.2	1.0	0.8	0.6	0.4	0.2
			Posterior estimated failure probabilities					
Patient	Dose (mg/h)	Response	0.02	0.05	0.1	0.2	0.25	0.5
1	0.8	Success	0.00	0.00	0.01	0.03	**0.04**	0.19
2	0.4	Success	0.00	0.00	0.00	0.01	0.01	**0.09**
3	0.2	Success	0.00	0.00	0.00	0.00	0.00	**0.04**
4	0.2	Failure	0.01	0.02	0.05	**0.11**	0.15	0.38
5	0.6	Failure	0.06	**0.12**	0.21	0.34	0.39	0.62
6	1	Failure	**0.24**	0.36	0.47	0.59	0.63	0.77
7	1.2	Success	**0.17**	0.27	0.38	0.52	0.56	0.73
8	1.2	Success	**0.13**	0.23	0.33	0.47	0.52	0.70
9	1.2	Failure	**0.27**	0.39	0.50	0.61	0.65	0.78
10	1.2	Success	**0.23**	0.34	0.45	0.58	0.62	0.76
11	1.2	Success	**0.20**	0.31	0.42	0.55	0.59	0.75
12	1.2	Failure	**0.29**	0.41	0.51	0.63	0.66	0.79
13	1.2	Failure	**0.37**	0.49	0.58	0.68	0.71	0.81
14	1.2	Success	**0.33**	0.45	0.55	0.66	0.69	0.80
15	1.2	Success	**0.30**	0.42	0.52	0.63	0.67	0.79
16	1.2	Failure	**0.36**	0.48	0.57	0.67	0.71	0.81
17	1.2	Success	**0.33**	0.45	0.55	0.66	0.69	0.80
18	1.2	Failure	**0.38**	0.50	0.59	0.69	0.72	0.81
19	1.2	Failure	**0.42**	0.54	0.62	0.71	0.74	0.83
20	1.2	Failure	**0.46**	0.57	0.65	0.73	0.75	0.84
21	1.2	Success	**0.43**	0.54	0.63	0.71	0.74	0.83
22	1.2	Failure	**0.47**	0.57	0.65	0.73	0.76	0.84
23	1.2	Failure	**0.49**	0.60	0.67	0.75	0.77	0.84
24	1.2	Success	**0.47**	0.58	0.66	0.73	0.76	0.84
25	1.2	Success	**0.45**	0.56	0.64	0.72	0.75	0.83

a fixed sample size of 25. Six different dose levels of nitroglycerin were studied, namely 0.2, 0.4, 0.6, 0.8, 1.0 and 1.2 mg/h. The associated initial guesses of failure probability were 0.5, 0.25, 0.2, 0.1, 0.05 and 0.02 respectively. The intercept parameters of the logistic model was fixed at 3 and a unit exponential prior for the model parameter was chosen. Table 10.6 displays the dose allocation and the sequential estimation of the mean posterior failure probability of each dose level. The last dose level (1.2 mg/h) that was administered consecutively from the 7th up to the 25th patient

Table 10.7 Sequential computation of the stopping criteria for the nitroglycerin trial.

Patient	Stopping criteria						
	SC1	SC3	SC5	SC6	SC7	SC8	SC9
	Stopping threshold						
	≥1.00	≥0.90	≤0.75	<0.05	<0.05	<0.05	<0.05
1	0.00	0.24	4.03	0.23	0.82	0.45	0.57
2	0.54	0.09	4.02	0.25	0.76	0.29	0.50
3	0.66	0.03	4.09	0.14	0.73	0.22	0.30
4	0.00	0.13	1.53	0.12	0.63	0.20	0.29
5	0.00	0.39	1.05	0.12	0.57	0.22	0.32
6	**1.00**	0.77	0.84	0.15	0.46	0.23	0.35
7	—	0.69	**0.74**	0.10	0.41	0.17	0.26
8	—	0.62	**0.69**	0.07	0.36	0.13	0.19
9	—	0.89	—	0.09	0.29	0.12	0.19
10	—	0.85	—	0.08	0.26	0.10	0.16
11	—	0.82	—	0.06	0.24	0.08	0.13
12	—	**0.95**	—	0.06	0.20	0.08	0.12
13	—	—	—	0.06	0.17	0.07	0.11
14	—	—	—	0.05	0.16	0.06	0.10
15	—	—	—	0.05	0.16	0.05	0.08
16	—	—	—	0.05	0.13	0.05	0.08
17	—	—	—	0.04	0.13	0.04	0.07
18	—	—	—	0.04	0.11	0.05	0.07
19	—	—	—	0.04	0.10	0.05	0.06
20	—	—	—	**0.04**	0.09	**0.04**	**0.05**
21	—	—	—	—	—	—	—
22	—	—	—	—	—	—	—
23	—	—	—	—	—	—	—
24	—	—	—	—	—	—	—
25	—	—	—	—	—	—	—

was estimated to be the MED and had an estimated mean posterior failure probability of 45 % (95 % credibility interval: 24–64 %), which is way above the target of 0.10.

As previously, we computed seven stopping criteria described above, with the stopping thresholds fixed at SC1 = 1.00, SC3 ≥ 0.90, SC5 ≤ 0.75 and SC6; SC7; SC8 and SC9 (three criteria from four) lower than 0.05 (Table 10.7).

The application of stopping rules would have been highlighted very early in the trial, since the inclusion of six patients and a mis-choice of dose levels (as indicated by the stopping criterion SC3) could have spared patients from being included in the trial at inefficacious dose levels. Moreover, this example illustrates that stopping criteria based on predictive gains (SC6, SC8 and SC9) require almost 20 patients to be fulfilled.

10.5 Conclusions

In this chapter, several stopping rules in the context of dose-finding studies, either in phase I or in phase II clinical trials, were presented. They should be distinguished according to their own stopping decision, either stopping for mis-range (SC3, SC4) of tested doses or stopping for suitable estimation of the MTD (or MED) (SC1, SC2, SC5–SC9).

From a practical point of view, several conclusive remarks could be made. Firstly, the rule SC1 based on the probability that dose allocation would not change subsequently and the rule SC3 based on the posterior probability that toxicity rates are too high (or efficacy rates too low) relative to expected rates, allow the early detection of a mis-definition of the tested dose levels, and should be applied since one or two cohorts of patients have been included. The other rules focus on the detection of a suitable estimation of the MTD (MED), based on either the credibility interval (SC5) or predictive gain of future responses (SC6–SC9), and appear to be more sensitive to the quantity of accumulated data throughout the trial.

Nevertheless, statisticians and clinicians who wish to apply stopping rules for a dose-finding trial should be able to do so. Although, as presented above, stopping rules were usually developed in the context of a particular dose-finding method, they can easily be adapted to other, nonnative, methods. For most stopping rules, softwares implementing these stopping rules are available, and can be download from researchers' websites (see Chapter 15). Finally, early stopping of dose-finding experiments is still a research open field, which only began to be explored in the last decade. Although new statistical approaches have been developed, only some of them propose stopping rules. Since the issue of sample size in dose-finding is an important point of interest, the applications of stopping rules should be investigated further in the future.

Acknowledgment

The author wishes to thank Professor Gérard Pons who allowed the Prantal trial data to be used.

References

1. P.C. O'Brien and T.R. Fleming (1979) A multiple testing procedure for clinical trials. *Biometrics*, **35**(3), 549–56.
2. T.R. Fleming (1982) One-sample multiple testing procedure for phase II clinical trials. *Biometrics*, **38**(1), 143–51.
3. S.J. Pocock (1982) Interim analyses for randomized clinical trials: the group sequential approach. *Biometrics*, **38**(1), 153–62.

4. J. Whitehead and I. Stratton (1983) Group sequential clinical trials with triangular contin-
    uation regions. *Biometrics*, **39**(1), 227–36.
5. C. Jennison and B.W. Turnbull (1984) Repeated confidence intervals for group sequential
    clinical trials. *Controlled Clin. Trials*, **5**(1), 33–45.
6. M.D. Hughes (1993) Stopping guidelines for clinical trials with multiple treatments. *Statis-
    tics in Medicine*, **12**(10), 901–15.
7. P.F. Thall and K.E. Russell (1998) A strategy for dose-finding and safety monitoring
    based on efficacy and adverse outcomes in phase I/II clinical trials. *Biometrics*, **54**(1),
    251–64.
8. J. O'Quigley and E. Reiner (1998) A stopping rule for the continual reassessment method.
    Biometrika, **85**, 741–8.
9. J.M. Heyd and B.P. Carlin (1999) Adaptive design improvements in the continual reassess-
    ment method for phase I studies. *Statistics in Medicine*, **18**(11), 1307–21.
10. S. Zohar and S. Chevret (2001) The continual reassessment method: comparison
    of Bayesian stopping rules for dose-ranging studies. *Statistics in Medicine*, **20**(19),
    2827–43.
11. J. O'Quigley (2002) Continual reassessment designs with early termination. *Biostatistics*,
    3(1), 87–99.
12. S. Zohar and S. Chevret (2003) Phase I (or phase II) dose-ranging clinical trials: proposal
    of a two-stage Bayesian design. *J. Biopharmaceutical Statistics*, **13**(1), 87–101.
13. P. Armitage (1969) Sequential analysis in therapeutic trials, *Ann. Rev. Medicine*, **20**, 425–
    30.
14. P. Armitage (1975) *Sequential Medical Trials*, 2nd edn, Blackwell Scientific Publications,
    Oxford.
15. S.J. Pocock (1978) Size of cancer clinical trials and stopping rules. *Br. J. Cancer*, **38**(6),
    757–66.
16. B. Freedman (1987) Equipoise and the ethics of clinical research. *N. Engl J. Medicine*,
    317(3), 141–5.
17. M. Baum, J. Houghton and K. Abrams (1994) Early stopping rules – clinical perspectives
    and ethical considerations. *Statistics in Medicine*, **13**, (13–14), 1459–69; discussion, 1471–
    2.
18. R.J. Lilford and J. Jackson (1995) Equipoise and the ethics of randomization. *J. R. Soc.
    Medicine*, **88**(10), 552–9.
19. C.R. Palmer and W.F. Rosenberger (1999) Ethics and practice: alternative designs for
    phase III randomized clinical trials. *Controlled Clin. Trials*, **20**(2), 172–86.
20. F. Gifford (2000) Freedman's 'clinical equipoise' and 'sliding-scale all-dimensions-
    considered equipoise'. *J. Med. Philosophy*, **25**(4), 399–426.
21. C. Weijer, S.H. Shapiro and K. Cranley Glass (2000) For and against: clinical equipoise
    and not the uncertainty principle is the moral underpinning of the randomised controlled
    trial. *Br. Med. J.*, **321**(7263), 756–8.
22. M.D. Hughes and S.J. Pocock (1988) Stopping rules and estimation problems in clinical
    trials. *Statistics in Medicine*, **7**(12), 1231–42.
23. N.L. Geller and S.J. Pocock (1987) Interim analyses in randomized clinical trials: ramifi-
    cations and guidelines for practitioners. *Biometrics*, **43**(1), 213–23.
24. E. Bellissant and J. Benichou and C. Chastang (1994) A comparison of methods for phase
    II cancer clinical trials: advantages of the triangular test, a group sequential method. *Lung
    Cancer*, **10** (Suppl.1), S105–15.

25. S. Todd, A. Whitehead, N. Stallard and J. Whitehead (2001) Interim analyses and sequential designs in phase III studies. *Br. J. Clin. Pharmacology*, **51**(5), 394–9.

26. J. Whitehead (1992) *The Design and Analysis of Sequential Clinical Trials*, 2nd edn, Ellis Horwood Limited, Chichester.

27. D.A. Berry and C.H. Ho (1988) One-sided sequential stopping boundaries for clinical trials: a decision-theoretic approach. *Biometrics*, **44**(1), 219–27.

28. E.L. Korn, K.F.Yu and L.L. Miller (1993) Stopping a clinical trial very early because of toxicity: summarizing the evidence. *Controlled Clin. Trials*, **14**(4), 286–95.

29. K.A. Cronin, L. S. Freedman, R. Lieberman, H. L. Weiss, S. W. Beenken and G. J. Kelloff (1999) Bayesian monitoring of phase II trials in cancer chemoprevention. *J. Clin. Epidemiology*, **52**(8), 705–11.

30. N. Stallard, J. Whitehead, S. Todd and A. Whitehead (2001) Stopping rules for phase II studies. *Br. J. Clin. Pharmacology*, **51**(6), 523–9.

31. D. J. Spiegelhalter, L. S. Freedman and M. K. Parmar (1993) Applying Bayesian ideas in drug development and clinical trials. *Statistics in Medicine*, **12**(15–16), 1501–11; discussion, 1513–7.

32. S.L. George, C. Li, D.A. Berry and M.R. Green (1994) Stopping a clinical trial early: frequentist and Bayesian approaches applied to a CALGB trial in non-small-cell lung cancer. *Statistics in Medicine*, **13**(13–14), 1313–27.

33. D.A. Berry, M.C. Wolff and D. Sack (1994) Decision making during a phase III randomized controlled trial. *Controlled Clin. Trials*. **15**(5), 360–78.

34. G.L. Rosner and D.A. Berry (1995) A Bayesian group sequential design for a multiple arm randomized clinical trial. *Statistics in Medicine*, **14**(4), 381–94.

35. S.J. Pocock and M.D. Hughes (1990) Estimation issues in clinical trials and overviews. *Statistics in Medicine*, **9**(6), 657–71.

36. L. S. Freedman and D. J. Spiegelhalter (1992) Application of Bayesian statistics to decision making during a clinical trial. *Statistics in Medicine*, **11**(1), 23–35.

37. P.F. Thall, R.M. Simon and E.H. Estey (1996) New statistical strategy for monitoring safety and efficacy in single-arm clinical trials. *J. Clin. Oncology*, **14**(1), 296–303.

38. D.J. Spiegelhalter, J.P. Myles, D.R. Jones and K.R. Abrams (2000) Bayesian methods in health technology assessment: a review. *Health Technol. Assess.*, **4**(38), 1–130.

39. E.L. Korn, D. Midthune, T.T. Chen, L.V. Rubinstein, M.C. Christian and R.M. Simon (1994) A comparison of two phase I trial designs. *Statistics in Medicine*, **13**(18), 1799–806.

40. J. O'Quigley, M. Pepe and L. Fisher (1990) Continual reassessment method: a practical design for phase I clinical trials in cancer. *Biometrics*, **46**(1), 33–48.

41. Y. Zhou and J. Whitehead (2002) Practical implementation of Bayesian dose-escalation procedures. Technical report, MPS.

42. T.B. Dougherty, V.H. Porche and P.F. Thall (2000) Maximum tolerated dose of nalmefene in patients receiving epidural fentanyl and dilute bupivacaine for postoperative analgesia. *Anesthesiology*, **92**(8), 1010–16.

43. M. de Spirlet, J.M. Treluyer, S. Chevret, E. Rey, M. Tournaire, D. Cabrol and G. Pons (2004) Tocolytic effects of intravenous nitroglycerin. *Fundamentals Clin. Pharmacology*, **18**(2), 207–13.

44. M.J. Ratain, R. Mick, R.L. Schilsky and M. Siegler (1993) Statistical and ethical issues in the design and conduct of phase I and II clinical trials of new anticancer agents. *J. Natl Cancer Inst.*, **85**(20), 1637–43.

45. S.G. Arbuck (1996) Workshop on phase I study design. Ninth NCI/EORTC New Drug Development Symposium, Amsterdam, March 12, 1996, *Ann. Oncology*, **7**(6), 567–73.

46. Y. Zhou (2004) Choice of designs and doses for early phase trials. *Fundamentals Clin. Pharmacology*, **18**(3), 373–8.

47. D. Faries (1994) Practical modifications of the continual reassessment method for phase I cancer clinical trials. *J. Biopharmaceutical Statistics*, **4**(2), 147–64.

48. S.N. Goodman, M.L. Zahurak and S. Piantadosi (1995) Some practical improvements in the continual reassessment method for phase I studies. *Statistics in Medicine*, **14**(11), 1149–61.

49. M. Gasparini and J. Eisele (2000) A curve-free method for phase I clinical trials. *Biometrics*, **56**(2), 609–15.

50. N. Ishizuka and Y. Ohashi (2001) The continual reassessment method and its applications: a Bayesian methodology for phase I cancer clinical trials. *Statistics in Medicine*, **20**(17–18), 2661–81.

51. D.M. Potter (2002) Adaptive dose finding for phase I clinical trials of drugs used for chemotherapy of cancer. *Statistics in Medicine*, **21**(13), 1805–23.

52. J.O'Quigley, M.D. Hughes and T. Fenton (2001) Dose-finding designs for HIV studies. *Biometrics*, **57**(4), 1018–29.

53. A. Ivanova (2003) A new dose-finding design for bivariate outcomes. *Biometrics*, **59**(4), 1001–7.

54. P.F. Thall, J.J. Lee, C.H. Tseng and E.H. Estey (1999) Accrual strategies for phase I trials with delayed patient outcome. *Statistics in Medicine*, **18**(10), 1155–69.

55. P.F. Thall, E.H. Estey and H.G. Sung (1999) A new statistical method for dose-finding based on efficacy and toxicity in early phase clinical trials. *Investigational New Drugs*, **17**(2), 155–67.

11

Dose-finding with delayed binary outcomes in cancer trials

Ying Kuen Cheung

Department of Biostatistics, Mailman School of Public Health, Columbia University, New York, USA

11.1 Introduction

This chapter reviews and discusses dose-finding methods for delayed toxicity outcomes in the context of phase I clinical trials in oncology, although the implications may also hold for efficacy endpoints and other diseases. A primary objective of a phase I clinical trial is to identify a maximum dose that is tolerated in a patient population. Storer and DeMets [1] define the maximum tolerated dose (MTD) as some percentile of the tolerance distribution with respect to some prespecified clinical toxicities. Since then, a wide range of phase I designs has been proposed to target this percentile interpretation of the MTD (e.g., see Storer [2], O'Quigley, Pepe and Fisher [3] and Babb, Rogatko and Zacks [4]. Cheung [5] discusses the practical advantages of using this MTD definition. Subsequently, Cheung and Chappell [6] acknowledge that such a percentile should be related to a given duration of time. This realization is important when late toxicities are expected. In treating cancer patients, late toxicities may arise on three occasions corresponding to the different natures of therapies:

Statistical Methods for Dose-Finding Experiments Edited by S. Chevret
© 2006 John Wiley & Sons, Ltd

1. *Toxicities during an extended chemotherapy.* To maximize therapeutic benefits, chemotherapy is often given over several courses, implying months of observations. This extended treatment strategy is crucial, for instance, in treating infants with leukemia to prevent relapse of the disease. To evaluate treatment safety that is relevant to further use of the regimen, we should control toxicity probability by the end of the entire treatment.

2. *Late-onset toxicities.* In radiation therapy for patients with localized prostate cancer or lung cancer, complications of normal tissues may occur several months after treatment. An adequate follow-up window for each patient should thus be allowed for observation of late-onset toxicities.

3. *Chronic or consequential toxicities.* Severe graft-versus-host disease (GVHD) is a major morbidity causing death after bone marrow transplantation. GVHD is said to be chronic if it is not resolved by day 100 after transplant. Thus, the evaluation of the chronic GVHD rate involves a time window of at least 100 days.

Existing phase I designs for cancer trials are outcome-adaptive in dose-escalation for ethical reasons because these trials are conducted in patients. The majority of these designs facilitate escalation (or de-escalation) based on binary toxic outcomes. As a result, accrual may be suspended until all current patients have been completely followed for the entire observation window. Apparently, repeated accrual suspension imposes excessive administrative burdens and an impractically long trial duration when toxicities are related to months of observations.

In Section 11.2, I will review some current approaches that deal with late toxicities. Among the several proposals, I will focus on the time-to-event approach in the rest of the article. In particular, Section 11.3 reviews the time-to-event continual reassessment method (TITE-CRM [6]). It is an extension of the continual reassessment method (CRM [3]). The CRM has proved to be efficient for dose-finding in cancer trials with short-term toxicities. More importantly, it has drawn attention in the medical community and has begun to impact on phase I practice. The original proposal of the TITE-CRM was intended to serve as a simple extension of the CRM so as to enhance its practicality. In Section 11.3, I will also describe an attempt to improve the method. To illustrate the operating characteristics of the TITE-CRM, I will present a numerical example in Section 11.4 and some simulation results in Section 11.5. Patient dropouts will also be considered in these illustrations.

Cheung and Chappell's [6] method is applicable to situations 1 and 2. For situations with chronic toxicities (3), implementation of the time-to-event approach follows the same principle of probability decomposition. Section 11.6 will outline the general approach. This chapter ends with a discussion in Section 11.7 and some bibliographic notes in Section 11.8.

11.2   Review of current practice

The standard practice in phase I trials follows the principle whereby three patients are treated at each nontoxic level and up to six at each level showing toxicity. Then the dose level immediately below the level with over 33 % toxicity estimates the MTD. A number of authors have pointed out that the standard design has poor statistical properties (e.g. reference [1]). Another problem in practice is a potentially long trial duration when late toxicities are of interest. The idea of continual reassessment is a breakthrough in phase I methodology; however, it does not address the timeliness problem. On the contrary, the CRM requires a longer trial duration than the standard method because it takes in one patient at a time, and hence potentially increases the number of interim suspension. This is indeed a major criticism of the method [7]. To evade the timeliness problem, investigators usually go about dose-escalation on the basis of short-term and acute toxicities. In a multicourse treatment, for example, it is common to increase the dose for the next three patients (in accord with the standard design) when there is no toxic outcome among the current group after their first course of treatment. By doing so, we underestimate the harm that a dose will incur when late toxicities are not negligible.

11.2.1   Group CRM

A simple remedy to the CRM is to accrue small groups of patients at a time. Goodman, Zahurak and Piantadosi [8] examine the performance of the group CRM. By using size 3, the group CRM will require comparable length to the standard design with minimal effects on accuracy. This approach is simple and often useful. However, the reduction in duration may not be adequate for practical purposes when the observation window is long. Suppose we plan to accrue 24 patients in groups of 3 patients, each of whom is to be followed for 6 months. Having to wait for complete follow-up of the current cohorts, the group CRM will require about 4 years to complete the trial.

11.2.2   Look-ahead methods

Thall et al. [9] study a look-ahead strategy used in conjunction with the CRM. The method enumerates all possible outcomes of current incompletely followed patients. If all outcomes point to the same recommendation for the next arriving patient, he (she) will be treated at the recommended dose; otherwise, the patient will be turned away. This further cuts down trial duration, although reduction due to grouping seems to be more substantial (see Figure 2 in reference [9]).

Hüsing et al. [10] formalize the look-ahead procedure via an excess recruitment function and apply it to shorten trial duration by the standard design. If the excess recruitment is evaluated to be larger than the number of needed patients in the current cohort, the new arriving patient will be admitted to the current cohort; otherwise, the patient will be turned away. In effect, the modified design follows the same escalation rules as the standard design with expanded cohort sizes. For an observation window of 6 months, the reduction in trial duration varies, and may be up to about 30 % relative to the standard method (see Table 2 in reference [10]).

11.2.3 Time-to-event methods

The contributions of Cheung and Chappell [6] are to define the MTD with respect to a time window and to recognize that toxicities occur randomly within the window. The authors thus introduce the TITE-CRM and use a weight function to incorporate time-to-toxicity of the patients in dose-escalation decisions during the trial. The weight is an increasing function of the follow-up time of the patient: a toxicity-free patient at his (her) fifth month is given a larger weight for a nontoxic outcome than another patient at his (her) first month. Likewise, a patient with a complete follow-up will be given a weight of 1. The following section will give the probabilistic interpretation of the weight function and outline the estimation procedure.

Finally, it may be noteworthy that Hüsing *et al.* [10] propose to evaluate the excess recruitment function based on the hazards ratio of the times-to-toxicity and the censoring process. Their approach differs from the TITE-CRM and considers a different set of decisions (i.e. accrual suspension or treatment at the current cohort). However, incorporation of the times-to-toxicity appears to be a natural approach to exploit the information available in a phase I trial.

11.3 Basic methods

11.3.1 The CRM

In a typical phase I trial setting, binary responses $\mathbf{Y}$ are observed at doses $d_1, \ldots, d_K$. The CRM assumes a single-parameter model $F(d, \beta)$ to describe the dose-toxicity relationship. With the first N observations, an estimate $\hat{\beta}_N$ of the model parameter is computed so that the next patient is assigned dose level $\arg\min_k |F(d_k, \hat{\beta}_N) - p_T|$, where p_T is the target probability of toxicity. An estimation of β can be based on the likelihood

$$\prod_{i=1}^{N} F(d_{k_i}, \beta)^{Y_i} \left[1 - F(d_{k_i}, \beta)\right]^{1-Y_i},$$

where Y_i is the indication of toxic response for the ith patient and k_i is the dose level assigned to him (her).

11.3.2 The TITE-CRM

The TITE-CRM considers a weighted dose-toxicity model $\hat{\omega} F(d; \beta)$ for $0 \leq \hat{\omega} \leq 1$, where $\hat{\omega}$ is a monotone increasing function of a patient's follow-up. Under this modeling framework, β can be estimated at any time based on the working likelihood

$$\prod_{i=1}^{N} \left[\hat{\omega}_{iN} F(d_{k_i}, \beta)\right]^{Y_{iN}} \left[1 - \hat{\omega}_{iN} F(d_{k_i}, \beta)\right]^{1-Y_{iN}}, \tag{11.1}$$

where Y_{iN} and $\hat{\omega}_{iN}$ are respectively the indication of toxic response for the ith patient and the weight assigned to this observation prior to the entry of the $(N + 1)$th patient. Suppose each patient is to be followed up to a fixed time window T. Let X_i be the time-to-toxicity of the ith patient and C_{iN} be the follow-up time. Then, for $C_{iN} \leq T$,

$$\Pr(X_i \leq C_{iN} | k_i) = \Pr(X_i \leq C_{iN} \mid X_i \leq T; k_i) \Pr(X_i \leq T | k_i) \equiv \omega_{iN} F(d_{k_i}, \beta);$$

(11.2)

i.e. the weight $\hat{\omega}_{iN}$ can be viewed as an estimate of the conditional distribution ω at time C_{iN} and the dose-response curve F is identified with the distribution function of X_i at time T. In other words, equation (11.1) is a likelihood function based on conditionally independent current status data.

Motivated by simplicity, Cheung and Chappell [6] focus on the linear weight function $\hat{\omega}_{iN}^{\text{lin}} = C_{iN}/T$ and show the consistency of the TITE-CRM under conditions that do not depend on the underlying distribution of time-to-toxicity X_i. The only additional assumption is that the number of incomplete observations is small when compared to the number of enrolled patients N. At small samples, simulation indicates that the linear weight is adequate in many situations.

Cheung and Chappell [6] also mention adaptive weighting schemes in brief; i.e. a functional form of the weight function is determined by accrued observations. In light of the probabilistic interpretation (11.2), a natural approach is to approximate the conditional probability ω_{iN} with the empirical quantity. We may further smooth out the empirical estimate with a prior, in order to avoid undue variation early in the trial when there are few observations. Thus, define an estimator for ω_{iN} as a weighted average of the empirical component and a prior component:

$$\hat{\omega}_{iN}^{\text{adp}} = \frac{m}{m + m_0} \left[\frac{\#\{j : X_j \leq C_{iN}, C_{jN} \geq T\}}{\#\{j : X_j \leq T, C_{jN} \geq T\}} \right] + \frac{m_0 \, \omega_{iN}^0}{m + m_0},$$

where $m = \#\{j : X_j \leq T, C_{jN} \geq T\}$ is the number of toxicities observed among completely followed patients. We may give the prior component ω_{iN}^0 a small weight by setting $m_0 = 1$. Generally, the linear weight serves as a reasonable prior component, i.e. $\omega_{iN}^0 = \hat{\omega}_{iN}^{\text{lin}}$. This type of estimator was used in Cheung and Thall [11].

11.3.3 A dose-adjusted weight

It is conceivable that toxicity may occur more rapidly with higher treatment intensity. To adjust for this dose effect in the estimation of ω_{iN}, one could apply $\hat{\omega}_{iN}^{\text{adp}}$ separately for each dose. However, this simple extension fails to borrow strength among doses. In addition, this approach is not feasible if a continuum of doses is to be used (cf. reference [12]). In the following, the steps to elicit dose-adjusted weights under mild assumptions are outlined.

Denote $\theta_k(s) = \Pr(X_i \leq s | k)$ so that $\omega_{iN} \equiv \theta_{k_i}(C_{iN})/\theta_{k_i}(T)$. Then assume for every given s that $\theta_k(s) \leq \theta_{k+1}(s)$ for $k = 1, \ldots, K - 1$. An implication on the times-to-toxicity of the doses is that their distribution functions do not cross, i.e. stochastic ordering of the times-to-toxicity. We do not impose other parametric assumptions on the relationship between dose and time-to-toxicity.

Define $U_i(s) = I(X_i \leq s)$ so that $E\{U_i(s)\} = \theta_{k_i}(s)$ and further let

$$U_k^+(s) = \sum_{k_i=k} U_i(s) I(C_{iN} \geq T) \quad \text{and} \quad n_k = \sum_{k_i=k} I(C_{iN} \geq T).$$

Under the stochastic ordering assumption, $\theta_k(s)$ can be estimated by the isotonic quantities $\theta_1(s) \leq \cdots \leq \hat{\theta}_K(s)$ based on $\{U_k^+(s), n_k\}$ for $k = 1, \ldots, K$. In particular, one could apply the pool-adjacent violators algorithm (PAVA) in Ayer *et al.* [13]:

1. If $U_1^+(s)/n_1 \leq \cdots \leq U_K^+(s)/n_K$, then $\hat{\theta}_k(s) = U_k^+(s)/n_k$ for $k = 1, \ldots, K$.

2. If $U_k^+(s)/n_k \geq U_{k+1}^+(s)/n_{k+1}$, then treat d_k and d_{k+1} as a combined dose by letting $\hat{\theta}_k(s) = \hat{\theta}_{k+1}(s)$. The ratios $U_k^+(s)/n_k$ and $U_{k+1}^+(s)/n_{k+1}$ are replaced in the sequence $\{U_j^+(s)/n_j\}_{j=1}^K$ by the single ratio $[U_k^+(s) + U_{k+1}^+(s)]/(n_k + n_{k+1})$, obtaining an ordered set of only $K - 1$ ratios.

3. Repeat until we obtain an ordered set of ratios that are monotone nondecreasing.

Consequently, we may estimate ω_{iN} with

$$\hat{\omega}_{iN}^{\text{adj}} = \frac{m_{k_i}}{m_{k_i} + m_0} \left[\frac{\hat{\theta}_{k_i}(C_{iN})}{\hat{\theta}_{k_i}(T)} \right] + \frac{m_0 \, \omega_{iN}^0}{m_{k_i} + m_0},$$

where m_k is the number of toxicities observed among completely followed patients at dose level k.

As a technical note, the dose-adjusted weight $\hat{\omega}_{iN}^{\text{adj}}$ is consistent for ω_{iN} as n_{k_i} grows large. Consequently, the TITE-CRM with these weights is consistent without requiring a small number of incomplete observations when compared to N (the proof is available from the author upon request). Thus, this adaptive weight is superior to the nonadaptive weight in an asymptotic sense. At small samples, on the other hand, extra variation induced due to estimation of ω_{iN} may undermine the benefit of adaptive weighting. Thus, it is important to evaluate various weight functions via simulation.

11.4   An example

11.4.1   Intensity modulated radiation therapy (IMRT)

Intensity modulated radiation therapy (IMRT) given to prostate cancer patients may cause morbidity at the rectum. An acute gastrointestinal (GI) toxicity is scored as grade 2 or higher if it occurs within 6 months of treatment completion and requires medication (see Storey *et al.* [14] for a detailed definition). Figure 11.1 gives a graphical summary of the acute GI toxicity experience of 63 patients treated at the Radiation Oncology Department at Columbia University between March 2000 and February 2002. The logistic regression fit on the left panel suggests a positive dose-toxicity relationship, although the 95 % pointwise confidence intervals are quite wide. All 63 patients were followed for at least 6 months after radiation

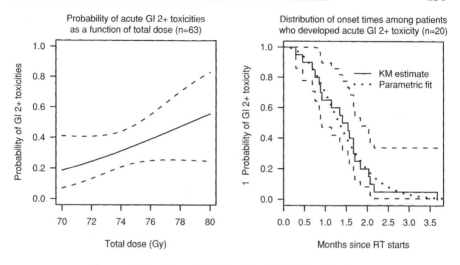

Figure 11.1   Parametric fit of the IMRT toxicity data.

therapy was complete; 20 patients experienced grade 2 or higher acute GI toxicities. The times to toxicity onset did not seem to depend on dose, provided that toxicity occurred; therefore, I summarized the 20 onset times with an empirical survival function (right panel). Taylor [15] also estimated the conditional distribution of times to morbidity without adjusting for the radiation dose in a mixture model. In addition, these 20 toxicity times were well fit by a three-parameter generalized odds rate model [16]: $\hat{\Pr}(X > t) = [1 + 0.275(t/1.48)^{2.46}]^{-1/0.275}$ (also shown in the right panel of Figure 11.1).

11.4.2   A single trial

In the following, the TITE-CRM will be illustrated in the context of an IMRT trial. The therapy lasts about 2 months for each patient. Thus, the historical data (Figure 11.1) suggests that if an acute GI toxicity occurs, it usually occurs during treatment, and rarely takes place beyond the 3 month window. However, in accord with the definition of acute toxicities, let us define the observation window $T = 8$ months since treatment begins. Based on clinicians' opinions, the MTD is defined to be the 40th percentile.

Five dose levels and the following model were considered:

$$F(d_k, \beta) = d_k^{\exp \beta}, \qquad \text{for } k = 1, \ldots, 5,$$

where $d_1 = 0.30$, $d_2 = 0.40$, $d_3 = 0.50$, $d_4 = 0.59$ and $d_5 = 0.67$. The prior distribution on the model parameter β is the standard normal. The posterior mean of β based on the working likelihood (11.1) is used to facilitate the dose assignment at every step. The doses d_k are scaled so that dose level 2 is the prior MTD and that the

Table 11.1 Current status of 18 patients on the arrival of patient 19 in a simulated trial.

Patient	Level	Toxic	Time	Follow-up	Weight			
i	k_i	$Y_{i,19}$	X_i	$C_{i,19}$	$\hat{\omega}_{i,19}^{\text{hist}}$	$\hat{\omega}_{i,19}^{\text{lin}}$	$\hat{\omega}_{i,19}^{\text{adp}}$	$\hat{\omega}_{i,19}^{\text{adj}}$
1	2	1	1.05	8.00	1.00	1.00	1.00	1.00
2	2	0	—	8.00	1.00	1.00	1.00	1.00
3	1	0	—	8.00	1.00	1.00	1.00	1.00
4	1	0	—	8.00	1.00	1.00	1.00	1.00
5	1	0	—	8.00	1.00	1.00	1.00	1.00
6	2	0	—	3.38	0.983	0.422	0.884	0.856
7	2	1	2.30	8.00	1.00	1.00	1.00	1.00
8	3	1	2.13	8.00	1.00	1.00	1.00	1.00
9	4	0	—	7.21	0.999	0.902	0.980	0.902
10	2	0	—	5.66	0.999	0.707	0.941	0.927
11	2	1	1.50	6.99	1.00	1.00	1.00	1.00
12	2	1	1.80	8.00	1.00	1.00	1.00	1.00
13	3	0	—	8.00	1.00	1.00	1.00	1.00
14	2	0	—	7.47	0.999	0.934	0.987	0.983
15	2	0	—	6.60	0.999	0.825	0.965	0.956
16	2	0	—	5.98	0.999	0.747	0.949	0.937
17	3	0	—	3.01	0.968	0.377	0.875	0.688
18	3	0	—	2.08	0.830	0.260	0.452	0.380

CRM (and TITE-CRM) will converge to a dose inside the 35–45th percentile range (see Cheung and Chappell [17] for a discussion on model sensitivity in the CRM).

Table 11.1 summarizes the partial outcomes of a simulated trial by the TITE-CRM with the historical weight based on the IMRT data: $\hat{\omega}_{iN}^{\text{hist}} = Q_{\text{hist}}(C_{iN})$, where

$$Q_{\text{hist}}(t) = \frac{1 - \left[1 + 0.275(t/1.48)^{2.46}\right]^{-1/0.275}}{1 - \left[1 + 0.275(T/1.48)^{2.46}\right]^{-1/0.275}}, \qquad \text{for } t \leq T.$$

While I deliberately chose this simulated trial so that the numerical examples will be illustrative, the outcome features of this trial are also typical in many simulation replicates. The trial starts at dose level 2. The toxicity outcomes and onset times are generated according to scenario 3A (Section 11.5) under which dose level 3 is the MTD and the times to toxicity follow Q_{hist} so that the historical weight function $\hat{\omega}_{iN}^{\text{hist}}$ is correctly specified.

Table 11.1 shows the current status of the first 18 patients upon the arrival of a new patient; the rest of the trial (size 30) stays at level 3 (the true MTD). Patient dropouts are allowed in the simulation (e.g. patient 10) and it is possible that a toxic outcome is observed before dropout (e.g. patient 11). Up to this point of the trial, most patients have been treated at level 2 because there are several toxic outcomes at level 2. This illustrates the large binomial variation when a relatively large toxicity probability ($p_T = 0.40$) is targeted; note that a binomial variance attains maximum at $p = 0.50$. In contrast, if we target at a lower percentile, we may anticipate with a higher probability that all outcomes are nontoxic at lower doses before reaching the target. Thus, with a higher toxicity tolerance (as long as $p_T < 0.50$), one will need a larger sample to attain comparable accuracy. More importantly, the TITE-CRM manages to escalate to level 3 by borrowing strength from the low toxicity rates at other doses. This example illustrates that the TITE-CRM is cautious and yet flexible in escalation.

11.4.3 Weight calculation

In the above simulated trial (Table 11.1), the dose assignment to patient 19 may change if we consider other weighting schemes than the historical weights $\hat{\omega}_{i,19}^{\text{hist}}$. When we look at the weights assigned to nontoxic patients, the adaptive schemes ($\hat{\omega}_{i,19}^{\text{adp}}$ and $\hat{\omega}_{i,19}^{\text{adj}}$) are quite close to the correct historical function, while the linear weight function gives much smaller weights. (Note that the weight assigned to a toxic outcome does not affect the likelihood estimation based on (11.1), and so is given a weight of 1 by convention.) As a result, using $\hat{\omega}_{i,19}^{\text{lin}}$ for escalation will result in a more cautious escalation plan than the other schemes; patient 19 would have received dose level 2 if the linear weight were used at this point in the simulated trial. The operating characteristics of the TITE-CRM with various weight functions will be further evaluated via simulation in a later section. Here, I will show the numerical steps to evaluate the adaptive weights. I will focus on patients 6 and 18 in Table 11.1.

Firstly, for the adaptive weight $\hat{\omega}_{i,19}^{\text{adp}}$ consider the linear weight $\hat{\omega}_{i,19}^{\text{lin}}$ as the prior component and set $m_0 = 1$. Since $C_{6,19} = 3.38$, $\#\{j : X_j \leq 3.38, C_{j,19} \geq 8\} = 4$ and $m = 4$, we obtain

$$\hat{\omega}_{6,19}^{\text{adp}} = \left(\frac{4}{4+1}\right)\left(\frac{4}{4}\right) + \left(\frac{1}{4+1}\right)(0.422) = 0.884.$$

In the same fashion, we have

$$\hat{\omega}_{18,19}^{\text{adp}} = \left(\frac{4}{4+1}\right)\left(\frac{2}{4}\right) + \left(\frac{1}{4+1}\right)(0.260) = 0.452.$$

Next, to calculate the dose-adjusted weights for patients 6 and 18, we need to evaluate the isotonic function $\hat{\theta}_k(s)$ at $s = C_{6,19}, C_{18,19}$ and T for each k involved. We may tabulate the steps, as follows:

s	$\dfrac{U_1^+(s)}{n_1}$	$\dfrac{U_2^+(s)}{n_2}$	$\dfrac{U_3^+(s)}{n_2}$		$\hat{\theta}_1(s)$	$\hat{\theta}_2(s)$	$\hat{\theta}_3(s)$
$C_{6,19} = 3.38$	0/3	3/4	1/2	PAVA	0/3	4/6	4/6
$C_{18,19} = 2.08$	0/3	2/4	0/2	$\Longrightarrow$	0/3	2/6	2/6
$T = 8.00$	0/3	3/4	1/2		0/3	4/6	4/6

Also, since $k_6 = 2$, $k_{18} = 3$, $m_2 = 3$ and $m_3 = 1$, we have

$$\hat{\omega}_{6,19}^{adj} = \left(\frac{3}{3+1}\right)\left(\frac{4/6}{4/6}\right) + \left(\frac{1}{3+1}\right)(0.422) = 0.856,$$

$$\hat{\omega}_{18,19}^{adj} = \left(\frac{1}{1+1}\right)\left(\frac{2/6}{4/6}\right) + \left(\frac{1}{1+1}\right)(0.260) = 0.380.$$

Although calculation of dose-adjusted weights introduces additional complexity in programming, the increase in computation intensity is trivial. Rather, the more important question is whether this weighting scheme will improve the performance of the TITE-CRM.

11.5 Simulation results

Simulation is a major tool to evaluate the operating characteristics of a design. In the following, some representative simulation results are presented to illustrate the features of various weight functions. Practical guidelines will be derived based on these results.

In the simulation, the CRM design setup was the same as the trial described in Section 11.4.2, except that different weight functions were used to incorporate times-to-toxicity into estimation. Specifically, I considered the linear weight $\hat{\omega}_{iN}^{lin}$, the adaptive weight $\hat{\omega}_{iN}^{adp}$ and the dose-adjusted weight $\hat{\omega}_{iN}^{adj}$, along with the respective correct weight functions in the following scenarios (see Figure 11.2).

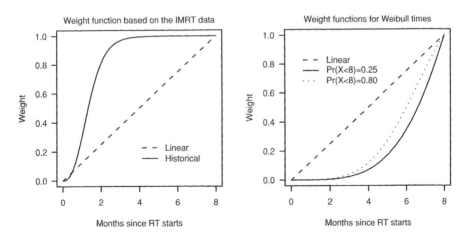

Figure 11.2   The correct weight functions under the two simulation scenarios.

11.5.1   The IMRT scenarios

In the first set of scenarios, the toxicity outcomes were generated based on the IMRT historical data. I first determined if a patient had a toxic response; if so, the toxicity onset would be generated according to Q_{hist}. Five toxicity probability configurations were considered in the simulation, designated as configuration kA, for $k = 1, \ldots, 5$. Dose level k was the true MTD (i.e. the 40th percentile) in configuration kA so that these five configurations encompassed all possibilities. The neighboring doses of the MTD were the 25th and the 55th percentiles. In light of the binomial variation and limited sample size ($N = 30$), identifying the correct dose was a rather challenging task.

I also considered the possibility of patient dropouts in each simulated trial: a dropout indicator was generated for each patient with a prespecified probability and, if applicable, a uniform variate on the interval $(0, 8)$ would be drawn as the time of dropout. Patient arrivals were simulated as a Poisson process with a rate of one per month.

Table 11.2 shows the distribution of the MTD recommendation based on 2000 replicates. The results for the CRM are also shown as references of accuracy, which should be interpreted in the light of timeliness: the TITE-CRM takes a median of 37 months to complete a trial of size 30, while the CRM needs about 20 years. A CRM with groups of 3 will take 80 months.

The accuracy of the TITE-CRM is competitive to that of the CRM under this scenario. When there is no dropout, the TITE-CRM with the correct historical weight $\hat{\omega}_{iN}^{\text{hist}}$ has virtually the same recommendation distributions and toxicity incidence as the CRM. The linear weight function is slightly inferior in terms of the proportion of correct recommendation, but induces fewer toxicities on average. Under this scenario, the linear weight function assigns less weights to the nontoxic outcomes than the historical weight (see the left panel of Figure 11.2), and thus results in a more conservative escalation plan, as illustrated in Section 11.4.3. The adaptive weight functions $\hat{\omega}_{iN}^{\text{adp}}$ and $\hat{\omega}_{iN}^{\text{adj}}$ seem to provide a good compromise of accuracy and toxicity under this scenario, although the former appears to be slightly better.

When using the CRM that considers binary toxic outcomes, an unbiased procedure to handle dropouts is to treat them as inevaluable and exclude them from analysis for escalation; i.e. if a patient has toxicity but leaves the study before the end of time T, this piece of information will not be used in reassessing the dose-toxicity curve. Apparently, this is inefficient because essential information is ignored. The simulation results confirm the notion: the accuracy of the CRM suffers under a 30 % dropout rate.

In contrast, the TITE-CRM accommodates patient dropouts naturally without artificially discarding information. With the historical weight, it maintains virtually the same accuracy as in the case of no dropout. There is loss in efficiency with the adaptive functions, but not as much as with the CRM, e.g. configuration 4A.

Under dropout, there is a noticeable decrease in accuracy for the linear weight under configurations 4A and 5A, where the higher doses are the MTD. In addition,

Table 11.2   The percentages of recommendation for each dose under five toxicity scenarios based on the IMRT data. The MTD is defined as the 40th percentile.

Dose level	Toxicity probability	No dropout					30 % dropout				
		crm	hist	lin	adp	adj	crm	hist	lin	adp	adj
Configuration 1A											
1	0.40	0.81	0.81	0.76	0.79	0.79	0.78	0.81	0.85	0.79	0.79
2	0.55	0.18	0.18	0.22	0.20	0.20	0.20	0.18	0.14	0.20	0.19
3	0.70	0.01	0.01	0.02	0.01	0.01	0.02	0.01	0.01	0.02	0.02
4	0.75	0.00	0.00	0.00	0.00	0.00	0.00	0.00	0.00	0.00	0.00
5	0.80	0.00	0.00	0.00	0.00	0.00	0.00	0.00	0.00	0.00	0.00
#toxicities		13.7	13.9	13.1	13.3	13.3	14.0	13.9	12.9	13.4	13.2
Configuration 2A											
1	0.25	0.23	0.25	0.18	0.20	0.20	0.28	0.24	0.28	0.21	0.20
2	0.40	0.56	0.55	0.54	0.56	0.56	0.51	0.55	0.53	0.55	0.54
3	0.55	0.20	0.20	0.26	0.23	0.22	0.20	0.20	0.18	0.23	0.24
4	0.70	0.01	0.01	0.02	0.01	0.02	0.01	0.01	0.01	0.02	0.01
5	0.80	0.00	0.00	0.00	0.00	0.00	0.00	0.00	0.00	0.00	0.00
#toxicities		12.0	12.2	10.9	11.5	11.2	12.1	12.1	10.3	11.1	10.8
Configuration 3A											
1	0.20	0.03	0.02	0.03	0.02	0.02	0.06	0.04	0.07	0.04	0.04
2	0.25	0.23	0.25	0.20	0.20	0.19	0.24	0.24	0.30	0.22	0.23
3	0.40	0.56	0.56	0.51	0.58	0.55	0.50	0.55	0.48	0.52	0.54
4	0.55	0.18	0.17	0.25	0.19	0.22	0.19	0.17	0.16	0.22	0.19
5	0.80	0.00	0.01	0.01	0.01	0.01	0.01	0.01	0.00	0.01	0.01
#toxicities		11.4	11.3	9.5	10.5	10.2	11.3	11.3	9.4	10.1	9.8
Configuration 4A											
1	0.15	0.00	0.00	0.00	0.00	0.00	0.01	0.00	0.01	0.00	0.01
2	0.20	0.03	0.03	0.05	0.03	0.04	0.06	0.04	0.09	0.05	0.05
3	0.25	0.24	0.24	0.22	0.22	0.24	0.27	0.24	0.29	0.24	0.25
4	0.40	0.55	0.53	0.50	0.54	0.51	0.45	0.52	0.45	0.51	0.49
5	0.55	0.18	0.20	0.23	0.21	0.21	0.21	0.20	0.17	0.20	0.20
#toxicities		10.6	10.4	9.9	9.5	9.1	10.3	10.4	8.5	9.1	8.7
Configuration 5A											
1	0.15	0.00	0.00	0.00	0.00	0.00	0.01	0.00	0.01	0.00	0.00
2	0.20	0.02	0.02	0.04	0.02	0.03	0.04	0.02	0.07	0.04	0.05
3	0.20	0.06	0.08	0.12	0.09	0.11	0.09	0.07	0.16	0.11	0.12
4	0.25	0.25	0.26	0.26	0.26	0.28	0.27	0.24	0.29	0.30	0.30
5	0.40	0.66	0.64	0.59	0.62	0.58	0.60	0.66	0.48	0.55	0.54
#toxicities		9.2	8.9	7.6	8.0	7.8	8.9	8.9	7.3	7.8	7.5

when we look closely at the recommendation distributions, there is a shift towards the lower doses. These again are due to the fact that the linear function underweighs (Figure 11.2) the nontoxic dropouts at the end of the trial.

11.5.2   The late-onset scenarios

The second set of simulation represents scenarios when toxicity tends to occur later in the observation window. As in Cheung and Chappell [6], I considered the Weibull model (shape 4) for times-to-toxicity: the scale parameters were chosen corresponding to the toxicity probabilities at $T = 8$ under the same set of five toxicity configurations, designated as configuration kB, for $k = 1, \ldots, 5$.

Under these scenarios, the correct weight function for dose d_k differs from others and depends on the scale parameter λ_k:

$$\hat{\omega}_{iN}^{\text{weib}} = \frac{1 - \exp\left(-\lambda_k C_{iN}^4\right)}{1 - \exp\left(-\lambda_k T^4\right)}.$$

Some examples are plotted in the right panel of Figure 11.2. Other than the onset time distribution and the correct weight functions, simulation and design parameters were the same as before. The results are shown in Table 11.3.

The correct weight function $\hat{\omega}_{iN}^{\text{weib}}$ does not guarantee a higher proportion of correct recommendations than other weighting schemes (configuration 5B). However, because it appropriately assigns small weights to early observations (Figure 11.2), the escalation plan is relatively conservative. With similar reasoning, using the linear weight results in more toxicities, and using the adaptive functions attenuates its agressiveness in escalation. Looking at Table 11.3 more closely, we see the trend that the TITE-CRM becomes less toxic in relation to the CRM as the scenario becomes less toxic. This trend holds even for the linear weight. Therefore, if the doses for a trial are selected in a somewhat conservative manner, which is usually the case in practice, the safety of the TITE-CRM is comparable to the CRM. In terms of accuracy, the CRM is slightly superior to the TITE-CRM. The advantage diminishes, however, if we anticipate patient dropouts during the trial.

11.5.3   Practical guidelines

The use of the correct weight function is advantageous for different reasons in different situations. When toxicity tends to occur early in the window (configurations A), it performs better than other weighting schemes in terms of accuracy, especially when there are dropouts. When there is a late-onset tendency (configurations B), it prevents erroneous escalation before any toxicities are seen. In reality, the shape of the onset time distribution may not be known. The simulation results suggest that the adaptive function $\hat{\omega}_{iN}^{\text{adp}}$ serves as a reasonable compromise between accuracy and safety. In the simulation, the adaptive weight is an average of an empirical component and the

Table 11.3 The percentages of recommendation for each dose under five toxicity scenarios with Weibull event times. The MTD is defined as the 40th percentile.

Dose level	Toxicity probability	No dropout					30 % dropout				
		crm	weib	lin	adp	adj	crm	weib	lin	adp	adj
Configuration 1B											
1	0.40	0.81	0.82	0.85	0.83	0.83	0.77	0.79	0.73	0.81	0.82
2	0.55	0.18	0.17	0.15	0.16	0.16	0.21	0.19	0.24	0.17	0.17
3	0.70	0.01	0.01	0.01	0.01	0.01	0.02	0.02	0.03	0.02	0.02
4	0.75	0.00	0.00	0.00	0.00	0.00	0.00	0.00	0.00	0.00	0.00
5	0.80	0.00	0.00	0.00	0.00	0.00	0.00	0.00	0.00	0.00	0.00
#toxicities		13.7	14.3	15.6	15.1	15.3	14.0	14.5	16.2	15.6	15.9
Configuration 2B											
1	0.25	0.23	0.25	0.34	0.29	0.32	0.29	0.28	0.26	0.33	0.36
2	0.40	0.57	0.55	0.51	0.52	0.52	0.49	0.48	0.48	0.46	0.47
3	0.55	0.20	0.20	0.15	0.18	0.16	0.20	0.22	0.23	0.20	0.16
4	0.70	0.01	0.02	0.01	0.01	0.01	0.02	0.02	0.02	0.02	0.01
5	0.80	0.00	0.00	0.00	0.00	0.00	0.00	0.00	0.00	0.00	0.00
#toxicities		12.1	12.2	13.8	13.1	13.4	12.1	12.1	14.6	13.5	14.0
Configuration 3B											
1	0.20	0.02	0.03	0.04	0.04	0.04	0.05	0.05	0.04	0.07	0.08
2	0.25	0.23	0.24	0.33	0.31	0.31	0.25	0.26	0.25	0.29	0.31
3	0.40	0.58	0.55	0.51	0.51	0.50	0.50	0.49	0.51	0.47	0.47
4	0.55	0.16	0.18	0.12	0.14	0.14	0.19	0.19	0.19	0.16	0.13
5	0.80	0.00	0.01	0.00	0.00	0.00	0.01	0.02	0.01	0.01	0.01
#toxicities		11.4	11.2	12.9	12.2	12.6	11.3	11.1	13.6	12.4	13.0
Configuration 4B											
1	0.15	0.00	0.00	0.00	0.00	0.00	0.01	0.01	0.00	0.01	0.01
2	0.20	0.03	0.04	0.04	0.04	0.03	0.05	0.06	0.03	0.06	0.06
3	0.25	0.25	0.26	0.28	0.26	0.27	0.27	0.25	0.21	0.26	0.28
4	0.40	0.54	0.51	0.51	0.51	0.51	0.45	0.47	0.48	0.46	0.46
5	0.55	0.18	0.20	0.17	0.19	0.18	0.21	0.22	0.28	0.22	0.19
#toxicities		10.7	9.7	11.4	10.8	11.1	10.4	9.5	11.7	10.8	11.3
Configuration 5B											
1	0.15	0.00	0.00	0.00	0.00	0.00	0.01	0.01	0.00	0.00	0.00
2	0.20	0.02	0.02	0.01	0.01	0.01	0.03	0.04	0.01	0.03	0.02
3	0.20	0.05	0.10	0.06	0.07	0.07	0.09	0.11	0.05	0.07	0.07
4	0.25	0.24	0.30	0.30	0.28	0.28	0.26	0.31	0.23	0.29	0.30
5	0.40	0.68	0.58	0.64	0.64	0.65	0.61	0.54	0.72	0.61	0.61
#toxicities		9.2	7.9	9.1	8.8	9.0	8.9	7.7	9.3	8.8	9.1

linear weight. If the investigators have certain expectations *a priori*, one may consider a more realistic prior component with a larger m_0.

The dose-adjusted weight $\hat{\omega}_{iN}^{adj}$, in theory the most flexible function, requires a moderate number of observations at each dose level before the data can take over to give a precise estimate for the true weight ω_{iN}. Therefore, it depends much on the prior component, at least with the typical sample size seen in a phase I trial. Besides, the adaptive function $\hat{\omega}_{iN}^{adp}$ is more comprehensible and easier to program.

This simulation study is intended to be comparative within a class of TITE-CRM, with the CRM as the referenced method. Certainly, more conservative dose-finding endeavor can be achieved by other logistical modifications, such as starting at the lowest dose [18] and adopting a two-stage design [6].

As a final note, the TITE-CRM reduces to the CRM when we look at short-term toxicities. With long-term toxicities, the TITE-CRM incorporates the likelihoods of toxicity for incompletely followed patients into estimation of the dose-toxicity curve. Recommended escalations based on such partial information may be erroneous at times and thus the TITE-CRM may be less accurate than the CRM with the same number of enrolled patients. As the simulation results suggest, the efficiency loss is not severe, even when the study time is reduced by over 80 % to a practical duration. Furthermore, if we anticipate patient dropouts, the incorporation of the time-to-toxicity seems to be the natural approach to preserve information. This aspect of the data may not be restored by other existing approaches such as grouping.

11.6 Chronic toxicities

This section outlines the formulation for chronic toxicity so as to illustrate the principle of the time-to-event approach. Readers who are interested in detailed development and generalization are referred to Cheung and Thall [11]. Let X be the onset time of toxicity and Z be the time when toxicity is resolved. A toxic outcome is classified as chronic if it is not resolved by a certain time T. In other words, a chronic toxicity is defined as a composite event $B = \{X \leq T < Z\}$. Let the nondecreasing function $F(d_k, \beta)$ of dose d_k model the probability of B. Thus, one may conduct dose-finding using the CRM by waiting for T time units to get a complete outcome for each patient. To incorporate time-to-toxicity, consider the probability decomposition, for $C_{iN} \leq T$:

$$\Pr(X_i \leq C_{iN} < Z_i | k_i) = \omega_{i1N} \Pr(B_i | k_i) + \omega_{i2N} \Pr(\bar{B}_i | k_i),$$

where $\bar{B}$ denotes the complement of B, and

$$\omega_{i1N} = \Pr(X_i \leq C_{iN} < Z_i | B_i, k_i) = \Pr(X_i \leq C_{iN} | B_i, k_i),$$
$$\omega_{i2N} = \Pr(X_i \leq C_{iN} < Z_i | \bar{B}_i, k_i) = \Pr(X_i \leq C_{iN} \leq Z_i \leq T | \bar{B}_i, k_i)$$

are the respective conditional probabilities of the observable event $\{X_i \leq C_{iN} < Z_i\}$, given that B_i and $\bar{B}_i$ would have occurred had follow-up of patient i been complete.

Define Y_{iN} as the indication of $\{X_i \leq C_{iN} < Z_i\}$ prior to the entry of the $(N + 1)$th patient, and let the weights $\hat{\omega}_{i1N}$ and $\hat{\omega}_{i2N}$ be respective estimates for ω_{i1N} and ω_{i2N}.

Then, model reassessment can be based on the working likelihood

$$\prod_{i=1}^{N} \Delta_{iN}(\beta)^{Y_{iN}} [1 - \Delta_{iN}(\beta)]^{1-Y_{iN}}, \tag{11.3}$$

where $\Delta_{iN}(\beta) = \hat{\omega}_{i1N} F(d_{k_i}, \beta) + \hat{\omega}_{i2N} [1 - F(d_{k_i}, \beta)]$. Estimation for ω_{i1N} and ω_{i2N} can be gone about analogously to $\hat{\omega}_{iN}^{adp}$: the empirical component is replaced by the corresponding observed proportion and the prior component by a simple function that respects certain constraints (see Cheung and Thall [11] for computation details).

11.7   Discussion

Patients eligible for phase I cancer trials are usually very sick, so it is realistic to accept patient dropouts. With incomplete observations, estimation with the working likelihoods of (11.1) and (11.3) is valid under the assumption that dropouts are independent of toxicity. If a patient is withdrawn for reasons due to intolerable toxicity, this outcome should be counted as toxic. It may appear that this complicates matters. However, the current practice (with a binary toxicity endpoint) to discard these patients as invaluable is implicitly imposing independence. The time-to-event approach provides a natural framework to use partial information from dropouts without an additional assumption.

Chronic toxicity is defined as a composite event that involves more than one time variable. Subsequently, a dose-toxicity model can be postulated for this composite event. This modeling strategy focuses on the parameter of interest, $\Pr(B|k)$, and circumvents joint estimation of the bivariate variables (X, Z). There is an increasing trend that dose-finding is based on composite endpoints that involve both efficacy and toxicity (e.g. reference [19]). The time-to-event approach can be applied to extend these methods when the endpoints require a long observation window.

To conclude, this chapter presents and demonstrates the TITE-CRM as a useful dose-finding method with late toxicities. It has three practical advantages:

1. substantial reduction in the study duration with minimal effects on accuracy and safety;

2. efficient use of information from dropouts;

3. flexibility in accommodating composite endpoints such as a chronic event.

In addition, the time-to-event approach is versatile in that it can be applied to other likelihood-based dose-finding methods for short-term toxicities, such as escalation with overdose control [4].

11.8   Bibliographic notes

Cheung and Thall [11] classify binary outcomes arising in clinical settings into three event cases. Late-onset toxicity discussed in the earlier sections is a case 1 simple event, while chronic toxicity (Section 11.6) is a case 2 composite event. The authors detail estimation in a general framework.

Authors who consider dose-finding with times to toxicity or longitudinal toxicity data include Hüsing *et al.* [10] and Legedza and Ibrahim [20]. Each works on different objectives: the former attempts to reduce the study time with the standard design, while the latter endeavors to identify individual MTDs and population MTDs at multiple time points.

References

1. B. Storer and D. DeMets (1987) Current phase I/II designs: are they adequate? *J. Clin. Res. Drug Development*, **1**, 121–30.
2. B.E. Storer (1989) Design and analysis of phase I clinical trial. *Biometrics*, **45**(3), 925–37.
3. J. O'Quigley, M. Pepe and L. Fisher (1990) Continual reassessment method: a practical design for phase I clinical trials in cancer. *Biometrics*, **46**(1), 33–48.
4. J. Babb, A. Rogatko and S. Zacks (1998) Cancer phase I clinical trials: efficient dose escalation with overdose control. *Statistics in Medicine*, **17**(10), 1103–20.
5. Y.K. Cheung (2000) Dose escalation strategies for phase I clinical trials with late-onset toxicities. PhD Dissertation, University of Wisconsin, Madison, Wisconsin.
6. Y.K. Cheung and R. Chappell (2000) Sequential designs for phase I clinical trials with late-onset toxicities. *Biometrics*, **56**(4), 1177–82.
7. E.L. Korn, D. Midthune, T.T. Chen, L.V. Rubinstein, M.C. Christian and R.M. Simon (1994) A comparison of two phase I trial designs. *Statistics in Medicine*, **13**(18), 1799–806.
8. S.N. Goodman, M.L. Zahurak and S. Piantadosi (1995) Some practical improvements in the continual reassessment method for phase I studies. *Statistics in Medicine*, **14**(11), 1149–61.
9. P.F. Thall, J.J. Lee, C.H. Tseng and E.H. Estey (1999) Accrual strategies for phase I trials with delayed patient outcome. *Statistics in Medicine*, **18**(10), 1155–69.
10. J. Hüsing, W. Sauerwein, K. Hideghéty and K.H. Jöckel (2001) A scheme for a dose-escalation study when the event is lagged. *Statistics in Medicine*, **20**(22), 3323–34.
11. Y.K. Cheung and P.F. Thall (2002) Monitoring the rates of composite events with censored data in phase II clinical trials. *Biometrics*, **58**(1), 89–97.
12. S. Piantadosi, J.D. Fisher and S. Grossman (1998) Practical implementation of a modified continual reassessment method for dose-finding trials. *Cancer Chemotherapy and Pharmacology*, **41**(6), 429–36.
13. M. Ayer, H.D. Brunk, G.M. Ewing, W.T. Reid and E. Silverman (1955) An empirical distribution function for sampling with incomplete information. *Ann. Math. Statistics*, **26**, 641–7.
14. M.R. Storey, A. Pollack, G. Zagars, L. Smith, J. Antolak and I. Rosen (2000) Complications from radiotherapy dose escalation in prostate cancer: preliminary results of a randomized trial. *Int. J. Radiation Oncology Biology Physics*, **48**(3), 635–42.
15. J.M. Taylor (1995) Semi-parametric estimation in failure time mixture models. *Biometrics*, **51**(3), 899–907.
16. D.M. Dabrowska and K.A. Doksum (1988) Estimation and testing in a two-sample generalized odds-rate model. *J. Am. Statistical Assoc.*, **83**, 744–9.

17. Y.K. Cheung and R. Chappell (2002) A simple technique to evaluate model sensitivity in the continual reassessment method. *Biometrics*, **58**(3), 671–4.

18. D. Faries (1994) Practical modifications of the continual reassessment method for phase I cancer clinical trials. *J. Biopharmaceutical Statistics*, **4**(2), 147–64.

19. P.F. Thall and K.E. Russell (1998) A strategy for dose-finding and safety monitoring based on efficacy and adverse outcomes in phase I/II clinical trials. *Biometrics*, **54**(1), 251–64.

20. A.T.R. Legedza and J.G. Ibrahim (2000) Longitudinal design for phase I clinical trials using the continual reassessment method. *Controlled Clin. Trials*, **21**(6), 574–88.

12

Dose-finding based on multiple ordinal toxicities in phase I oncology trials

B. Nebiyou Bekele and Peter F. Thall

M. D. Anderson Cancer Center, Department of Biostatistics and Applied Mathematics, The University of Texas, Houston, Texas, USA

12.1 Introduction

This chapter describes a method for designing a phase I trial of presurgical gemcitabine with external beam radiation (EBR) for patients with soft tissue sarcoma. We planned the trial with a team of three oncologists who share responsibility for trial conduct. Each patient receives a fixed dose of 50 cGy EBR and one of 10 doses of gemcitabine, 100, 200, ... or 1000 mg/m^2. In most oncology chemotherapy trials, the patient is at risk of several different types of toxicity, each occurring at several possible severity levels, or 'grades'. The toxicities used as a basis for dose-finding in the sarcoma trial are summarized in Table 12.1.

The 'severity weight' listed beside each grade of each toxicity will play a central role in all that follows. Because toxicity evaluation may take up to six weeks, to facilitate trial conduct the cohort size is allowed to vary between three and four. If the first three patients in a cohort have had all of their toxicities evaluated before the next is accrued, then that cohort is considered complete, the next dose is chosen and treatment of the next cohort at that dose is begun. The safety constraint is imposed

Statistical Methods for Dose-Finding Experiments Edited by S. Chevret
© 2006 John Wiley & Sons, Ltd

Table 12.1 Toxicities and elicited severity weights used in the sarcoma trial.

	Type of toxicity	Grade	Severity weight
1	Myelosuppression without fever	3	1.0
		4	1.5
	Myelosuppression with fever	3	5.0
		4	6.0
2	Dermatitis	3	2.5
		4	6.0
3	Liver	2	2.0
		3	3.0
		4	6.0
4	Nausea/vomiting	3	1.5
		4	2.0
5	Fatigue	3	0.5
		4	1.0

that no untried dose may be skipped when escalating. The planned sample size is 36 patients.

The methodology that we developed for dose-finding in the sarcoma trial was motivated by several concerns. The oncologists requested that the dose-finding method account for the fact that the toxicities that they had identified are not equally important and do not occur independently. For example, fatigue and nausea/vomiting are likely to occur together, as are myelosuppression and fever. It was also requested that the method utilize the information that a low-grade toxicity observed at a given dose, while not dose-limiting, is a warning that a higher grade of that toxicity is more likely to occur at a higher dose.

Most phase I oncology trials require multiple toxicities to be monitored. These often include transient conditions such as fatigue, nausea/vomiting, myelosuppression, thrombocytopenia, fever, infection, organ dysfunction and irreversible toxicities such as permanent organ damage or death. In general, the different toxicities do not occur independently. Most phase I protocols define 'toxicity' as the occurrence at grade 3 or 4 of several listed toxicities. While it is convenient to reduce each toxicity to the binary variable, typically calling grades 0, 1 or 2 'no toxicity' and grades 3 or 4 'toxicity', this discards useful information. For example, if several patients experience a grade 2 toxicity at dose level k, then a typical method based on the above binary variable would escalate to level $k + 1$ as if no toxicities had occurred at level k. We will use a probability model that distinguishes between grades 0, 1 and 2, rather than combining them as the event 'no toxicity', in order to obtain a more reliable basis for predicting the jump from grade 2 to grade 3 or higher as the dose is increased from k to $k + 1$. Moreover, if each type of toxicity is defined as a binary variable, defining 'toxicity' as the maximum of these indicators implicitly assumes that the different toxicities are equally important. For example, this definition does not distinguish between a patient with grade 3 fatigue and a patient who has suffered complete kidney failure.

To develop a dose-finding method for the sarcoma trial addressing all of these issues, we characterized patient outcome as a vector of correlated, ordinal-valued toxicities by applying the multivariate ordinal probit regression model of Chen and Dey [1], extended to allow the different toxicities to have different numbers of severity levels. To address the oncologists' concern that different toxicities may not be equally important, we elicited numerical weights to characterize the clinical importance of each severity level of each type of toxicity. We defined a patient's total toxicity burden to be the sum of the weights of all toxicities experienced by that patient. Given the elicited weights, we identified a target total toxicity burden by constructing a set of hypothetical dose-toxicity scenarios and asking the physicians, in each scenario, whether they would escalate, repeat the same dose, or de-escalate for the next cohort. Our method assigns each cohort the dose having the posterior mean total toxicity burden closest to the target.

We developed the methodology during several meetings with the oncologists. Initially, they specified five toxicities, myelosuppression (M), fever, dermatitis (D), nausea/vomiting (N) and fatigue (F), as binary variables. We defined 'toxicity' conventionally as the maximum of these five indicators, and we constructed a continual reassessment method (CRM) design [2] with a target toxicity rate of 30 %. At the second meeting the issues arose that M is positively associated with fever and that M with fever (M^+) is a much more severe event than M without fever (M^-). This led us to combine M and fever into the five-level ordinal toxicity $M_0 < M_3^- < M_4^- < M_3^+ < M_4^+$, where the grade is denoted by a subscript and M_0 denotes no M of grade > 2. This also motivated the physicians to refine the other toxicities, making D, N and F each a trinary variable, and they also added liver toxicity (L), defined as a four-level variable (Table 12.1). We next elicited numerical weights to quantify the clinical importance of each level of each type of toxicity. We repeated this process over the course of several meetings, until the algorithm made decisions that the oncologists considered clinically sensible under all of the scenarios. Additional details are given in reference [3].

12.2 Probability model

For the sarcoma trial, since the decision is which dose to give the next cohort, we required a model characterizing how the probabilities of the severity levels of each type of toxicity vary with dose, while also accounting for association among the toxicities. Since we use computer simulation of the trial design to examine its operating characteristics and calibrate its parameters before actual trial conduct, and this requires the model to be fit thousands of times, computational tractability is also an essential requirement. To obtain a model with all of these properties for the sarcoma trial, we applied the Bayesian multivariate ordinal probit model of Chen and Dey [1]. This belongs to the general class of models, developed by Albert and Chib [4] and Chib and Greenberg [5], that uses a vector of correlated latent Gaussian variables to induce association among discrete outcomes.

Let $Y = (Y_1, \ldots, Y_J)$ denote the vector of ordinal toxicities. The jth type of toxicity, Y_j, takes on one of the $C_j + 1$ values $\{y_{j,0}, y_{j,1}, \ldots, y_{j,C_j}\}$, where $y_{j,k}$ is the kth most severe level for $k = 0, \ldots, C_j$. In the sarcoma trial, $J = 5$. For example, if Y_j is dermatitis then $C_j = 2$, $y_{j,0}$ denotes grade 0, 1 or 2, $y_{j,1}$ denotes grade 3 and $y_{j,2}$ denotes grade 4. Binary Y_j corresponds to $C_j = 1$. We replaced each raw gemcitabine dose d by $x = \log(d/1000)$, and we will refer to x as the 'dose'. Association among the Y_j values is induced by the vector $\mathbf{Z}^{J \times 1} = (Z_1, \ldots, Z_J)$ of correlated latent variables, assumed to be multivariate normal with $E(Z_j) = \beta_{j,0} + x\beta_{j,1}$ for each j, all variances equal to 1 and correlation matrix $\mathbf{\Omega}$. Thus, $E(\mathbf{Z}) = \mathbf{X}\boldsymbol{\beta}$, where $\mathbf{X}^{J \times 2J}$ is the block diagonal matrix with the jth block $(1\ x)$ and $\boldsymbol{\beta}^{2J \times 1} = (\beta_{1,0}, \beta_{1,1}, \ldots, \beta_{J,0}, \beta_{J,1})$. The latent variable vector $\mathbf{Z}$ determines the observed vector $\mathbf{Y}$ as follows:

$$Y_j = y_{j,k} \text{ if } \gamma_{j,k} \leq Z_j < \gamma_{j,k+1} \text{ for } k = 0, 1, \ldots, C_j \text{ and } j = 1, \ldots, J,$$

where the cut-off parameters $\boldsymbol{\gamma}_j^{C_j \times 1} = (\gamma_{j,1}, \ldots, \gamma_{j,C_j})$ satisfy the constraint $-\infty = \gamma_{j,0} < \gamma_{j,1} < \cdots < \gamma_{j,C_j} < \gamma_{j,C_j+1} = +\infty$. Denote $A_{j,k} = (\gamma_{j,k}, \gamma_{j,k+1}]$ and $\boldsymbol{\gamma}^{C_+ \times 1} = (\gamma_1, \ldots, \gamma_J)$, where $C_+ = C_1 + \cdots + C_J$. The variance–covariance matrix $\mathbf{\Omega}$ of $\mathbf{Z}$ must be its correlation matrix to ensure identifiability of the posteriors, which also requires that $\gamma_{j,1} \equiv 0$. Since $\gamma_{j,0} = -\infty$, $\gamma_{j,C_j+1} = +\infty$ and $\gamma_{j,1} = 0$, if $C_j > 1$ there are only $C_j - 1$ random cut-point parameters. Thus, while $\boldsymbol{\gamma}$ has C_+ entries, it actually contains only $\Sigma_{j=1}^{J} \mathbf{1}(C_j > 1)(C_j - 1)$ parameters, where $\mathbf{1}(A)$ indicates the event A. Denoting the vector of all model parameters by $\boldsymbol{\theta}$, the marginal distribution of Y_j for a patient treated with dose x is

$$
\begin{aligned}
\pi_{j,k}(x, \boldsymbol{\theta}) &= \Pr(Y_j = y_{j,k} \mid x, \boldsymbol{\theta}) \\
&= \Phi\{\gamma_{j,k+1} - (\beta_{j,0} + \beta_{j,1}x)\} - \Phi\{\gamma_{j,k} - (\beta_{j,0} + \beta_{j,1}x)\}, \quad (12.1)
\end{aligned}
$$

where Φ is the standard normal cumulative distribution function (CDF). Denote $\boldsymbol{\pi}_j(x, \boldsymbol{\theta}) = (\pi_{j,1}(x, \boldsymbol{\theta}), \ldots, \pi_{j,C_j}(x, \boldsymbol{\theta}))$ for each $j = 1, \ldots, J$ and $\boldsymbol{\pi}(x, \boldsymbol{\theta}) = (\boldsymbol{\pi}_1(x, \boldsymbol{\theta}), \ldots, \boldsymbol{\pi}_J(x, \boldsymbol{\theta}))$. Let $\phi_{\mathbf{W}}(\cdot \mid \boldsymbol{\mu}, \boldsymbol{\Sigma})$ denote the probability distribution function (PDF) of a multivariate normal random vector $\mathbf{W}$ with mean vector $\boldsymbol{\mu}$ and variance–covariance matrix $\boldsymbol{\Sigma}$, and write $\mathbf{W} \sim N(\boldsymbol{\mu}, \boldsymbol{\Sigma})$. For a given vector $k = (k_1, \ldots, k_J)$ of toxicity severity levels, the corresponding outcome is $y(k) = (y_{1,k_1}, \ldots, y_{J,k_J})$. This would arise from the J-dimensional set $A(k, \boldsymbol{\gamma}) = A_{1,k_1} \times \cdots \times A_{J,k_J}$ of $\mathbf{Z}$ values. A single patient's likelihood contribution may be written as

$$
\mathcal{L}(\mathbf{Y} \mid \boldsymbol{\gamma}, \boldsymbol{\beta}, \boldsymbol{\Omega}, x) = \prod_{k_1=0}^{C_1} \cdots \prod_{k_J=0}^{C_J} \left\{ \int_{A(k, \boldsymbol{\gamma})} \phi_Z(z \mid \mathbf{X}\boldsymbol{\beta}, \boldsymbol{\Omega}) \, dz \right\}^{\mathbf{1}[Y=y(k)]}. \quad (12.2)
$$

This shows how $\mathbf{Z}$ induces association among the elements of $\mathbf{Y}$ through $\boldsymbol{\Omega}$. Let $x_{(i)}$ denote the ith patient's dose and $\mathbf{X}_i$ the corresponding matrix. The likelihood for n patients is obtained by substituting $\mathbf{Y} = \mathbf{Y}_i$, $x = x_{(i)}$ and $\mathbf{X} = \mathbf{X}_i$ in equation (12.2) and taking the product over $i = 1, \ldots, n$.

Denote the $J(J-1)/2$ unique off-diagonal elements of $\boldsymbol{\Omega}$ by $\rho = (\rho_{1,2}, \rho_{1,3}, \ldots, \rho_{J-1,J})$ and the cut-point parameter vector by $\boldsymbol{\gamma}$, so that the model parameter vector is $\boldsymbol{\theta} = (\boldsymbol{\beta}, \boldsymbol{\gamma}, \boldsymbol{\rho})$. *A priori*, we assume that $\boldsymbol{\beta} \sim N(\boldsymbol{\mu}, \boldsymbol{\Sigma})$ and require $\Pr(\beta_{j,1} > 0) = 1$ for all $j = 1, \ldots, J$. Thus, the prior of $\boldsymbol{\beta}$ is $2J$-variate normal with J entries truncated at 0, but $\boldsymbol{\mu}$ and $\boldsymbol{\Sigma}$ correspond to the untruncated $2J$-variate normal. This ensures that $\Pr(Y_j > y_{j,k} \mid x) = 1 - \Phi\{\gamma_{j,k} - (\beta_{j,0} + \beta_{j,1}x)\}$ increases with x for each j and $k > 1$, so that toxicity severity increases with dose. For each j with $C_j > 1$, we will assume that $\{\gamma_{j,2}, \ldots, \gamma_{j,C_j}\}$ follow independent, uninformative priors on $[0, 10]$, with each $g(\boldsymbol{\gamma}_j) \propto 1$, subject to the constraint $0 < \gamma_{j,2} < \gamma_{j,3} < \cdots < \gamma_{j,C_j}$. The upper limit 10 on the support of the distribution of the $\gamma_{j,k}$ values is chosen for numerical convenience, since the probability mass beyond 10 is negligible. We assume that the elements of $\boldsymbol{\rho}$ are iid (independent and identically distributed) $N(0, 1000)$, truncated to the support $[-1, +1]$, with $\boldsymbol{\Omega}$ positive definite. A method for eliciting a prior on $\boldsymbol{\beta}$ will be described in Section 12.4.

12.3 Dose-finding algorithm

If doses are to be chosen based on multivariate toxicity data, inevitably some form of dimension reduction must be carried out to obtain a real-valued criterion to use as a basis for deciding whether to escalate, stay at the same dose or de-escalate. The following dose-finding method incorporates medical knowledge into the dimension reduction process. The method requires positive-valued numerical severity weights, characterizing the importance of each level of each type of toxicity, and these must be elicited from the physicians. For each $j = 1, \ldots, J$, denote the elicited weight of toxicity type j at severity level $y_{j,k}$ by $w_{j,k}$, and denote $\boldsymbol{w}_j = (w_{j,1}, \ldots, w_{j,C_j})$ and $\boldsymbol{w}^{C_+ - J \times 1} = (\boldsymbol{w}_1, \ldots, \boldsymbol{w}_J)$, subject to the admissibility requirement $0 = w_{j,0} < w_{j,1} < w_{j,2} < \cdots < w_{j,C_j}$. If the physicians assign the same weights to adjacent severity levels $w_{j,k} = w_{j,k+1}$, then levels k and $k + 1$ of Y_j should be combined. The numerical domain of the $w_{j,k}$ values is arbitrary since the method is invariant to the weights' multiplicative scale, and we used the interval 0 to 10 in the sarcoma trial because the physicians were comfortable with this range.

The severity weight of Y_j for a patient given dose x is the random variable W_j taking on the value $w_{j,k}$ with probability $\pi_{j,k}(x, \boldsymbol{\theta})$. This replaces the observed toxicity Y_j with the weight-valued variable W_j, by assigning the severity category probabilities of Y_j to the corresponding elicited weights. The patient's total toxicity burden is $\mathrm{TTB} = \sum_{j=1}^{J} W_j$. The dose-finding algorithm is based on the posterior expected TTB at each dose, which takes the following form:

$$\psi(\boldsymbol{w}, x, \text{data}) = E\{E(\mathrm{TTB} \mid x, \boldsymbol{\theta}) \mid \text{data}\} = \sum_{j=1}^{J} \sum_{k=1}^{C_j} w_{j,k} E\{\pi_{j,k}(x, \boldsymbol{\theta}) \mid \text{data}\}.$$

(12.3)

It is easy to show [3] that $\psi(\boldsymbol{w}, x, \text{data})$ is increasing in x. We use $\psi(\boldsymbol{w}, x, \text{data})$ as a basis for dose-finding by eliciting a fixed target TTB value, ψ^*, from the physicians, and assigning each successive cohort the dose currently having $\psi(\boldsymbol{w}, x, \text{data})$ closest to ψ^*. For simplicity, suppress j and consider one toxicity. If $Y = y_k$ is observed at x, then the posterior of $\{\pi_1(x, \boldsymbol{\theta}), \ldots, \pi_C(x, \boldsymbol{\theta})\}$ must shift probability mass towards $\pi_k(x, \boldsymbol{\theta})$. If y_k is a high-level toxicity, i. e. if k is high in the range $1, \ldots, C$, since the w_k values are increasing in k, it follows that $\sum_{k=1}^{C} w_k \pi_k(x, \boldsymbol{\theta})$ must increase stochastically; hence it must increase in expectation given the data. By the monotonicity of $\psi(\boldsymbol{w}, x, \text{data})$ in x, this tends to decrease the next selected dose. Similarly, observation of low-level toxicities will on average increase the chosen dose.

12.4   Elicitation process

To implement the method, the physicians must specify the cohort size, c, sample size, N, doses, $\boldsymbol{d} = (d_1, \ldots, d_K)$, the toxicities to be monitored and their severity levels. Since there will be N/c cohorts available to search among the K doses, it is useful to study several feasible values of N in the computer simulations, and choose N on that basis. The physicians must specify a numerical severity weight for each level of each toxicity, within some given positive-valued numerical range, with 0 corresponding to no toxicity. The method is invariant to the particular numerical range of severity weights, so the main criterion is that the physicians should use a range with which they are comfortable. This establishes $\boldsymbol{w}$. This process may also lead the physicians to modify the toxicities, and this is a natural part of the process of establishing toxicities and severity weights.

To establish a target TTB given $\boldsymbol{d}$, Y and $\boldsymbol{w}$, ask the physicians to specify several hypothetical J-variate toxicity outcomes for m hypothetical cohorts, with the severities of the toxicities varying widely between cohorts, from 'very toxic' to 'not toxic at all'. The number of hypothetical cohorts should be large enough to obtain a reasonable representation of the range of possible toxicities and severities, but not so large that the elicitation process becomes unduly burdensome to the physicians. Toxicities having larger numbers of levels should be included in more cohorts than toxicities having fewer levels, and no single type of toxicity should be the only contributor to all of the 'very toxic' cohorts. The statisticians may suggest additional cohorts, but these must make sense clinically to the physicians. Denote the outcomes of the m hypothetical cohorts by $\boldsymbol{y}_1^* = (\boldsymbol{y}_{1,1}^*, \ldots, \boldsymbol{y}_{1,c}^*), \ldots, \boldsymbol{y}_m^* = (\boldsymbol{y}_{m,1}^*, \ldots, \boldsymbol{y}_{m,c}^*)$. For each hypothetical cohort, $r = 1, \ldots, m$, first ask the physicians whether observation of $\boldsymbol{y}_r^* = (\boldsymbol{y}_{r,1}^*, \ldots, \boldsymbol{y}_{r,c}^*)$ in the first cohort of the trial would cause them to repeat the same dose ($D_r = \text{repeat}$), escalate to a higher dose ($D_r = \text{escalate}$), or de-escalate to a lower dose ($D_r = \text{de-escalate}$) for the next cohort. Next, ask what dose, $d_r^* = d(\boldsymbol{y}_r^*)$, they would consider most likely to produce the outcomes $\boldsymbol{y}_r^*$ of that hypothetical cohort. Let $\boldsymbol{w}_{r,l}^*$ denote the severity weight vector corresponding to $\boldsymbol{y}_{r,l}^*$, for $r = 1, \ldots, m$ and $l = 1, \ldots, c$. The mean total toxicity burden of the rth hypothetical cohort is

$$\overline{\text{TTB}}_r^* = \frac{1}{c} \sum_{l=1}^{c} \sum_{j=1}^{J} w_{r,l,j}^*.$$

Denote the m ordered mean hypothetical TTB values by $\overline{\mathrm{TTB}}^*_{(1)} \leq \cdots \leq \overline{\mathrm{TTB}}^*_{(m)}$, and the corresponding vector of decisions in this order of increasing TTB values by $D_{(1)}, \ldots, D_{(m)}$. An admissible sequence of decisions ordered in this way is one consisting of a string of escalations, followed by a string of repeats, followed by a string of de-escalations. If the m decisions are not admissible then, working with the physicians, one must modify the hypothetical outcomes, elicited decisions, weights or possibly other portions of the underlying structure as appropriate. Once an admissible set of decisions is established, the target TTB is defined to be the mean of the elicited $\overline{\mathrm{TTB}}^*_r$ values for which the physicians' decision was to repeat the same dose, formally

$$\psi^* = \frac{\sum_{r=1}^m \overline{\mathrm{TTB}}^*_r \, \mathbf{1}(D_r = \mathrm{repeat})}{\sum_{r=1}^m \mathbf{1}(D_r = \mathrm{repeat})}.$$

Because ψ^* is determined from the physicians' subjective input, it is analogous to a fixed target toxicity probability specified by the physicians in the simpler case of one binary toxicity.

Since we assume vague priors on γ and ρ, only the hyperparameters μ and Σ of the prior on β must be specified. The doses $d_1^*, \ldots, d_m^*$ obtained as answers to the second question may also be used to construct a prior on β, as follows. Beginning with a vague $N(\mu^o, \Sigma^o)$ prior on β, with $\mu_{j,0}^o = 0$, $\mu_{j,1}^o = 1$, $\mathrm{var}^o(\beta_{j,0}) = \mathrm{var}^o(\beta_{j,1}) = 10\,000$ for each j, compute the posterior of β given the hypothetical data $\{d_1^*, \mathbf{y}_1^*, \ldots, d_m^*, \mathbf{y}_m^*\}$. We modified this distribution by multiplying each variance by m, the number of hypothetical cohorts, and setting each off-diagonal element of Σ equal to 0. This yielded the prior on β used at the start of the trial. As a check for internal consistency, one may assume in turn that each hypothetical cohort is the first cohort in the trial. If the algorithm's decisions are the same as those made by the physicians, then one may proceed; otherwise, the prior or possibly some other aspect of the model or design must be modified, as appropriate, so that the method properly reflects clinical practice.

12.5 Application to the sarcoma trial

The oncologists specified toxicity severity weights ranging from 0 (no clinical importance) to 6 (Table 12.1). The elicited toxicity severity weights are illustrated in Figure 12.1. Table 12.2 summarizes the 16 hypothetical cohorts used in the elicitation process for the sarcoma trial, with no toxicities of any type denoted by NT. Each toxicity is subscripted by its grade. For example, the first patient in hypothetical cohort 3, with outcomes denoted by $\mathrm{M}_3^- + \mathrm{D}_3 + \mathrm{N}_3$, experienced grade 3 myelosuppression without fever, grade 3 dermatitis and grade 3 nausea/vomiting. The description of each cohort is followed by the corresponding empirical mean TTB, the elicited decision for the next cohort and the dose considered by the physicians to be most likely to have caused the cohort's outcomes. Using the elicitation method described in Section 12.4, the three cohorts for which the decision was to repeat the same dose were 1, 9 and 16, giving a target per patient TTB of $\psi^* = (3.00 + 3.12 + 3.00)/3 = 3.04$.

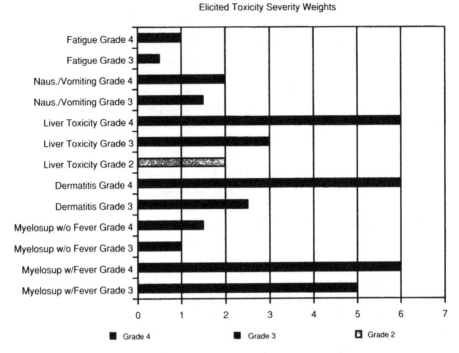

Figure 12.1   Elicited toxicity severity weights identified as clinically important by the investigators (Naus., Nausea; Myelosup, Myelosuppression).

At this writing, 18 patients have been treated and evaluated. Table 12.3 summarizes their outcomes and TTBs. The third cohort included only three patients because the toxicities of all of these three patients were evaluated before a fourth patient was available to be accrued. The first cohort was treated at 400 mg/m^2. Although $\psi(\boldsymbol{w}, 700, \text{data}_4) = 3.24$ is closest to the target $\psi^* = 3.04$, because no untried dose may be skipped when escalating, the second cohort received 500 mg/m^2. Incorporating the second cohort's data, since $\psi(\boldsymbol{w}, 600, \text{data}_8) = 2.85$ is closest to 3.04, the third cohort received 600 mg/m^2. Since $\psi(\boldsymbol{w}, 700, \text{data}_{11}) = 3.24$, the fourth cohort received 700 mg/m^2. Since $\psi(\boldsymbol{w}, 700, \text{data}_{15}) = 3.19$, the trial stayed at 700 mg/m^2. The last cohort of patients resulted in $\psi(\boldsymbol{w}, 700, \text{data}_{18}) = 3.14$, resulting in a decision to again stay at 700 mg/m^2.

For this trial, conventional dose-finding methods typically would define one binary 'toxicity' as the maximum of the indicators $\mathbf{1}$ (myelosuppression grade ≥ 3), $\mathbf{1}$ (dermatitis grade ≥ 3), $\mathbf{1}$ (liver toxicity grade ≥ 3), $\mathbf{1}$ (nausea/vomiting grade ≥ 3), $\mathbf{1}$ (fatigue grade ≥ 3). Thus, for example, a conventional method would consider a patient with grade 2 liver toxicity (TTB = 2.5) to have 'no toxicity' and a patient with grade 4 fatigue (TTB = 1) to have 'toxicity'. Furthermore, conventional methods would not distinguish the latter patient from a patient with grade 4 myelosuppression

Table 12.2 Hypothetical cohorts used to elicit the target TTB for the sarcoma trial. Myelosuppression, dermatitis, liver toxicity, fatigue and nausea/vomiting are denoted by M, D, L, F and N respectively, with the grade represented by a subscript. With myelosuppression, the presence and absence of fever are denoted by superscripted $^+$ and $^-$. NT denotes no toxicities of any type and d^* is the dose considered by the physicians most likely to have caused the cohort's outcomes.

Cohort	Outcomes	$\overline{\mathrm{TTB}}^*$	Decision	d^*
1	M_4^+, D_4, NT, NT	3.00	Repeat	400
2	M_4^-, L_3, F_4, N_4	1.88	Escalation	200
3	$M_3^- + D_3 + N_3, M_3^-, M_3^-, M_3^-$	2.00	Escalation	300
4	D_4, D_4, L_2, L_2	4.00	De-escalation	600
5	$M_3^- + F_3, M_3^- + F_3, L_2 + F_3, N_3$	2.25	Escalation	300
6	M_4^+, L_4, D_4, NT	4.50	De-escalation	700
7	D_3, D_3, NT, NT	1.25	Escalation	100
8	M_3^-, D_3, F_3, F_3	1.25	Escalation	200
9	D_3, D_4, L_2, L_2	3.12	Repeat	400
10	$M_3^+ + N_3, M_3^+ + D_3 + N_3,$ $D_3 + F_3 + N_3, F_3 + N_3$	5.50	De-escalation	800
11	$M_3^- + D_3 + F_3, F_3, F_2, N_4$	2.12	Escalation	300
12	L_3, L_3, NT, NT	1.50	Escalation	200
13	$M_3^+ + D_3 + F_4, M_3^+ + D_3 + F_4,$ $M_3^- + F_4, D_3 + F_4$	5.62	De-escalation	900
14	$M_3^- + N_3, F_4, L_2, D_3 + N_3$	2.38	Escalation	300
15	$D_4 + F_4, L_3 + F_4, L_2 + N_4, N_4$	4.25	De-escalation	600
16	$M_3^- + F_4, L_2 + F_3, M_3^- + D_3 + N_4, L_2$	3.00	Repeat	500

with fever, grade 4 dermatitis, and grade 4 liver toxicity (TTB = 18). The proposed algorithm based on the TTB with target 3.04 for $\psi(\boldsymbol{w}, x, \text{data})$ makes more sensible decisions. For example, three of the four patients in the first cohort had grade 3 myelosuppression without fever and one also has grade 3 nausea and grade 3 dermatitis, for TTB values $\{5, 1, 1, 0\}$ and empirical mean TTB = 1.75. As noted above, $\psi(\boldsymbol{w}, 700, \text{data}_4) = 3.24$ so the algorithm escalated to 500 mg/m^2. In contrast, a conventional method would score three toxicities in these four patients and de-escalate to a lower dose.

12.6 Simulation study and sensitivity analyses

12.6.1 Simulation study design

This section describes a simulation study of the sarcoma trial to assess the method's average behavior. In order to obtain a manageable set of dose-toxicity scenarios for

Table 12.3 Patient-by-patient illustration of the method in the sarcoma trial. Toxicities for the first 18 patients enrolled in the trial.

Patient	Dose	Myelosuppression	Dermatitis	Liver	Fatigue	Nausea	TTB
1	400	Gr. 3 w/o fever	Gr. 3	None	None	Gr. 3	5.0
2	400	Gr. 3 w/o fever	None	None	None	None	1.0
3	400	Gr. 3 w/o fever	None	None	None	None	1.0
4	400	None	None	None	None	None	0
5	500	None	Gr. 3	None	None	None	2.5
6	500	None	None	None	None	None	0
7	500	Gr. 3 w/o fever	Gr. 3	None	None	None	3.5
8	500	Gr. 4 w/o fever	None	Gr. 2	None	None	3.5
9	600	None	Gr. 3	None	None	None	2.5
10	600	None	None	Gr. 3	None	None	2.0
11	600	None	Gr. 3	None	None	None	2.5
12	700	Gr. 3 w/o fever	None	None	None	None	1.0
13	700	None	None	Gr. 3	None	None	3.0
14	700	None	None	None	Gr. 3	None	0.5
15	700	Gr. 4 w/o fever	Gr. 3	Gr. 2	Gr. 3	None	6.5
16	700	None	None	Gr. 3	None	None	3.0
17	700	Gr. 3 w/o fever	None	Gr. 3	None	Gr. 3	5.5
18	700	None	None	None	None	None	0

the simulations, we considered only cases where the target TTB occurred at 200, 500 or 800 mg/m^2, and we categorized the main source of toxicity as being either those having high severity (HS) weights ($w \geq 5$) or greater, or low severity (LS) weights ($w \leq 2$). The remaining toxicities, grade 3 dermatitis ($w = 2.5$) and grade 3 liver toxicity ($w = 3$), were considered intermediate and were included in either group. For each simulation scenario, the fixed probabilities were $p_{j,1,d}, \ldots,$ $p_{j,C_j,d}$, for $j = 1, \ldots, 5$ and $d = 100, \ldots, 1000$, where $p_{j,k,d} = \Pr(Y_j = y_{j,k} \mid d)$ and $p_{j,0,d} = 1 - \sum_{k=1}^{C_j} p_{j,k,d}$. These probabilities were chosen nonparametrically to satisfy $\sum_j \sum_k w_{j,k} p_{j,k,d} = 3.04$ for $d = 200$ under scenarios 1 and 2, $d = 500$ under scenarios 3 and 4 , and $d = 800$ under scenarios 5 and 6. Figure 12.2 summarizes the six scenarios graphically in terms of the TTB as a function of dose. Association among the elements of each simulated $(Y_1, \ldots, Y_5)$ was induced by first generating a sample of standard normal random variables $\mathbf{Z}^{5 \times 1}$ with specified correlation matrix, then defining the correlated uniform(0, 1) random variates $\mathbf{U}^{5 \times 1} = (\Phi(Z_1), \ldots, \Phi(Z_5))$ and then denoting $P_{j,k,d} = \sum_{r=0}^{k} p_{j,r,d}$ for $k = 0, \ldots, C_j$ and $P_{j,-1,d} = 0$, defining

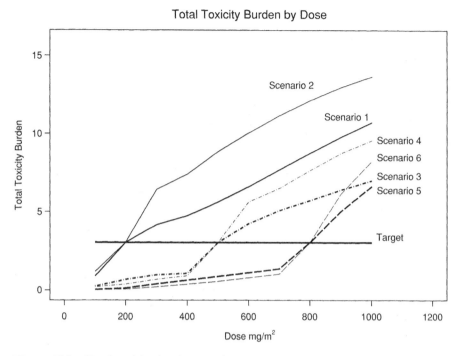

Figure 12.2 Total toxicity burden as a function of dose under each of the six dose-toxicity scenarios considered in the simulation study.

$Y_j = y_{j,k}$ if $P_{j,k-1,d} \leq U_j < P_{j,k,d}$. The correlations were elicited from the physicians in terms of the underlying toxicities. The trial was simulated 1000 times under each scenario, and each reported value is the average over these replications. We followed the computational framework developed by Albert and Chib [4] for one polytomous outcome, extended by Chib and Greenberg [5] to accommodate correlated binary outcomes and by Chen and Dey [1] to the correlated ordinal case.

For the simulation study, we evaluated the MCMC algorithm's performance using standard convergence diagnostics. A burn-in of 1000 and a chain of length 30 000, retaining every 15th sample, provided adequate convergence. Additional details are provided in Bekele and Thall (Section 12.6.1) [3].

12.6.2 Simulation results

Table 12.4 summarizes the simulation results. Under scenarios 1 and 2, where the target $\psi^* = 3.04$ is achieved at 200 mg/m^2, the starting dose of 400 mg/m^2 is unacceptably toxic. Under scenario 1, most of the toxicity is due to LS events such as L$_2$, F or N. Under scenario 2, most of the toxicity burden is due to HS toxicities such as M$^+$ or L$_4$.

Table 12.4   Simulation results for the sarcoma trial under six dose-toxicity scenarios. (LS = low severity toxicities, HS = high severity toxicities, Psel = % selected, Npats = number of patients treated).

Scenario	Main toxicities		Gemcitabine dose (mg/m²)									
			100	200	300	400	500	600	700	800	900	1000
			$\psi^* = 3.04$ at 200 mg/m²									
1	LS	Psel	1.6	93.7	4.7	0.0	0.0	0.0	0.0	0.0	0.0	0.0
		Npats	2.2	21.8	5.3	5.6	1.1	0.0	0.0	0.0	0.0	0.0
2	HS	Psel	4.1	92.0	3.8	0.0	0.0	0.0	0.0	0.0	0.0	0.0
		Npats	4.5	22.0	4.5	4.6	0.4	0.0	0.0	0.0	0.0	0.0
			$\psi^* = 3.04$ at 500 mg/m²									
3	LS	Psel	0.0	0.0	0.0	5.6	85.4	9.0	0.0	0.0	0.0	0.0
		Npats	0.0	0.0	0.0	5.6	18.5	9.7	2.1	0.1	0.0	0.0
4	HS	Psel	0.0	0.1	0.0	5.2	86.9	7.8	0.0	0.0	0.0	0.0
		Npats	0.0	0.0	0.1	6.6	20.6	7.8	1.0	0.0	0.0	0.0
			$\psi^* = 3.04$ at 800 mg/m²									
5	LS	Psel	0.0	0.0	0.0	0.0	0.0	0.3	10.4	80.7	8.3	0.2
		Npats	0.0	0.0	0.0	4.0	4.0	4.0	5.6	11.4	5.9	1.0
6	HS	Psel	0.0	0.0	0.0	0.0	0.0	0.1	13.3	80.3	6.2	0.0
		Npats	0.0	0.0	0.0	4.0	4.0	4.0	5.7	11.7	5.8	0.7

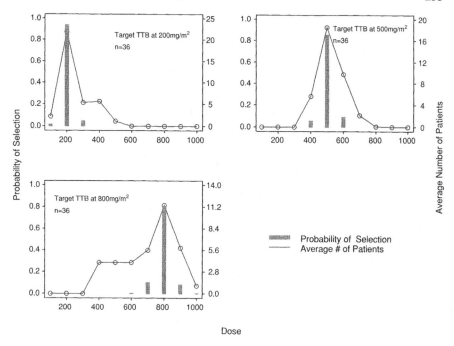

Figure 12.3   Graphical display of simulation results for the sarcoma trial under scenarios 1, 3 and 5.

Under either of these scenarios, the method chooses the best dose, 200 mg/m^2, over 90 % of the time, and on average treats 22 (61 %) of the 36 patients at this dose. The algorithm appears to perform well regardless of whether most of the toxicity burden arises from low or high severity toxicities. For scenarios 3 and 4, the target TTB is achieved at 500 mg/m^2, with most of the TTB due to LS toxicities under scenario 3 and HS toxicities under scenario 4. The method is insensitive to the source of the toxicities, with an 85–87 % correct selection rate and most of the 36 patients treated at or within one level of the selected MTD. For each of scenarios 5 and 6, where $\psi^* = 3.04$ at 800 mg/m^2, the correct selection rate is about 80 %, slightly lower than the other cases. This is due primarily to the 'do-not-skip' rule, which requires that at least one cohort be treated at each dose level when escalating, so that at least 16 of the 36 patients must be treated at doses below 800 mg/m^2 and few patients are available for evaluation at the higher dose levels. The selection probabilities and sample sizes are illustrated in Figure 12.3.

12.6.3   Sensitivity analyses

To address the method's robustness to the severity weights, we performed a sensitivity analysis by randomly perturbing the elicited weight vector, $\boldsymbol{w} = (\boldsymbol{w}_1, \ldots, \boldsymbol{w}_J)$, to obtain hypothetical weights. For each type of toxicity, we randomly perturbed the maximum weight, w_C, of its most severe level by multiplying it by a uniform [0.5, 1.5] random variable, and then we randomly perturbed the lower weights $w_1 < w_2 < \cdots < w_{C-1}$ while still maintaining their order. The hypothetical $\boldsymbol{w}^{(h)}$ obtained in this way determines a TTB target, $\psi^{(*,h)}$, and given fixed outcome probabilities, $\{p_{j,k,d}\}$, as defined in Section 12.6.1, where $\boldsymbol{w}^{(h)}$ determines the best dose, $d^{(*,h)}$, among the 10 doses $\{100, \ldots, 1000\}$, having the TTB closest to $\psi^{(*,h)}$. Independently generating 10 000 such $\boldsymbol{w}^{(h)}$ vectors, the distribution of the corresponding $\psi^{(*,h)}$ values has (2.5, 50, 97.5)th percentiles (1.76, 2.97, 4.67). To examine the distribution of the corresponding $d^{(*,h)}$ values, e.g. under scenario 4, where $d = 500$ has the TTB closest to the elicited $\psi^* = 3.04$, $d^{(*,h)} = 400, 500$ and 600 mg/m^2 with probabilities 0.051, 0.875 and 0.071. Thus, despite the fact that $\boldsymbol{w}^{(h)}$ is obtained as a rather severe perturbation of $\boldsymbol{w}$, under scenario 4 the targeted dose under $\boldsymbol{w}^{(h)}$ is nearly certain to be within one dose level of the dose (500 mg/m^2) targeted by the elicited $\boldsymbol{w}$, and 87.5 % of the time the targeted dose is the same. Similar results were obtained under the other scenarios. Thus, the targeted dose appears to be robust to the elicited weights.

To examine the sensitivity of the dose-finding method to $\boldsymbol{w}$, we simulated the trial under scenario 4 using each of 16 hypothetical weight vectors, $\boldsymbol{w}^{(h,1)}, \ldots, \boldsymbol{w}^{(h,16)}$. We chose these to reflect the distribution of $d^{(*,h)}$ noted above, so that the targeted doses were $d^{(*,h,1)} = 400$, $d^{(*,h,2)} = \cdots = d^{(*,h,15)} = 500$ and $d^{(*,h,16)} = 600$. For the rth hypothetical weight vector, $\boldsymbol{w}^{(h,r)}$, denote the percentage absolute deviation of the selected dose, d_{sel}, from $d^{(*,h,r)}$ by $\text{dev}_r = 100 |d_{\text{sel}} - d^{(*,h,r)}| / d^{(*,h,r)}$. In all 16 cases, d_{sel} was within one level of $d^{(*,h,r)}$ over 99.9 % of the time. For $d^{(*,h,1)} = 400$, doses (300, 400, 500) were selected (1.7, 60.6, 37.7) % of the time, and on average dev_1 was 10.4 %. In 13 of the 14 cases where $d^{(*,h,r)} = 500$, this target dose was selected between 80.6 % and 86.5 % of the time, and in one case 500 was selected 73.2 % of the time. The mean values of $\text{dev}_2, \ldots, \text{dev}_{15}$ varied from 2.9 % to 5.5 %. In the 16th case, (500, 600, 700) were selected (43, 54, 3) % of the time, and on average dev_{16} was 12.1 %. Thus, the method appears to be robust to the elicited weights in terms of changes in the targeted dose, correct selection percentage and deviation of the selected dose from the targeted dose.

Using the elicited severity weights, we also examined the method's sensitivity to cohort size, sample size, starting dose and ψ^*. Simulations examining the effects of cohort size and sample size were conducted under scenario 4. For cohort sizes (1, 2, 3, 4, 5), with starting dose 400 and sample size 36, the corresponding correct selection percentages were (89, 86, 89, 87, 86). Since the range of these values is well within what would be expected from simulation variation, the method appears to be insensitive to cohort size. For sample sizes (28, 32, 36, 40, 44), with the cohort size fixed at 4 and starting dose 400 mg/m^2, the correct selection percentages were (82, 84, 87, 88, 89). Thus, the method's reliability improves with larger sample size. We examined the effect of changing the starting dose from 400 mg/m^2 to 100 mg/m^2 under scenarios 2, 4 and 6, where the target TTB is achieved at 200 mg/m^2, 500 mg/m^2 and 800 mg/m^2 respectively. In these cases the correct selection percentages were 92 % when the target is 200 mg/m^2, 84 % when the target is 500 mg/m^2 and 42 % when the target is 800 mg/m^2. The comparatively low value in the last case is as expected, since the 'do-not-skip rule' with starting dose 100 mg/m^2 requires that 28 of the 36 patients be treated at doses below 800 mg/m^2, which leaves at most two cohorts to treat at the correct dose. If this rule is dropped, then the correct selection percentage in this case is 80 %. To examine the effect of higher correlation among the toxicities on the correct selection rate, we changed the correlations so that there was high correlation between fatigue and nausea/vomiting (0.60), low correlation between fatigue and dermatitis (0.20) and moderate correlation between fatigue and myelosuppression (0.40). Under scenarios 2, 4 and 6, with this correlation structure the correct selection percentages were 92 % when the target TTB was achieved at 200 mg/m^2, 86 % at 500 mg/m^2 and 79 % at 800 mg/m^2. Since these are nearly identical to the values in Table 12.4 obtained with the original correlation structure, it appears that this degree of association among the toxicities does not alter the method's behavior, on average.

We assessed the method's sensitivity to ψ^* by simulating the trial with target $\psi^*(\Delta) = \psi^* \pm \Delta$, for $\Delta = \pm 0.25$ and ± 0.50, i.e. $\psi^*(\Delta) = 2.54, 2.79, 3.29$ and 3.54, under each of scenarios 2, 4 and 6. Defining the 'best' dose d among the 10 levels studied as that at which $\sum_j \sum_k w_{j,k} p_{j,k,d}$ is closest to $\psi^*(\Delta)$, in each of these cases the best dose is identical to that for which $\Delta = 0$. The percentages of selecting the best dose for $\Delta = (-0.50, -0.25, 0, +0.25, +0.50)$ are $(68, 76, 92, 75, 65)$ under scenario 2, $(77, 82, 87, 85, 80)$ under scenario 4 and $(55, 67, 80, 79, 75)$ under scenario 6. However, the method selects a dose within one level, i.e. within ± 100 mg/m^2, of the best dose over 99.5 % of the time in all of these cases.

12.7   Concluding remarks

The dose-finding method used for the sarcoma trial accommodates several different toxicities having severity levels of varying clinical importance. Our simulation study shows that, on average, the algorithm performs well under a wide variety of circumstances. The method requires substantially more effort to implement than conventional dose-finding methods, including close interaction with the physicians to establish the toxicities, severity weights and target TTB, as well as a simulation study of the design.

The method is much easier to implement in the case of one ordinal toxicity, which still provides a substantial advantage over methods based on one binary toxicity. A single ordinal Y takes on one of $C + 1$ severity values $y_0 < y_1 < \ldots, y_C$, there is one latent variable $Z \sim N(\beta_0 + \beta_1 x, 1)$ with $(Y = y_k) = (\gamma_k \leq Z < \gamma_{k+1})$ and $\pi_k(x, \boldsymbol{\theta}) = \Pr(Y = y_k \mid x, \boldsymbol{\theta}) = \Phi\{\gamma_k - (\beta_0 + \beta_1 x)\} - \Phi\{\gamma_{k+1} - (\beta_0 + \beta_1 x)\}$ for $k = 0, \ldots, C$, where $0 = \gamma_1 < \gamma_2 < \cdots < \gamma_C$. Only one vector of severity weights, $(w_1, \ldots, w_k)$, is elicited, the TTB $= W$, where W is univariate with $\Pr(W = w_k) = \pi_k(x, \boldsymbol{\theta})$ and ψ^* is the elicited target for $E(W \mid \text{data}) = \sum_{k=1}^{C} w_k E\{\pi_k(x, \boldsymbol{\theta}) \mid \text{data}\}$. For example, if a single ordinal toxicity is defined in terms of grades 0, 1, 2, 3, 4 but has elicited severity weights 0, 1, 2, 3, 6, and if $\boldsymbol{\pi}^{(a)}(x) = (0.50, 0.10, 0.10, 0.20, 0.10)$ and $\boldsymbol{\pi}^{(b)}(x) = (0.10, 0.10, 0.50, 0.10, 0.20)$ for a given dose x, then both of these probability vectors yield the same conventionally used criterion $\Pr(Y \geq 3 \mid x) = 0.30$ for dose-limiting (grade 3 or 4) toxicity, whereas $\pi^{(a)}(x)$ has $E^{(a)}(\text{TTB}) = 1.5$ while $\pi^{(b)}(x)$ has $E^{(b)}(\text{TTB}) = 2.6$. This illustrates the fact that, even with only one toxicity, accounting for multiple severity levels and eliciting severity weights provides a more informative evaluation of toxicity.

References

1. M.H. Chen and D.K. Dey (2000) Bayesian analysis for correlated ordinal data models, in *Generalized Linear Models: A Bayesian Perspective* (eds S.K. Ghosh, D.K. Dey and B.K. Mallick), Marcel Dekker, New York, PP. 133–57.
2. J. O'Quigley, M. Pepe and L. Fisher (1990) Continual reassessment method: a practical design for phase I clinical trials in cancer. *Biometrics*, **46**, 33–48.
3. B.N. Bekele and P.F. Thall (2004) Dose-finding based on multiple toxicities in a soft tissue sarcoma trial. *J. Am. Statistical Assoc.*, **99**, 26–35.
4. J.H. Albert and S. Chib (1993) Bayesian analysis of binary and polytomous response data. *J. Am. Statistical Assoc.*, **88**, 669–79.
5. S. Chib and E. Greenberg (1998) Analysis of multivariate probit models. *Biometrika*, **85**, 347–61.

13

A two-stage design for dose-finding with two agents

Peter F. Thall

M.D. Anderson Cancer Center, Department of Biostatistics and Applied Mathematics, The University of Texas, Houston, Texas, USA

13.1 Introduction

Potential new anticancer agents typically are broadly cytotoxic, in that they destroy normal cells as well as cancer cells. Thus, higher doses of a cytotoxic agent are better in that they are more likely to kill more cancer cells, and also worse in that they are more likely to cause adverse events or even death. For example, busulfan is used as a preparative regimen in bone marrow transplantation for treating leukemia because it very effectively ablates the patient's marrow prior to transplant. Consequently, increasing the dose of busulfan without limit would very likely eradicate all of the patient's leukemia cells, but it would also kill the patient. Thus, in general, the first step in clinically evaluating a potential new cytotoxic anticancer agent is to determine a dose that has acceptable toxicity. Such dose-finding is done in a phase I clinical trial. Typically, toxicity is defined as any of several adverse events that, if sufficiently severe, constitute a practical limitation to the delivery of treatment. The particular events, and the severity level at which each adverse event is considered a 'toxicity', vary substantially with the clinical setting. Because toxicity is a random event, inevitably dose-finding is based on the probability of toxicity as a function of dose. Beyond its monotonicity, in practice little is known *a priori* about the dose-toxicity curve. Most

Statistical Methods for Dose-Finding Experiments   Edited by S. Chevret
© 2006 John Wiley & Sons, Ltd

phase I trials are conducted adaptively, with the dose for each successive patient cohort chosen using the dose-toxicity data from patients treated previously in the trial. Both ethically and scientifically, phase I trials are difficult because decisions must be based on very small sample sizes, and this problem is especially acute early in the trial.

When two agents are tested in combination for the first time in a particular patient-disease group, the phase I goal is to determine an acceptable dose-pair, $x = (x_1, x_2)$. The problem of constructing an algorithm for choosing doses sequentially in this case is more difficult than the analogous single-agent problem. Although prior knowledge of each agent's individual dose-toxicity curve typically is available from previous phase I trials, such information is of limited use for predicting the probability of toxicity as a function of x when the two agents are used together. This is because biological effects of the combination may be quite complex and unpredictable, and the dose-toxicity probability surface may depend on unknown interactions between the two agents. Simon and Korn [1] provide a detailed discussion of this problem. From a practical viewpoint, even a reasonably small two-dimensional region of potential x pairs is a much larger set in which to do dose-finding than the usual line segment or finite set of doses considered in a single-agent phase I trial. Because an exhaustive search of the two-dimensional domain of x is not feasible in phase I due to the limited sample size and ethical constraints, other strategies must be adopted.

This chapter describes a two-stage Bayesian design, proposed by Thall $et\ al.$ [2], for finding one or more acceptable dose-pairs in the two-agent setting. The method relies on a parametric model for the probability of toxicity, $\pi(x, \theta)$, as a function of x and a parameter vector, $\theta = (\theta_1, \theta_2, \theta_3)$. The subvectors θ_1 and θ_2 parameterize the two single-agent toxicity probabilities, $\pi_1(x_1, \theta_1)$ and $\pi_2(x_2, \theta_2)$, while θ_3 accounts for interaction between the two agents. The design exploits the facts that $\pi(x, \theta)$ is increasing in each of x_1 and x_2, and that the single-dose toxicity curves $\{\pi(x, \theta) : x_2 = 0,\ x_1 \geq 0\}$ and $\{\pi(x, \theta) : x_1 = 0,\ x_2 \geq 0\}$ on the edges of the dose-pair toxicity surface $\{\pi(x, \theta) : x_1 \geq 0,\ x_2 \geq 0\}$ must coincide with the respective single-agent dose-toxicity curves, $\{\pi_1(x_1, \theta_1) : x_1 \geq 0\}$ and $\{\pi_2(x_2, \theta_2) : x_2 \geq 0\}$. Thus, while prior knowledge about the two single-agent curves cannot predict interactions, i.e. values of $\pi(x, \theta)$ where both $x_1 > 0$ and $x_2 > 0$, it provides useful information about the edges of the dose-toxicity surface.

Implementation of the method requires the statistician to collaborate closely with the physician(s). One must elicit the definition of dose-limiting toxicity, hereafter 'toxicity', a fixed target toxicity probability, π^*, and prior information characterizing the dose-toxicity curve of each single agent. This information is used to construct informative priors on θ_1 and θ_2. Given π^*, an acceptable dose (AD) is defined as any pair x having posterior mean toxicity probability

$$E\{\pi(x, \theta) \mid \text{data}\} = \pi^*. \tag{13.1}$$

In contrast with the single-agent setting, when x is two-dimensional, equation (13.1) does not have one solution but rather is satisfied by all x on the random contour

$$L_2(\pi^*, \text{data}) = \{x : E\{\pi(x, \theta) \mid \text{data}\} = \pi^*\} \tag{13.2}$$

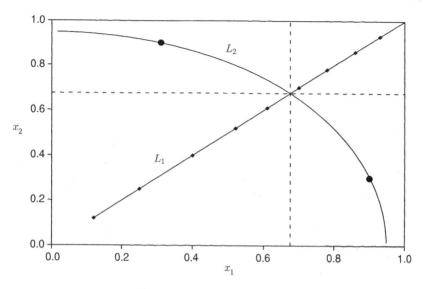

Figure 13.1   The fixed line L_1 and random contour L_2 of the dose-finding algorithm.

in the two-dimensional domain of x. Refer to Figure 13.1. The design chooses values of x from the plane for successive patient cohorts by first restricting dose-finding to a fixed-line diagonal segment, L_1, in stage 1. The search in stage 2 chooses doses from L_2 (π^*, data) subject to additional optimality criteria. At the end of the trial, several ADs may be selected for study in a subsequent trial.

The method will be illustrated by a trial of gemcitabine (Gem) and cyclophosphamide (CTX), a combination that may have several clinical indications [?]. For a variety of reasons, it is anticipated that these two agents are likely to exhibit synergistic effects. The goal of the trial is to determine three acceptable dose combinations for study in a subsequent phase II trial: one that is mostly Gem, one that is mostly CTX and one that is roughly an even mixture of the two agents.

13.2   Dose-toxicity model

13.2.1   Toxicity probabilities

Given a dose d_i and single-agent AD, d_i^*, for agent i, we formulate the dose-toxicity probability model in terms of the standardized doses $x_i = d_i/d_i^*$, for $i = 1, 2$. This ensures that x_1 and x_2 will have similar domains, with most values between 0 and 1, and hence that model parameters corresponding to the two doses will have similar numerical scales, which in turn stabilizes numerical computations. The ADs d_1^* and d_2^* may be elicited from the physician(s) along with the priors on θ_1 and θ_2 while planning the trial. A method for eliciting the single-agent priors and ADs is described below.

For any $\boldsymbol{\theta}$, the toxicity probabilities $\pi(x, \boldsymbol{\theta})$, $\pi_1(x_1, \boldsymbol{\theta}_1)$ and $\pi_2(x_2, \boldsymbol{\theta}_2)$ must satisfy the following admissibility conditions:

(a) $\pi(x_1, 0, \boldsymbol{\theta}) = \pi_1(x_1, \boldsymbol{\theta}_1)$ for all x_1 and $\pi(0, x_2, \boldsymbol{\theta}) = \pi_2(x_2, \boldsymbol{\theta}_2)$ for all x_2;

(b) $\pi(x_1, x_2, \boldsymbol{\theta})$ is increasing in both x_1 and x_2;

(c) $\pi_1(0, \boldsymbol{\theta}_1) = 0$ and $\pi_2(0, \boldsymbol{\theta}_2) = 0$.

Conditions (a) and (b) together imply that each $\pi_i(x_i, \boldsymbol{\theta}_i)$ is increasing in x_i, and consequently that $\pi(x_1, x_2, \boldsymbol{\theta}) > \max\{\pi_1(x_1, \boldsymbol{\theta}_1), \pi_2(x_2, \boldsymbol{\theta}_2)\}$ for all $x_1 > 0$ and $x_2 > 0$. This says that adding any amount of agent 2 to a given amount of agent 1 must increase the probability of toxicity. Properties (a) and (c) together imply that $\pi(0, 0, \boldsymbol{\theta}) = 0$, which says that a patient who receives no amount of either agent has no risk of toxicity.

Many models satisfy the above conditions. Because the sample size is small in phase I, especially early in the trial, the model must be parsimonious. At the same time, the model must be sufficiently flexible to allow a wide variety of possible shapes that the dose-toxicity probability surface may assume. A model that provides a practical compromise between these two requirements is given by

$$
\pi(x, \theta) = \frac{\alpha_1 x_1^{\beta_1} + \alpha_2 x_2^{\beta_2} + \alpha_3 \left(x_1^{\beta_1} x_2^{\beta_2} \right)^{\beta_3}}{1 + \alpha_1 x_1^{\beta_1} + \alpha_2 x_2^{\beta_2} + \alpha_3 \left(x_1^{\beta_1} x_2^{\beta_2} \right)^{\beta_3}}, \tag{13.3}
$$

with $\theta_i = (\alpha_i, \beta_i)$, for $i = 1, 2, 3$, and each entry of the parameter vector $\theta = (\theta_1, \theta_2, \theta_3) = (\alpha_1, \beta_1, \alpha_2, \beta_2, \alpha_3, \beta_3)$ positive real-valued. Denoting $\eta_i(x_i, \boldsymbol{\theta}_i) = \log(\alpha_i) + \beta_i \log(x_i)$, for $i = 1, 2$, it follows that $\pi_i(x_i, \boldsymbol{\theta}_i) = \text{logit}^{-1}\{\eta_i(x_i, \boldsymbol{\theta}_i)\}$. It is easy to verify that this model satisfies the admissibility conditions.

Denote the dose combinations and toxicity indicators of the first n patients in the trial by $Z_n = \{(x_k, Y_k), k = 1, \ldots, n\}$. The likelihood is the usual product of binary outcome terms

$$
f(Z_n \mid \theta) = \prod_{k=1}^{n} \pi(x_k, \theta)^{Y_k} \{1 - \pi(x_k, \theta)\}^{1 - Y_k}. \tag{13.4}
$$

Denoting the prior on θ at the start of the trial by $f(\theta)$, given current data Z_n decisions will be based on the posterior $f(\theta \mid Z_n) \propto f(Z_n \mid \theta) f(\theta)$. Because integrals to obtain the posterior here are analytically intractable, numerical integration is required. This is described below.

13.2.2 Establishing priors

The dose-finding algorithm begins with independent informative priors $f_1(\boldsymbol{\theta}_1)$ and $f_2(\boldsymbol{\theta}_2)$ on $\boldsymbol{\theta}_1$ and $\boldsymbol{\theta}_2$ and a vague prior $f_3^0(\boldsymbol{\theta}_3)$ on $\boldsymbol{\theta}_3$. The informative priors may be obtained either using historical data from previous single-agent studies or by elicitation from the physician(s). In either case, we assume that each parameter follows a gamma prior, with the gamma distribution with mean ab and variance ab^2 denoted by $G(a, b)$.

If dose-toxicity data are available from previous single-agent studies, they may be used to obtain priors on θ_1 and θ_2 for use in the planned trial. For each $i = 1, 2$, the likelihood of the historical data, $\mathcal{Z}^{(i)}$, takes the same general form as equation (13.4), but in terms of the single-agent probabilities $\pi_i(x_i, \theta_i)$. Starting with a non-informative prior f_i^0 on θ_i that may be assumed before the historical data are observed, as usual the posterior of θ_i given $\mathcal{Z}^{(i)}$ is $f_i(\theta_i \mid \mathcal{Z}^{(i)}) \propto f_i(\mathcal{Z}^{(i)} \mid \theta_i) f_i^0(\theta_i)$, and the prior we use at the start of the two-agent trial is

$$f(\theta \mid \mathcal{Z}^{(1)}, \mathcal{Z}^{(2)}) = f_1(\theta_1 \mid \mathcal{Z}^{(1)}) f_2(\theta_2 \mid \mathcal{Z}^{(2)}) f_3^0(\theta_3). \qquad (13.5)$$

In practice, historical single-agent data on individual patients may not be available. In this case, informative priors $f_1(\theta_1)$ and $f_2(\theta_2)$ must be elicited from the physician(s). The particular elicitation method may be tailored to the particular setting at hand. The following method was employed in the Gem/CTX trial and worked quite well. For simplicity, temporarily restrict attention to one agent and suppress subscripts, so that the two parameters of interest are α and β, and $\alpha x^\beta = \pi(x, \theta)/\{1 - \pi(x, \theta)\}$. Assume that $\alpha \sim G(a_1, a_2)$ and $\beta \sim G(b_1, b_2)$, so that each single-agent prior is characterized by the four hyperparameters (a_1, a_2, b_1, b_2). The following four questions pertain to the agent's toxicity probability curve, and require that one should first clearly establish the definition of 'toxicity' and the target probability π^*. The physician's answer to these questions will yield four equations in $\{a_1, a_2, b_1, b_2\}$, and the solution yields the prior on θ.

1. What is the highest dose that is almost certain to be toxic in less than 5 % of patients?

2. What is the dose that will have on average $100\pi^*$ % toxicities?

3. What dose has a prohibitively high toxicity rate, say 60 %?

4. What is the smallest dose that you are almost certain has a toxicity rate above the targeted value $100\pi^*$ %?

The physician(s) may use numerical values different from those given above, say replacing the 5 % in question 1 with some other small percentage or, similarly, replacing the 60 % in question 3 with a different large percentage. This is perfectly acceptable, as the above is an illustration of the elicitation questions that were used with Dr R. Millikan in the Gem/CTX trial. Denoting $z_j = d^{(j)}/d^*$ and $g(\eta) = \eta/(1 + \eta)$, the doses $d^{(1)}$, $d^{(2)}$, $d^{(3)}$ and $d^{(4)}$ given as answers to these questions yield the following four equations:

$$\Pr\{g(\alpha z_1^\beta) < 0.05\} = 0.99, \qquad (13.6)$$

$$E(\alpha) = a_1 a_2 = \pi^*/(1 - \pi^*), \qquad (13.7)$$

$$E(\alpha z_3^\beta) = a_1 a_2 E(z_3^\beta) = 0.60/0.40, \qquad (13.8)$$

$$\Pr\{g(\alpha z_4^\beta) > \pi^*\} = 0.99. \qquad (13.9)$$

Table 13.1   Elicited doses (mg/m^2) and priors for gemcitabine and
cyclophosphamide as single agents.

	Gemcitabine		Cyclophosphamide	
	Elicited dose	Median (π)	Elicited dose	Median (π)
d_1	600	0.002	350	0.006
$d_2 = d^*$	1200	0.258	600	0.269
d_3	1400	0.542	700	0.546
d_4	2000	0.936	800	0.768
	Mean	Variance	Mean	Variance
α	0.429	0.105	0.429	0.079
β	7.649	5.714	7.802	3.993

These equations may be solved numerically for a_1, a_2, b_1, b_2. This process must be
carried out twice, once for each single agent. Table 13.1 summarizes the elicited
values for Gem and CTX.

Because nothing is known *a priori* about interactions between the two agents,
vague priors on α_3 and β_3 should be used. A sensitivity analysis of the priors on
α_3 and β_3 showed that either large values of $E(\beta_3)$ or values of $E(\alpha_3)$ far from 1
give highly skewed, overly informative priors on $\pi(x, \theta)$ that cause the dose-finding
algorithm to behave pathologically. The effects of the variances are less pronounced
for values ≥ 3, and the range 3–10 gives very reasonable behavior. We thus used
$E(\beta_3) = 0.05$, $E(\alpha_3) = 1$ and var(α_3) = var(β_3) = 3, and we recommend these or
similar values for general application.

13.3   A two-stage dose-finding algorithm

13.3.1   Geometry of L_1 and L_2

Dose-finding in stage 1 is restricted to the fixed line segment, L_1, illustrated in
Figure 13.1. To determine L_1, the physician(s) first must choose a lowest dose-pair,
$x^{(1)}$, the least toxic dose-pair considered in stage 1. The criteria for choosing $x^{(1)}$ are
that its prior mean toxicity probability, $E\{\pi(x^{(1)}, \theta)\}$, should be low relative to π^*,
but not so low that it is very unlikely to be therapeutically effective. If $d_{i,1}$ is the dose
of agent i elicited by question 1 in section 13.2.2, hence thought to have negligible
toxicity, one may choose $x^{(1)} = (d_{1,1}/d_1^*, \, d_{2,1}/d_2^*)$. To decide on the highest dose-pair
on L_1, given prior single-agent ADs $x_{0,1}^*$ and $x_{0,2}^*$, the combination $x_0^* = (x_{0,1}^*, x_{0,2}^*)$
is likely to be unacceptably toxic. Thus, a safety requirement is that $x_1^{(1)} < x_{0,1}^*$ and
$x_2^{(1)} < x_{0,2}^*$, and in practice $x_i^{(1)}$ should be well below $x_{0,i}^*$ for each $i = 1, 2$. We

define L_1 to be the straight-line segment from $x^{(1)}$ to x_0^*. Given L_1, the physician(s) must specify a set of dose-pairs, $D_1 = \{x^{(1)}, \ldots, x^{(k)}\}$, on L_1 for dose-finding in stage 1.

Because $\pi(x, \theta)$ is monotone in x, $\overline{\pi}_n(x) = E\{\pi(x, \theta) \mid Z_n\}$ is monotone increasing in x_1 and x_2, and hence is monotone increasing as x moves up L_1. The physician(s) may decide to treat the first cohort at $x^{(1)}$, or at $x^{(2)}$ or possibly $x^{(3)}$, with $x^{(1)}$ included as a fall-back option if the starting dose turns out to be unexpectedly toxic. The elements of D_1 may be equally spaced along L_1 with $x^{(k)} = (x_{0,1}^*, x_{0,2}^*)$, or possibly with $x^{(k)}$ a pair of smaller values. Denoting $L_{2,n} = L_2(\pi^*, Z_n)$, let $x_n^* = L_1 \cap L_{2,n}$ be the unique point on L_1 having mean posterior toxicity probability π^*. Unlike the L_1, which is fixed, $L_{2,n}$ changes randomly as the data from each new cohort are incorporated into Z_n. Since $\pi(x, \theta)$ and hence $\overline{\pi}_n(x)$ is increasing in both x_1 and x_2, it follows that $L_{2,n}$ lies entirely within the upper left and lower right quadrants of the Cartesian plane having origin x_n^*. Denote the respective portions of $L_{2,n}$ in these quadrants by $L_{2,n}^{\uparrow \text{left}}$ and $L_{2,n}^{\downarrow \text{right}}$. Dose-finding in stage 2 will be restricted to these two random contours.

13.3.2 Dose-finding algorithm

To implement the method, one must first establish (a) informative priors on θ_1 and θ_2, (b) a noninformative prior on θ_3, (c) the design parameters $\{n_1, n_2, c, \pi^*\}$, where $c =$ cohort size, and (d) L_1 and D_1. The goal of the following two-stage algorithm is to choose one or more acceptable dose combinations.

Stage 1

Treat the first cohort at the starting dose in D_1 specified by the physicians(s). Treat each successive cohort at the dose $x^{(j)} \in D_1$ minimizing

$$|\overline{\pi}_n(x^{(j)}) - \pi^*|, \tag{13.10}$$

subject to the constraint that no untried dose-pair in D_1 may be skipped when escalating. Once the first toxicity is observed, say at $x^{(r)}$, expand D_1 to D_1^* by adding doses midway between the consecutive pairs above $x^{(r)}$, and also all doses below $x^{(r)}$. As before, choose the dose minimizing (13.10), with no untried dose-pair in D_1^* skipped when escalating. When n_1 patients have been treated, proceed to stage 2.

Stage 2

Treat successive cohorts at dose combinations selected alternately from $L_{2,n}^{\uparrow \text{left}}$ and $L_{2,n}^{\downarrow \text{right}}$. Stop when a total of $N = n_1 + n_2$ patients have been treated.

Since L_1 is one-dimensional, stage 1 is similar to a conventional single-agent phase I trial. As in most single-agent phase I trials, to reduce the likelihood of overdosing patients untried dose-pairs may not be skipped in stage 1. The stage 1 sample size should be large enough to obtain a reasonable idea of how high the contour $L_{2,n}$ is likely to be on the $\pi(x, \theta)$ surface. This motivated our choice of $n_1 = 20$ in the Gem/CTX trial. The risk of overdosing is less of a concern in stage 2, since all patients are treated at doses on $L_{2,n}$, where all dose-pairs have a posterior expected risk of toxicity π^*.

13.3.3   Criteria for stage 2

Based on the toxicity criterion (13.1) alone, all dose-pairs $x \in L_{2,n}$ are equally acceptable. Thus, additional criteria are needed to determine how to choose doses on $L_{2,n}$ in stage 2. The algorithm described here alternates between $L_{2,n}^{\uparrow\text{left}}$ and $L_{2,n}^{\downarrow\text{right}}$, using the following two criteria to pick specific doses. Clinically, it is desirable to choose a dose combination to maximize the potential to kill cancer cells, while still maintaining the posterior mean toxicity rate at π^*. Statistically, it is desirable to maximize the amount of information about $\pi(x, \theta)$ obtained from each new cohort's data. To formalize the first goal, assume that λ is the potential cancer-killing effect of one unit change in x_1 relative to one unit change in x_2. Thus, the amount of potential increase in the cancer-killing effect obtained by moving from x_n^* to x on $L_{2,n}$ is proportional to

$$\mathcal{K}_n(x, x_n^*) = \lambda(x_1 - x_{n,1}^*) + (x_2 - x_{n,2}^*). \tag{13.11}$$

Any dose-pair $x \in L_{2,n}^{\uparrow\text{left}} - \{x_n^*\}$ must satisfy the inequalities $x_1 - x_{n,1}^* < 0 < x_2 - x_{n,2}^*$ and, similarly, any $x \in L_{2,n}^{\downarrow\text{right}} - \{x_n^*\}$ must satisfy $x_1 - x_{n,1}^* > 0 > x_2 - x_{n,2}^*$. This says that the two summands of $\mathcal{K}_n(x, x_n^*)$ must have opposite signs. It follows that choosing x from either $L_{2,n}^{\uparrow\text{left}}$ or $L_{2,n}^{\downarrow\text{right}}$ to maximize the cancer-killing potential compared to x_n^* amounts to choosing x so that the negative summand of $\mathcal{K}_n(x, x_n^*)$ is small relative to its positive summand. This is similar to the idea of a total equivalent dose used by Simon and Korn [1]. The amount of information obtained by treating the next cohort at $x \in L_{2,n}$ may be obtained from the Fisher information matrix. Since the likelihood for one patient treated at x is $\pi(x, \theta)^Y [1 - \pi(x, \theta)]^{1-Y}$, denoting $\pi(x, \theta)^{(j)} = \partial \pi(x, \theta)/\partial \theta_j$ where θ_j is the jth entry of θ, the Fisher information matrix associated with this patient's data is

$$\mathcal{I}(x, \theta)^{(6 \times 6)} = \left[\frac{\pi(x, \theta)^{(j)} \pi(x, \theta)^{(k)}}{\pi(x, \theta)\{1 - \pi(x, \theta)\}} \right]. \tag{13.12}$$

A statistical criterion for choosing a dose on $L_{2,n}$ is the maximum posterior expectation of the log determinant of the Fisher information matrix given the current data:

$$\mathcal{I}_n(x) = E\left[\log\{\det \mathcal{I}(x, \theta)\} \mid Z_n \right]. \tag{13.13}$$

To address the problem that $\mathcal{K}_n(x, x_n^*)$ and $\mathcal{I}_n(x)$ take on values on different scales, we first choose the optimal dose-pair under each criterion and then average these two doses. Specifically, if the next cohort in stage 2 is to be treated at a dose in $L_{2,n}^{\uparrow\text{left}}$, denoting the dose-pair that maximizes the cancer-killing criterion function $\mathcal{K}_n(x, x_n^*)$ by $x(\mathcal{K}_n, L_{2,n}^{\uparrow\text{left}})$ and the dose-pair that maximizes the information criterion function $\mathcal{I}_n(x)$ by $x(\mathcal{I}_n, L_{2,n}^{\uparrow\text{left}})$, the next cohort is treated at the dose, $x(\mathcal{K}_n, \mathcal{I}_n, L_{2,n}^{\uparrow\text{left}})$, which is midway between $x(\mathcal{K}_n, L_{2,n}^{\uparrow\text{left}})$ and $x(\mathcal{I}_n, L_{2,n}^{\uparrow\text{left}})$ on $L_{2,n}^{\uparrow\text{left}}$. The dose $x(\mathcal{K}_n, \mathcal{I}_n, L_{2,n}^{\downarrow\text{right}})$ chosen from $L_{2,n}^{\downarrow\text{right}}$ is defined similarly.

Based on the final data, Z_N, at the end of the trial, we select three dose combinations: $x_N^{\downarrow\text{right}} = x(\mathcal{K}_n, \mathcal{I}_N, L_{2,N}^{\downarrow\text{right}})$, $x_N^{\uparrow\text{left}} = x(\mathcal{K}_n, \mathcal{I}_N, L_{2,N}^{\uparrow\text{left}})$ and the unique combination $x_N^{\text{middle}} = L_1 \cap L_{2,N}$. Roughly speaking, x_N^{middle} contains substantial quantities of both agents, $x_N^{\downarrow\text{right}}$ contains more of agent 1 and less of agent 2 and $x_N^{\uparrow\text{left}}$ contains more of agent 2 and less of agent 1. These three combinations may be studied in a subsequent randomized trial.

13.3.4 Computing

The method is computationally intensive since it requires repeatedly calculating the posterior mean toxicity surface, $\{\overline{\pi}_n(x) : 0 < x_1 < 1, 0 < x_2 < 1\}$, after each new cohort has been evaluated. Consequently, the use of computationally efficient algorithms is critical for a successful implementation. We use Markov chain Monte Carlo simulation [3, 4], accelerated by the use of the maximum *a posteriori* estimate as an initial starting point and an asymptotic posterior approximation to define transition probabilities in the Markov chain. Additional details are given in Thall *et al.* [2].

13.4 Application

In the Gem/CTX trial, $c = 2$, $n_1 = 20$ and $n_2 = 40$. The line L_1 was defined to connect the standardized doses $x^{(1)} = (0.12, 0.12)$ and $(x_{0,1}^*, x_{0,2}^*) = (1,1)$, which correspond to the raw (Gem, CTX) dose-pairs (144, 72) and (1200, 600) mg/m². Ten dose-pairs were used for stage 1, with eight intermediate doses on L_1 chosen so that anticipated toxicity probabilities were dominated by the corresponding prior means. Specifically, $D_1 = \{(x, x) : x = 0.12, 0.25, 0.40, 0.52, 0.61, 0.70, 0.78, 0.86, 0.93, 1\}$. The first cohort was treated at (0.25, 0.25). Although we did not do so in the Gem/CTX trial, one may also impose an additional safety rule to stop the trial if the lowest dose is too toxic, e.g. if $\Pr\{\pi(x^{(1)}, \theta) > \pi^* \mid \text{data}\}$ exceeds an upper probability bound, such as 0.95.

Figure 13.2 gives the 30 successive dose-pairs chosen by this design in a hypothetical example, including the final $L_{2,N}$ based on the data from all $N = 60$ patients. Each cohort is numbered by the order in which its patients were treated in the trial. The sequence of locations of the dose-pairs 11 through 30, chosen in stage 2 of the

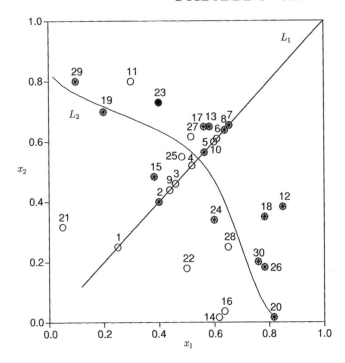

Figure 13.2   Illustrative example of a hypothetical trial. Cohorts are numbered consecutively, from 1 to 30, with 0/2, 1/2 and 2/2 toxicities denoted by an open circle, a
circle enclosing a star and a filled circle respectively.

trial, as well as their variability, illustrate the manner in which L_2 changes as the data
from successive cohorts are obtained and the posterior is updated.

To assess average behavior, we simulated the trial under each of five dose-toxicity
scenarios. These are illustrated in terms of their contours of constant toxicity probability in Figure 13.3. Table 13.2 summarizes the selected dose-pairs x_N^{middle}, $x_N^{\downarrow right}$
and $x_N^{\uparrow left}$, corresponding values of the true $\pi(x)$ and the posterior mean, $\overline{\pi}_n(x)$, at
each selected dose-pair.

The values $x_{n_1}^{middle}$ and x_N^{middle} together show how much the selected dose on L_1
changes by carrying out the second stage. The desired contour under scenario 1 is
the diagonal line in the middle of the x domain, running roughly from (1,0) to (0,1),
and the toxicity probability surface in not very steep. Under scenario 2, the desired
dose-pairs lie on a contour with one or both doses very close to their maximum values;
scenario 3 is the opposite case, with all acceptable dose-pairs having one or both doses
very close to their minimum values. Scenario 4 is the most complex, with S-shaped
contours for π at or near the target 0.30. To examine the method's robustness, we

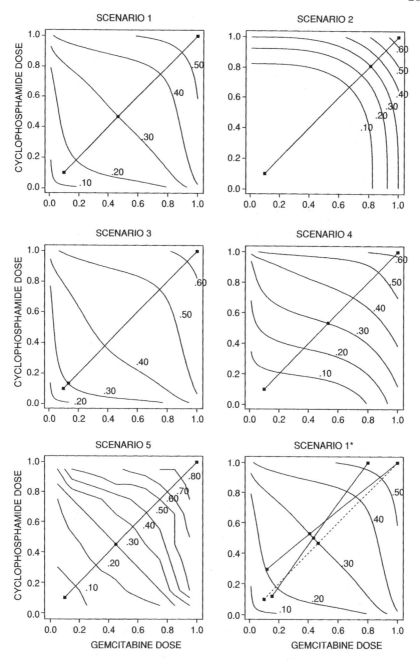

Figure 13.3   Scenarios for the probability of toxicity as a function of the cyclophosphamide and gemcitabine doses in the prostate cancer trial. For each agent, the doses are given in standard units on the domain from 0 to 1.

Table 13.2 Dose combinations selected for the Gem/CTX. Standard deviations are given as subscripts.

	$x_{n_1}^{\text{middle}}$	x_N^{middle}	$x_N^{\downarrow\text{right}}$	$x_N^{\uparrow\text{left}}$
			Scenario 1	
Selected dose x	$(0.47_{0.16}, 0.47_{0.16})$	$(0.50_{0.10}, 0.50_{0.10})$	$(0.66_{0.11}, 0.24_{0.19})$	$(0.34_{0.13}, 0.67_{0.10})$
$\bar{\pi}_n(x)$, true $\pi(x)$	$0.30_{0.05}, 0.30_{0.06}$	$0.30_{0.01}, 0.31_{0.04}$	$0.30_{0.01}, 0.28_{0.07}$	$0.30_{0.01}, 0.32_{0.04}$
			Scenario 2	
Selected dose x	$(0.81_{0.04}, 0.81_{0.04})$	$(0.80_{0.03}, 0.80_{0.03})$	$(0.92_{0.05}, 0.72_{0.05})$	$(0.58_{0.12}, 0.86_{0.05})$
$\bar{\pi}_n(x)$, true $\pi(x)$	$0.30_{0.01}, 0.30_{0.08}$	$0.30_{0.01}, 0.28_{0.05}$	$0.29_{0.01}, 0.35_{0.05}$	$0.30_{0.01}, 0.22_{0.05}$
			Scenario 3	
Selected dose x	$(0.28_{0.14}, 0.28_{0.14})$	$(0.23_{0.17}, 0.23_{0.17})$	$(0.46_{0.21}, 0.07_{0.17})$	$(0.10_{0.14}, 0.40_{0.22})$
$\bar{\pi}_n(x)$, true $\pi(x)$	$0.37_{0.07}, 0.36_{0.05}$	$0.30_{0.02}, 0.33_{0.08}$	$0.29_{0.02}, 0.29_{0.08}$	$0.30_{0.02}, 0.31_{0.08}$
			Scenario 4	
Selected dose x	$(0.57_{0.12}, 0.57_{0.12})$	$(0.56_{0.07}, 0.56_{0.07})$	$(0.70_{0.10}, 0.38_{0.15})$	$(0.39_{0.10}, 0.68_{0.08})$
$\bar{\pi}_n(x)$, true $\pi(x)$	$0.29_{0.05}, 0.32_{0.07}$	$0.30_{0.01}, 0.32_{0.04}$	$0.30_{0.005}, 0.26_{0.08}$	$0.30_{0.01}, 0.34_{0.04}$
			Scenario 5	
Selected dose x	$(0.47_{0.11}, 0.47_{0.11})$	$(0.45_{0.09}, 0.45_{0.09})$	$(0.67_{0.13}, 0.17_{0.16})$	$(0.29_{0.13}, 0.63_{0.11})$
$\bar{\pi}_n(x)$, true $\pi(x)$	$0.31_{0.03}, 0.33_{0.10}$	$0.30_{0.01}, 0.32_{0.10}$	$0.30_{0.01}, 0.27_{0.13}$	$0.30_{0.01}, 0.32_{0.10}$

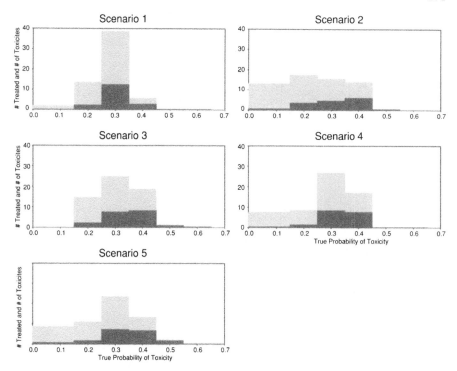

Figure 13.4 Number of patients treated (light shaded bars) and and number of toxicities (dark shaded bars) by true probability of toxicity, under each of the five hypothetical scenarios.

simulated the design under scenario 5, which does not correspond to the underlying probability model.

The algorithm has very accurate behavior under scenarios 1, 3 and 4, choosing dose-pairs with both $\pi(x)$ and posterior mean $\overline{\pi}_n(x)$ on average very close to the target 0.30. The largest deviation is the mean 0.22 of $\pi(x^{\uparrow \text{left}})$ under scenario 2. This is reasonable, given that the toxicity surface rises very rapidly with x_1 and x_2 in this case, and thus the contours where $0.20 \leq \pi(x) \leq 0.40$ are very close together. The fact that the average toxicity probability is below, rather than above, the target in this dangerous case is reassuring, in terms of the procedure's safety. The largest differences between $\{\pi(x), \overline{\pi}_{n_1}(x)\}$ for $x = x_{20}^{\text{middle}}$, at the end of stage 1, and the final values for $x = x_{60}^{\text{middle}}$ are seen under scenario 3. This is reasonable, given that the desired contour is located at very low dose values in this case.

Figure 13.4 gives histograms of the number of patients treated and number of toxicities under each scenario. Under scenarios 1 to 4, on average between 36 (60 %) and 52 (87 %) of the 60 patients are treated at a dose with $\mid \pi(x) - 0.30 \mid < 0.10$,

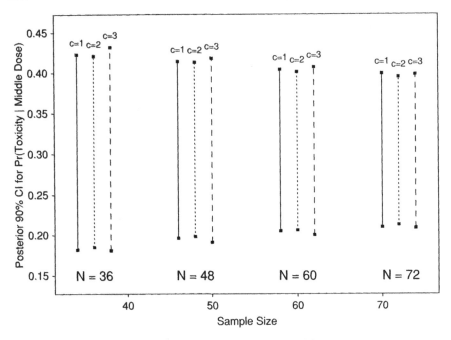

Figure 13.5   Posterior 90 % credible intervals for $\pi(x_N^{\text{middle}})$ as a function of cohort size and sample size. Intervals are given by solid lines for cohort sizes $c = 1$, dotted lines for $c = 2$ and dashed lines for $c = 3$.

at most 19 (15 %) are treated at a dose with $0.41 \leq \pi(x) \leq 0.50$, only 1.4 patients are treated at a dose with $0.51 \leq \pi(x) \leq 0.70$, with none at a more toxic dose. The dispersion of patients over the range of true toxicity probabilities is slightly higher under scenario 5, with on average 9.5 patients (16 %) treated at doses with toxicities above 0.40, although most of these were in the range 0.41–0.50. The algorithm thus appears to be very safe.

Scenario 5 is a more dangerous case, since the target contour where $\pi(x) = 0.30$ is similar to that in scenario 1 but the toxicity probability surface is much steeper. Table 13.2 indicates that the algorithm's ability to select doses with $\pi(x)$ close to the target is quite good in this case, although the variability (not tabled) is greater. The average posterior mean and true $\pi(x)$ at the selected doses are all between 0.27 and 0.33, results nearly identical to those under scenario 1.

To examine the method's sensitivity to the placement of L_1, we used two additional, different versions of L_1, illustrated as solid lines in the lowest right corner graph (scenario 1*) in Figure 13.3, with the original version of L_1 given as a dotted line. The first new line, L_1^a, is steeper, running from (0.155, 0.12) to (0.80, 1.0), with D_1 consisting of these points plus eight intermediate points on L_1^a having the same x_2

entries as those used previously. This might be motivated by the desire to decrease the upper limit on the dose of the first agent during stage 1. In this case the highest dose of Gem on L_1 is decreased from 1200 mg/m^2 to 960 mg/m^2. We also considered the less steep line, L_1^b, running from (0.12, 0.296) to (1.0, 1.0), with D_1 having the same x_1 entries as those used previously. This might be motivated by the desire to increase the lower limit on the dose of the second agent during stage 1, in this case increasing the lowest CTX dose on L_1 from 72 mg/m^2 to 178 mg/m^2. Simulations of these two modified versions of the algorithm under scenario 1 showed that, with either L_1^a or L_1^b, all mean values of $\overline{\pi}_n(x)$ and $\pi(x)$ at the selected dose-pairs were between 0.29 and 0.31, and each entry of each selected dose differed from the corresponding value under the original L_1 by 0.01 to 0.06. The method thus appears to be insensitive to the placement of L_1.

A simulation study of the method's sensitivity to N and c showed that average values of $|\overline{\pi}(x_N) - 0.30|$ are insensitive to both parameters. These deviations equal 0.01 for x_N^{middle} and 0.02 to 0.04 for $x_N^{\uparrow\text{left}}$ or $x_N^{\downarrow\text{right}}$. In contrast, for both types of dose-pair, $|\overline{\pi}(x_N) - \text{true } \pi(x)|$ on average decreases with N, as expected, but increases sharply as c increases from 2 to 3. This is due to the fact that, as c increases for given N, the total number of cohorts, N/c, decreases, and hence information is available on fewer dose-pairs. Figure 13.5 gives posterior 90 % credible intervals for $\pi(x_N^{\text{middle}})$ as a function of N and c. It appears that, in this setting, $c = 1$ or 2 provides a more reliable dose-pair selection than $c = 3$.

13.5   Discussion

This chapter has described a model-based, adaptive, two–stage Bayesian method for determining several acceptable dose-pairs of two agents used together in a phase I cancer chemotherapy trial. Simulation results indicate that the method is both safe and reliable. Because this dose-finding problem arises frequently in clinical oncology, the method should be broadly applicable. An important advantage of the method is that it is rooted in actual clinical practice. The requirement of informative priors on θ_1 and θ_2, the prior elicitation algorithm and the goal of choosing several dose-pairs are all motivated by practical experience with the Gem/CTX trial. While the method is computationally intensive, in our experience this did not present any substantive problems.

References

1. R. Simon and E.L. Korn (1990) Selecting drug combinations based on total equivalent dose (dose intensity). *J. Natl Cancer Inst.*, **82**(18), 1469–76.
2. P.F. Thall, R.E. Millikan, P. Mueller and S.J. Lee (2003) Dose-finding with two agents in Phase I oncology trials. *Biometrics*, **59**(3), 487–96.

3. A.E. Gelfand and A.F.M. Smith (1990) Sampling based approaches to calculating marginal densities. *JASA*, **85**, 398–409.

4. W.R. Gilks, D.G. Clayton, D.J. Spiegelhalter, N.G. Best, A.J. McNeil, L.D. Sharples and A.J. Kirby (1993) Modelling complexity: applications of Gibbs sampling in medicine. *JRSS B*, **55**, 39–52.

14

Using both efficacy and toxicity for dose-finding

Peter F. Thall and John D. Cook

M.D. Anderson Cancer Center, Department of Biostatistics and Applied Mathematics, The University of Texas, Houston, Texas, USA

14.1 Introduction

In this chapter, we describe an outcome-adaptive Bayesian method [1] that uses both efficacy (E) and toxicity (T) to choose doses of an experimental agent for successive patient cohorts in a clinical trial. This is an example of a 'phase I/II' clinical trial design, since it includes both dose-finding and efficacy evaluation. Denote the probabilities of E and T for a patient given dose x by $\pi(x, \theta) = \{\pi_E(x, \theta), \pi_T(x, \theta)\}$, where θ denotes the model parameter vector. The method is based on a family of contours in the two-dimensional set of π pairs that characterize trade-offs between π_E and π_T. The contours are constructed from target values of π elicited from the physician, similarly to the method of Thall, Sung and Estey [2]. Each contour has a numerical value associated with it that quantifies the desirability of each pair (π_E, π_T) on it, and all pairs on the same contour are considered equally desirable. This construction provides a basis for the ordering of the two-dimensional set of π values in terms of their desirabilities, which in turn induces an ordering on the doses. Each time a dose must be chosen based on the current interim data, $\mathcal{D}$, the desirability of each x is defined to be the desirability of the contour containing the pair $E\{\pi(x, \theta) \mid \mathcal{D}\} = (E\{\pi_E(x, \theta) \mid \mathcal{D}\}, E\{\pi_T(x, \theta) \mid \mathcal{D}\})$, and the next cohort is given the most desirable dose.

Statistical Methods for Dose-Finding Experiments Edited by S. Chevret
© 2006 John Wiley & Sons, Ltd

The method accommodates settings with trinary outcomes, $\{E, T, (E \cup T)^c\}$, where E and T are disjoint and it is also possible that neither event may occur, and trials with bivariate binary outcomes, where the patient may experience both events. To simplify the presentation here, we will focus on the bivariate binary outcome case. We will illustrate the method with a phase I/II trial of a treatment for graft-versus-host disease in allogeneic bone marrow transplantation. A computer simulation study in the context of this trial is described.

14.2 Illustrative trial

Patients undergoing allogeneic blood or bone marrow stem cell transplantation from an HLA-matched donor (allotx) for treatment of hematologic malignancies are at substantial risk of graft-versus-host disease (GVHD). This occurs when the transplanted cells successfully engraft and repopulate the patient's bone marrow, but the engrafted cells then attack the patient's organs in an autoimmune reaction. GVHD varies in severity, but it often is life-threatening. When GVHD occurs but cannot be brought into remission through conventional steroid therapy, a different, 'salvage' therapy typically is used in an attempt to save the patient. In a trial of Pentostatin as a salvage therapy for steroid-refractory GVHD conducted at M.D. Anderson Cancer Center, up to $N = 36$ patients are treated in cohorts of size $c = 3$. The scientific goal is to find the best dose among the four doses $(0.25, 0.50, 0.75, 1.00)$ mg/m^2, which we will refer to as levels 1, 2, 3 and 4. For the purpose of dose-finding, within a 2-week evaluation period, toxicity (T) is defined as an infection that cannot be resolved by antibiotics, or death, and response (E) is defined as a decrease in the GVHD severity level by at least one grade. These events are defined within a 2-week evaluation period from the start of Pentostatin therapy. In particular, a patient who responds to therapy and is alive but has an unresolved infection at 2-weeks has both E and T.

14.3 Dose-outcome models

14.3.1 Bivariate binary probability distributions

In the sequel, dose is coded as $x_j = \log(d_j) - \text{mean}\{\log(d)\}$, where $d_1, \cdots, d_J$ are the raw dose values. Let $Y = (Y_E, Y_T)$ be the binary indicators of E and T, with the bivariate distribution $\pi_{a,b}(x, \theta) = Pr(Y_E = a, Y_T = b \mid x, \theta)$ for $a, b \in \{0, 1\}$. There are numerous bivariate binary regression models (cf. reference [3]). Let g be a link function appropriate for a binary outcome regression model, such as the logit, probit or complementary log–log [4]. To facilitate model interpretation and prior elicitation, and to ensure that the model will be numerically tractable, we formulate $\pi_{a,b}(x, \theta)$ in terms of the marginal probabilities

$$\pi_T(x, \theta) = \pi_{1,1}(x, \theta) + \pi_{0,1}(x, \theta) = g^{-1}\{\eta_T(x, \theta)\}$$

and

$$\pi_E(x, \theta) = \pi_{1,1}(x, \theta) + \pi_{1,0}(x, \theta) = g^{-1}\{\eta_E(x, \theta)\},$$

and one real-valued parameter, ψ, characterizing association. For toxicity, we assume that $\eta_T(x, \boldsymbol{\theta}) = \mu_T + x\beta_T$, with $\beta_T > 0$ to ensure that $\pi_T(x, \boldsymbol{\theta})$ is monotone increasing in dose. For efficacy, it is important that the model allows a wide variety of possible dose-response relationships, including nonmonotone functions. To achieve this, we use the quadratic form $\eta_E(x, \boldsymbol{\theta}) = \mu_E + x\,\beta_{E,1} + x^2\,\beta_{E,2}$, which is quite flexible. In particular, this allows the method to be used for trials of biologic agents, where $\pi_E(x, \boldsymbol{\theta})$ may initially increase in x and then vary very little or possibly decrease for higher doses. Thus, $\boldsymbol{\theta} = (\mu_T, \beta_T, \mu_E, \beta_{E,1}, \beta_{E,2}, \psi)$. We will use the so-called 'Morgenstern' or 'Gumbel' model given by

$$\pi_{a,b} = (\pi_E)^a (1 - \pi_E)^{1-a} (\pi_T)^b (1 - \pi_T)^{1-b}$$
$$+ (-1)^{a+b} \pi_E (1 - \pi_E) \pi_T (1 - \pi_T) \left(\frac{e^\psi - 1}{e^\psi + 1} \right), \qquad (14.1)$$

where $a, b \in \{0, 1\}$ and ψ is real-valued.

The likelihood for a patient treated at dose x is

$$\mathcal{L}(\boldsymbol{Y}, x \mid \boldsymbol{\theta}) = \pi_{1,1}(x, \boldsymbol{\theta})^{Y_E Y_T} \pi_{1,0}(x, \boldsymbol{\theta})^{Y_E(1-Y_T)}$$
$$\times \pi_{0,1}(x, \boldsymbol{\theta})^{(1-Y_E)Y_T} \pi_{0,0}(x, \boldsymbol{\theta})^{(1-Y_E)(1-Y_T)},$$

where $\pi_{0,0} = 1 - (\pi_{1,1} + \pi_{1,0} + \pi_{0,1})$. Denote the data for the first n patients in the trial by $\mathcal{D}_n$ for $1 \leq n \leq N$, where N is the maximum sample size in the trial. The likelihood based on $\mathcal{D}_n$ is

$$\mathcal{L}_n(\mathcal{D}_n \mid \boldsymbol{\theta}) = \prod_{i=1}^{n} \mathcal{L}(\boldsymbol{Y}_i, x_{(i)} \mid \boldsymbol{\theta}), \qquad (14.2)$$

where $\boldsymbol{Y}_i$ and $x_{(i)}$ denote the ith patient's outcome and dose.

14.3.2 Priors and posteriors

The family of phase I/II clinical trials considered here falls within the larger class of trials that may be characterized as being small-scale, with model-based Bayesian adaptive decision making. In such settings, the prior must give a reasonable representation of the physician's uncertainty, provide a reliable basis for making sensible decisions early in the trial, but be sufficiently vague so that the accumulating data dominate the posterior and hence the decisions later in the trial. We assume that each component θ_l of $\boldsymbol{\theta}$ is normally distributed with mean μ_l and standard deviation (SD) σ_l, which we denote by $\theta_l \sim N(\mu_l, \sigma_l)$. Let $\boldsymbol{\xi} = (\mu_1, \sigma_1, \mu_2, \sigma_2, \ldots, \mu_p, \sigma_p)$ denote the $2p$-vector of hyperparameters, with all prior covariances set equal to 0, and let $\phi_p(\boldsymbol{\theta} \mid \boldsymbol{\xi})$ denote the p-variate normal prior of $\boldsymbol{\theta}$. For each dose x_j, $j = 1, \ldots, J$, let $m_{E,j}$ and $s_{E,j}$ denote the prior mean and SD of $\pi_E(x_j, \boldsymbol{\theta})$ and let $m_{T,j}$ and $s_{T,j}$ be the prior mean and SD of $\pi_T(x_j, \boldsymbol{\theta})$. Initially, for each x_j, we elicit the means of $\pi_E(x_j, \boldsymbol{\theta})$ and $\pi_T(x_j, \boldsymbol{\theta})$, which we denote by $\hat{m}_{E,j}$ and $\hat{m}_{T,j}$, that the physician expects *a priori* at that dose. We also specify values of $\hat{s}_{E,j}$ and $\hat{s}_{T,j}$ in the range 0.29–0.50, corresponding to beta distributions with parameters having a sum of at most 2; i.e. we allow the marginal prior of each $\pi_y(x_j, \boldsymbol{\theta})$ to have roughly as much information as at most two data points. Given $\{\hat{m}_{E,j}, \hat{m}_{T,j}, \hat{s}_{E,j}, \hat{s}_{T,j}, j = 1, \ldots, J\}$, we numerically solve for the value of $\boldsymbol{\xi}$ that best fits the target means and variances. Specifically, we solve for $\boldsymbol{\xi}$ that minimizes the objective function

$$h(\boldsymbol{\xi}) = \sum_{y=E,T} \sum_{1 \le j \le J} \left\{ (m_{y,j} - \hat{m}_{y,j})^2 + (s_{y,j} - \hat{s}_{y,j})^2 \right\} + c \sum_{1 \le j < k \le J} (\sigma_j - \sigma_k)^2. \quad (14.3)$$

The second term in $h(\boldsymbol{\xi})$ is included so that the solution will distribute the prior variance more evenly among the components of $\boldsymbol{\theta}$, with c a small positive constant, e.g. $c = 0.15$. We intentionally elicit more pieces of prior information than hyperparameters, with $4J > 2p$, and obtain $\boldsymbol{\xi}$ as the least-squares solution to the $4J$ equations in $2p$ unknowns.

The dose-finding method described here is computationally intensive because it requires that the posterior $p(\boldsymbol{\theta} \mid \mathcal{D})$ be computed repeatedly each time $\mathcal{D}$ is updated by incorporating the data from the most recent cohort. Many computations based on each posterior must be carried out, including evaluation of $E\{\pi_y(x_j, \boldsymbol{\theta}) \mid \mathcal{D}\}$ for each x_j and $y = E$ and T, as well as additional dose acceptability criteria, described below. A simulation study of the design requires that all of these computations be carried out many times; thus, establishing the method's average behavior in this way is computationally intensive at an even deeper level. To compute posteriors, numerical integration of $\mathcal{L}_n(\mathcal{D}_n \mid \boldsymbol{\theta})\phi_p(\boldsymbol{\theta} \mid \boldsymbol{\xi})$ with respect to $\boldsymbol{\theta}$ is required, since this integral cannot be evaluated analytically. An accurate and time-efficient method for carrying out this computation is described by Thall and Cook [1].

14.4   The dose-finding algorithm

14.4.1   Acceptability limits

The dose-finding algorithm will utilize two types of criteria, both based on the most recent posterior $p(\boldsymbol{\theta} \mid \mathcal{D})$. The first criterion consists of a pair of probabilities for determining the set of acceptable doses and the second is a geometric method for choosing the best acceptable dose. Let $\underline{\pi}_E$ and $\overline{\pi}_T$ be fixed lower and upper limits on the probabilities of E and T specified by the physician, and let p_E and p_T be fixed probability cut-offs. The following definition is motivated by the desire to control the risk of treating patients at a dose that is unacceptable due to either high toxicity or low efficacy.

Definition

A dose x has acceptable efficacy if

$$\Pr\{\pi_E(x, \boldsymbol{\theta}) > \underline{\pi}_E \mid \mathcal{D}\} > p_E \quad (14.4)$$

and x has acceptable toxicity if

$$\Pr\{\pi_T(x, \boldsymbol{\theta}) < \overline{\pi}_T \mid \mathcal{D}\} > p_T. \quad (14.5)$$

Given current data $\mathcal{D}$, a dose x is acceptable if x satisfies both (14.4) and (14.5), or if x is the lowest untried dose above the starting dose and it satisfies (14.5).

We denote the current set of acceptable doses, given $\mathcal{D}$, by $\mathcal{A}(\mathcal{D})$. Note that the lowest untried dose is acceptable if it has acceptable toxicity, but the efficacy requirement (14.4) is not imposed. Thus, if the predicted safety of the lowest untried dose is acceptable, then it may be used to treat patients regardless of its predicted efficacy. The effect of this extension is that the algorithm is likely to treat patients at higher, untried doses, provided that patient safety is still protected, and hence it is likely to discover a higher dose having superior efficacy.

14.4.2 Trade-off contours

The following geometric construction will provide a basis for choosing the best among several acceptable doses. This will be done by defining the desirability of the pair $\pi(x, \theta)$ in the two-dimensional domain, $\Pi = [0, 1]^2$, of possible values of π. We first construct a target efficacy-toxicity trade-off contour, $\mathcal{C}$, in Π by fitting a curve to target values of π elicited from the physician. The target contour is then used to construct a family of trade-off contours such that all π on the same contour are equally desirable. Because the family of contours partitions Π, this construction provides a basis for comparing doses in terms of their posterior means, $E\{\pi(x, \theta) \mid \mathcal{D}\}$. The contour is determined by three elicited target probability pairs, $\{\pi_1^*, \pi_2^*, \pi_3^*\}$, that the physician considers equally desirable (refer to Figure 14.1).

To obtain these, first elicit a desirable trade-off target, $\pi_1^* = (\pi_{1,E}^*, \pi_{1,T}^*) = (\pi_{1,E}^*, 0)$, in the case where $\pi_T = 0$; i.e. $\pi_{1,E}^*$ is the smallest efficacy probability that the physician considers to be desirable if toxicity were impossible. Next, elicit $\pi_2^* = (\pi_{2,E}^*, \pi_{2,T}^*) = (1, \pi_{2,T}^*)$, having the same desirability as π_1^* by asking the physician what the maximum value of π_T may be if $\pi_E = 1$. Given these two equally desirable extremes, elicit a third pair, π_3^*, that is equally desirable but is intermediate between π_1^* and π_2^*. Plot each target as it is elicited and, once π_3^* is specified, draw the target efficacy-toxicity trade-off contour, $\mathcal{C}$, determined by $\{\pi_1^*, \pi_2^*, \pi_3^*\}$. In practice, it is easiest to elicit the targets $\{\pi_1^*, \pi_2^*, \pi_3^*\}$ at the same time one elicits prior parameter values and the other design parameters. One may obtain $\mathcal{C}$ by fitting a continuous, strictly increasing function, $\pi_T = f(\pi_E)$ to the three target points and defining $\mathcal{C} = \{(\pi_E, \pi_T) : \pi_{1,E}^* \leq \pi_E \leq 1, \pi_T = f(\pi_E)\} \cap \Pi$, as illustrated by the thick curved line in Figure 14.1. Any tractable function $\pi_T = f(\pi_E)$ may be used, provided that it increases continuously over the domain of π_E where $\pi_{1,E}^* \leq \pi_E \leq 1$. In practice, the elicitation process is iterative, and the physician will usually modify the target points on the basis of the plot of $\pi_T = f(\pi_E)$ on π_E.

Once $\mathcal{C}$ is established, it may be used to generate a family of contours, as follows. Again, refer to Figure 14.1. For any $q \in \Pi$, let $L(q)$ denote the straight line through q and the ideal probability pair $(1,0)$, and denote the Euclidean distance from q to $(1,0)$ by $\rho(q)$. For $p \in \mathcal{C}$ and $z > 0$, we define the homotopy $h_z(p) = q$ if $q \in L(p)$ and $\rho(p)/\rho(q) = z$, which implies that $h_z(p) = [1 - (1 - p_E)/z, p_T/z]$. While the range $h_z(\mathcal{C}) = \{h_z(p) : p \in \mathcal{C}\}$ of h_z may not be a subset of Π for some z, and possibly

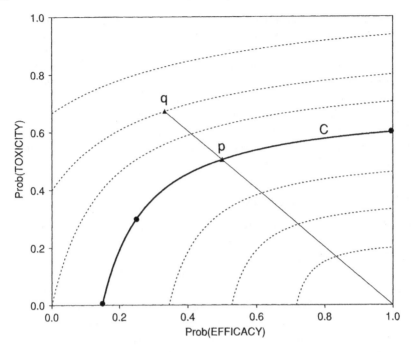

Figure 14.1 Efficacy–toxicity trade-off contours for the Pentostatin trial. The target
contour C is given by the thick solid line. Six other trade-off contours are given by
dashed lines. The three elicited target points that determine C are given by round dots.
The two triangular points illustrate the homotopy $h_{0.75}(p) = q$, and all points on the
contour containing q have $\delta = 0.75$.

may lie entirely outside Π, since we are only interested in contours inside Π, we
define $C_z = \{h_z(C)\} \cap \Pi$. Thus, aside from values of z such that C_z is empty, C_z is
the contour in Π obtained by shifting each $p \in C$ along $L(p)$ to the point q such
that $\rho(p)/\rho(q) = z$; *i.e.* the ratio of the distances to (1,0) equals z. Since values of
q closer to (1,0) are more desirable, we define the desirability of a given $q \in \Pi$ to
be the number $\delta(q) = z - 1$ such that $q \in C_z$. We subtract 1 from z to standardize
the desirability of points on the elicited contour, $C = C_1$, to equal 0. In particular,
$\delta(q) > 0$ for q inside the region in Π between C and (1,0), and $\delta(q) < 0$ for q outside
the region. Since the contours are ordered by their desirabilities and the set of all C_z is
a partition of the two-dimensional set Π, the contours induce an ordering on Π. The
following definition exploits this structure to induce an ordering on the set of doses.

Definition

Given $\mathcal{D}$ and x, the desirability, $\delta(x, \mathcal{D})$, of x is the desirability of the posterior mean
$E\{\pi(x, \theta) \mid \mathcal{D}\}$.

In practice, after the most recent cohort's data have been incorporated into $\mathcal{D}$, for each x, $q = E\{\pi(x, \theta) \mid \mathcal{D}\}$ is first computed, then $p = L(q) \cap \mathcal{C}$ is obtained algebraically and the desirability of x is then given by $\delta(x, \mathcal{D}) = \rho(p)/\rho(q) - 1$. We require $f(\pi_E)$ to be strictly increasing to ensure that, given $(\pi_E, \pi_T) \in \mathcal{C}$ and $\epsilon > 0$, provided that $(\pi_E + \epsilon, \pi_T) \in \Pi$, it must be the case that $(\pi_E + \epsilon, \pi_T)$ is on a contour below $\mathcal{C}$ and hence is more desirable than (π_E, π_T). Similarly, a pair $(\pi_E, \pi_T + \epsilon) \in \Pi$ must be on a contour above $\mathcal{C}$ and hence less desirable than (π_E, π_T). In particular, the rectangular boundary comprised of the line segments from $(\underline{\pi}_E, \overline{\pi}_T)$ to $(\underline{\pi}_E, 0)$ and from $(\underline{\pi}_E, \overline{\pi}_T)$ to $(1, \overline{\pi}_T)$ is not admissible. We used the convenient function $\pi_T = f(\pi_E) = a + b/\pi_E + c/\pi_E^2$ in the applications described here, although several other functions should work as well.

14.4.3   The algorithm

To establish the underlying structure required by the method, the physician must specify a set of doses, a starting dose for the first cohort, N, c, the acceptability limits $\underline{\pi}_E$ and $\overline{\pi}_T$, and the trade-off targets $\{\pi_1^*, \pi_2^*, \pi_3^*\}$. Given the structure determined by this information, the trial is conducted as follows:

1. Treat the first cohort at the starting dose specified by the physician.

2. For each cohort after the first, no untried dose may be skipped when escalating.

3. If $\mathcal{A}(\mathcal{D}) \neq \phi$, then treat the next cohort at the $x \in \mathcal{A}(\mathcal{D})$ maximizing $\delta(x, \mathcal{D})$.

4. If $\mathcal{A}(\mathcal{D}) = \phi$, then terminate the trial and do not select any dose.

5. If the trial is not stopped early and $\mathcal{A}(\mathcal{D}_N) \neq \phi$ at the end of the trial, then select the dose in $\mathcal{A}(\mathcal{D}_N)$ that maximizes $\delta(x, \mathcal{D}_N)$.

14.5   Simulation studies

The following computer simulation study provides an empirical evaluation of algorithm's average behavior. We simulated the Pentostatin trial under the four scenarios given in Table 14.1 and illustrated by Figure 14.2.

In each of these scenarios, we assumed initially that $\psi = 0$, so that E and T occurred independently according to the fixed values of (p_E, p_T) at each dose given in Table 14.1. The trial design parameters in the simulations were those actually being used to conduct the trial, with $c = 3$, $N = 36$, $\underline{\pi}_E = 0.20$, $\overline{\pi}_T = 0.40$, $p_E = p_T = 0.10$, starting at dose level 1, and $\mathcal{C}$ determined by fitting the curve $p_T = a + b/p_E + c/p_E^2$ to the elicited trade-off points $(p_E, p_T) = (0.15, 0), (0.25, 0.30), (1, 0.60)$. The means and SDs of the Gaussian prior parameters were $(-0.619, 0.941)$ for μ_T, $(0.587, 1.659)$ for β_T, $(-1.496, 1.113)$ for μ_E, $(1.180, 0.869)$ for $\beta_{E,1}$, $(0.149, 1.192)$ for $\beta_{E,2}$ and $(0.00, 1.00)$ for ψ.

These simulation results show that, in all four scenarios, the method makes a correct decision, namely selecting an acceptable dose or stopping early when no

Table 14.1   Selection percentage, followed by the number of patients treated in parentheses, by dose, of the new algorithm under the bivariate binary model, for the GVHD prophylaxis trial.

Scenario		\multicolumn{5}{c}{Pentostatin dose (mg/m^2)}				
		0.25	0.50	0.75	1.00	None
1	(p_E, p_T)	(0.02, 0.05)	(0.30, 0.12)	(0.55, 0.30)	(0.65, 0.80)	
	δ	−0.16	0.16	0.35	−0.45	
		0.0 (3.0)	17.3 (8.7)	80.3 (20.8)	2.4 (3.4)	0.0
2	(p_E, p_T)	(0.02, 0.05)	(0.28, 0.10)	(0.50, 0.16)	(0.80, 0.22)	
	δ	−0.16	0.14	0.38	0.59	
		0.0 (3.0)	0.5 (3.6)	13.6 (7.7)	86.0 (21.7)	0.0
3	(p_E, p_T)	(0.25, 0.05)	(0.65, 0.15)	(0.50, 0.42)	(0.05, 0.65)	
	δ	0.11	0.55	0.18	−0.38	
		5.2 (5.8)	81.3 (21.0)	13.1 (7.8)	0.2 (1.3)	0.2
4	(p_E, p_T)	(0.05, 0.50)	(0.25, 0.75)	(0.50, 0.85)	(0.70, 0.87)	
	δ	−0.26	−0.41	−0.55	−0.58	
		3.5 (8.0)	1.4 (5.6)	0.3 (2.6)	0.3 (1.2)	94.5

doses are acceptable, at least 94 % of the time, and relatively few patients are treated at undesirable doses. Under scenario 1, dose level 1 is efficacious, dose level 4 is too toxic and of the two acceptable levels, 2 and 3, the latter is more desirable, as shown by Figure 14.3 and the numerical values of δ in Table 14.1. In this case, the method chooses the best dose 80 % of the time and chooses an acceptable dose level 98 % of the time. Under scenario 2, where toxicity is acceptable for all four doses levels but $p_E(x)$ increases with the dose, the best dose level 4 is chosen 86 % of the time. Under scenario 3, where $p_E(x)$ increases and then sharply decreases with x, the method very reliably detects this pattern and selects the best dose, level 2, 81 % of the time. In each of scenarios 1 to 3, the proportions of patients treated at each dose closely reflect their desirabilities. In scenario 4, where no dose is acceptable, the trial is correctly stopped early with no dose selected 94 % of the time, and the mean sample size is 17 patients.

To assess the method's sensitivity to association between E and T, we simulated extended versions of scenario 2 with fixed values of ψ equal to $\{-2.049, -0.814, 0, +0.814, +2.0486\}$, which correspond to $p_{E|T}$ at 0.50 mg/m^2 equal to $\{0.14, 0.21, 0.28, 0.35, 0.42\}$. This range of association corresponds to varying $p_{E|T}$ at 0.50 mg/m^2 from 0.5 p_E to 1.5 p_E. For each value of ψ and each dose x, the simulation probabilities $\{p_{a,b}(x) : a, b = 0, 1\}$ were obtained from formula (14.1) using ψ and the fixed marginal values of (p_E, p_T) given in Table 14.1 for scenario 2. As a basis for comparison, in the case where E and T are independent ($\psi = 0$), given in Table 14.1, dose levels 3 or 4 are selected 13.6 % and 86.0 % of the

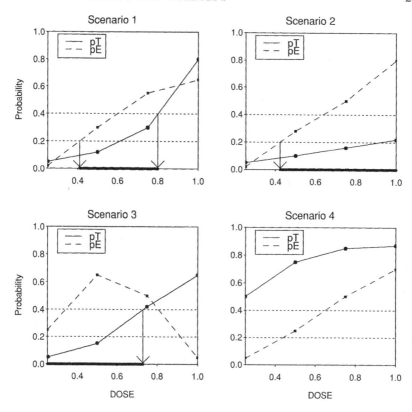

Figure 14.2 Plots of $\pi_E(x)$ (dashed line) and $\pi_T(x)$ (solid line) for each of the four scenarios in the simulation study. The dashed horizontal lines represent the acceptability limits $\overline{\pi}_T = 0.40$ and $\underline{\pi}_E = 0.20$. The domain of doses having both acceptable toxicity and acceptable efficacy is given by the thick line on the horizontal axis.

time. These two percentages become (64 %, 36 %) for $\psi = -2.049$, (69 %, 30 %) for $\psi = -0.814$, (40 %, 41 %) with no dose chosen 18 % of the time for $\psi = +0.814$ and (82 %, 16 %) for $\psi = +2.049$. These results are as expected, for the following reasons. If $p_{E|T}(x) < p_E(x)$, then the occurrence of T at x reduces the posterior values of the marginal probability $\pi_E(x, \theta)$ and hence makes it less likely that x will satisfy the efficacy acceptability criterion (14.4). If $p_{E|T}(x) > p_E(x)$ then, by Bayes' law, $p_{T|E}(x) > p_T(x)$ and the occurrence of E at x increases the marginal posterior values of $\pi_T(x, \theta)$ and hence makes it less likely that x will satisfy the toxicity acceptability criterion (14.5). Thus, either strong positive association or strong negative association between Y_E and Y_T reduces the likelihood of acceptability for all doses. Given the goals of controlling $\pi_T(x, \theta) < \overline{\pi}_T$ and $\pi_E(x, \theta) > \underline{\pi}_E$, this is a desirable property of the method, provided that ψ does not vary with x. If this is not the case, then one may use an extended model, say with $\psi = \mu_\psi + \beta_{\psi,1}x + \beta_{\psi,2}x^2$.

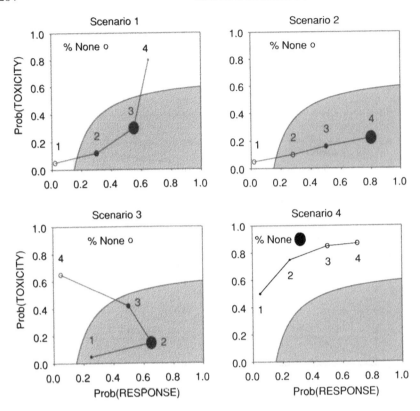

Figure 14.3   Decision percentages for the Pentostatin trial for each of the dose-outcome scenarios given in Table 14.1. The doses of Pentostatin are labeled 1,2,3, and 4. The area of each disc equals the probability that the dose having (p_E, p_T) located as its center is selected.

14.6   Discussion

Several other authors have investigated the problem of dose-finding based on both response and toxicity. Gooley *et al.* [5] also considered two dose-outcome curves and also proposed using computer simulation in the process of designing a clinical trial. O'Quigley, Hughes and Fenton [6] and Braun [7] proposed methods that extend the continual reassessment method for toxicity alone [8] to accommodate efficacy and toxicity.

The dose-finding methodology described here is somewhat more structured than most dose-finding methods, and it requires substantial efforts from both the statistician and the physician to implement. We feel that this extra effort is well warranted by the scientific and ethical advantages of accounting for both efficacy and toxicity, as well as the method's attractive operating characteristics. This methodology also requires reliable, user-friendly computer programs for both simulation during the design process and trial conduct. A software package called EffTox is freely available at http://biostatistics.mdanderson.org/SoftwareDownload for this purpose.

References

1. P.F. Thall and J.D. Cook (2004) Dose-finding based on efficacy-toxicity trade-offs, *Biometrics*, **60**(3), 684–693. Technical report 006-03, M.D. Anderson Cancer Center, Department of Biostatistics, University of Texas, Houston, Texas.
2. P.F. Thall, H.G. Sung and E.H. Estey (2002) Selecting therapeutic strategies based on efficacy and death in multi–course clinical trials, *J. Am. Statistical Assoc.*, **97**(457), 29–39.
3. H. Joe (1997) *Multivariate Models and Dependence Concepts*, Chapman and Hall, London.
4. P. McCullagh and J.A. Nelder (1989) *Generalized Linear Models*, 2nd edn, Chapman and Hall, New York.
5. T.A. Gooley, P.J. Martin, L.D. Fisher and M. Pettinger (1994) Simulation as a design tool for phase I/II clinical trials: an example from bone marrow transplantation, *Controlled Clin. Trials*, **15**(6), 450–62.
6. J. O'Quigley, M.D. Hughes and T. Fenton (2001) Dose-finding designs for HIV studies, *Biometrics*, **57**(4), 1018–29.
7. T. Braun (2002) The bivariate continual reassessment method: extending the CRM to phase I trials of two competing outcomes, *Controlled Clin. Trials*, **23**(3), 240–56.
8. J. O'Quigley, M. Pepe and L. Fisher (1990) Continual reassessment method: a practical design for phase I clinical trials in cancer, *Biometrics*, **46**(1), 33–48.

Part V

Conclusions

15

Websites and software

Sarah Zohar

Département de Biostatistique et Informatique Médicale, U717 Inserm
Hôpital Saint-Louis, Paris, France

15.1 Introduction

The development and application of methods for dose-finding clinical trials were gratefully helped by recent advances in computer technology. Statisticians and medical researchers today have easy access to statistical software. However, most commercial statistical software do not have in their native release any package or macro dealing with dose-finding (menu options or interactive system). Users have either to use software or programs developed by other researchers which are available on their websites (commercial or free) or to write their own program. Firstly, this chapter will provide in the next sections some guidelines for researchers who want to develop their own application in common statistical software (SAS version 8.2,[1] S-PLUS version 6.2,[2] R version 2.1[3]) via an example. Secondly, statistical software developed by researchers to increment published methods will be presented and some examples on how to use them will be provided. Finally, the software issues will be discussed in a last section.

---

[1] Copyright © SAS Institute Inc., SAS Campus Drive, Cary, North Carolina, USA.
[2] Copyright © Insightful Corporation, Seattle, Washington, USA.
[3] The R Foundation for Statistical Computing, Vienna, Austria.

Statistical Methods for Dose-Finding Experiments   Edited by S. Chevret
© 2006 John Wiley & Sons, Ltd

15.2   Computation methods using statistical software

Most common commercial statistical software give all mathematical functions in order to write and implement dose-finding analysis. Integration functions, for Bayesian methods or the maximum likelihood function, are often available and easy to use. Nevertheless, statisticians need to have some minimal knowledge and practice in programming language. In this chapter, a simple S program is presented where the continual reassessment method (CRM) is implemented (for S-PLUS 6.2 and R 2.1) [1]. This method was chosen for the increased number of publications that deal with it and applications in dose-finding clinical trials [2–5, 7–10]. In this example the used dose-response model is a power function, α_i^a (with $i = 1, \ldots, k$), where k is the number of dose levels and a is random with a unit exponential prior distribution [4]. The original CRM is a Bayesian method (Chapter 6), so it requires an integration function. Firstly, the function to be integrated needs to be defined:

```
crmh <- function(x){(exp(-x)*vcrm(x))}
crmht <-function(x){x*(exp(-x)*vcrm(x))}
```

with vcrm the likelihood function:

```
vcrm <- function(a){
v <- 1
for(i in (1:length(x1p)))
{v <- v*((x1p[i]^a)^y1p[i])*(((1-x1p[i]^a)^(1-y1p[i])))}
return(v)}
```

Then, the CRM function is defined by

```
crm <- function(n,prior,target,tox,dose){

### function parameters initializing
ptox <- matrix(NA,nrow=n,ncol=length(prior))
dcrm <- x1p <- y1p <- rep(0,n)

### dose allocation procedure
for (i in 1:n)
{
### x1p and y1p are global variable needed for the integration
x1p <<- c(prior[dose[1:i]])
y1p <<- tox[1:i]

### ptox is the matrix of the estimated probabilities of
   responses
ptox[i,]<- prior^(integrate(crmht,0,Inf)[[1]]/integrate
   (crmh,0,Inf)[[1]])
```

```
### dcrm is the vector of the sequential recommended dose level
dcrm[i] <-which(abs(ptox[i,]-target)==min(abs(ptox[i,]-
    target)))
}
### results printing
cat("N","\t","Dose","\t","Tox","\t", paste("pt",seq(1,length
    (prior))), "\t","Recommended dose","\n")
for (i in 1:n){
cat(i,"\t",dose[i],"\t",tox[i],"\t",round(ptox[i,],3),"\t",
    dcrm[i],"\n")}
}
```

The input of the crm function is the following:

1. "n" is the number of patients to be included in the trial for which observations are available.

2. "prior" is the vector of prior response probabilities associated with each dose level.

3. "target" is the toxicity target.

4. "tox" is the vector of patient's observations (1 = toxicity and 0 = no toxicity).

5. "dose" is the vector of dose levels attributed to each patient included in the trial.

To run the program[4] under either (a) R software, where the user has to load the functions vcrm, crmh, crmht and crm by writing the following commande source(file="my save path/crm.r"), or (b) S-SPLUS software, where the user has to go to the menu option "script" and select "run". For example, for a dose-finding where 10 patients were included, the execution commands for the two software are respectively:

```
crm(n=10,prior=c(0.04,0.07,0.2,0.35,0.55,0.7),target=0.2,
tox=c(0,1,0,0,0,1,0,0,0,0),dose=c(1,3,2,2,2,3,2,2,2,2))
```

Figure 15.1 represents the output of the program where (a) "N" is the patient rank, (b) "Dose" is the given dose level to those patients, (c) "Tox" is the patient observation, (d) "Pt1, ..., Pt6" are the sequential estimation of the probabilities of response at each dose level and (e) "Recommended dose" is the dose level recommended by the CRM. In this example, after the inclusion of 10 patients the

---

[4]This program can be downloaded at: http://dbim.chu-stlouis.fr/soft.html.crm.r for R software and crm.ssc for S-PLUS software.

N	Dose	Tox	pt 1	pt 2	pt 3	pt 4	pt 5	pt 6	Recommended dose
1	1	0	0.019	0.037	0.137	0.273	0.477	0.643	3
2	3	1	0.168	0.229	0.409	0.559	0.718	0.820	2
3	2	0	0.111	0.163	0.334	0.489	0.665	0.784	2
4	2	0	0.082	0.126	0.286	0.442	0.628	0.758	2
5	2	0	0.064	0.103	0.253	0.408	0.600	0.737	3
6	3	1	0.133	0.189	0.365	0.518	0.688	0.800	2
7	2	0	0.111	0.162	0.333	0.488	0.664	0.784	2
8	2	0	0.094	0.142	0.307	0.463	0.645	0.770	2
9	2	0	0.082	0.126	0.286	0.442	0.628	0.758	2
10	2	0	0.072	0.114	0.268	0.424	0.613	0.747	3

Figure 15.1   CRM output.

recommended dose level for the next patient is the third dose level with the associated response probability of 0.268 (closest to the target of 0.3).

The lcrm program uses a frequentist framework by estimating the response probabilities associated with each dose level with a maximum likelihood method. The log likelihood is as follows:

```
lvcrm <- function(a=1){-sum(y1p*log(x1p^a)+(1-y1p)
   *log(1-x1p^a))}

lcrm  <- function(n,prior,target,tox,dose,initial){

ptox   <- matrix(NA,nrow=n,ncol=length(prior))
dcrm   <- x1p <- y1p <- rep(0,n)

for (i in initial:n)
{
x1p <<- c(prior[dose[1:i]])
y1p <<- tox[1:i]
### maximum likelihood estimation
ptox[i,]<-prior^(optim (1,1vcrm, method="L-BFGS-
   B",lower=10^(−3))$par)
dcrm[i] <-which(abs(ptox[i,]-target)==min(abs(ptox[i,]-
   target)))
}
cat("N","\t","Dose","\t","Tox","\t", paste("pt",seq(1,length
   (prior))),  "\t","Recommended dose","\n")
for (i in initial:n){
cat(i,"\t",dose[i],"\t",tox[i],"\t",round(ptox[i,],3),"\t",
   dcrm[i],"\n")}
}
```

In this program one input was added, which is "initial" the patient number from which at least one toxicity and one no toxicty were observed.

These scripts can be written into SAS software by using SAS/IML for the integration procedure. In order to program dose-finding methods, one should be able to know how to use computational software and have a good knowledge of the mathematical method. Unfortunately, most users do not have the skill or the time to do so. In the next section are presented available software for dose-finding for users who do not wish to program their own application.

15.3   Phase I or phase II dose-finding software

In this section are presented software that are free to download or commercial software that allow dose-finding clinical trials to be simulated, planned, conducted and analyzed. For several software some examples of simulated phase I dose-finding clinical trials will be provided. In order to be able to compare and present the software functionalities one option was chosen, i.e. the conduction and analysis of a clinical trial.

The same simulated data, which came from a random number generated from R software (see the Appendix), were used for the examples, but they differ in the treatment allocation procedure associated with different applied methods. The applications shared several common features. We considered a phase I dose-finding aimed at estimating, among six dose levels (1, 2, 3, 4, 5 and 6 mg), the dose level associated with the probability of response closest to the target of 0.3. The true underlying dose-response probabilities were 0.1, 0.15, 0.2, 0.3, 0.45 and 0.5, which were associated with initial guesses of response probabilities of 0.05, 0.1, 0.3, 0.5, 0.6 and 0.65 respectively. The maximal number of patients to be included in the trial was 25 and the cohort size per dose level was 1. Unless the dose level used to assign to the first cohort was not specified, the first dose level was given. If needed, some additional particular features associated with a specific method, not specified above, are presented. Finally, for all applications, a table of the dose allocation procedure is given and the output files or windows are detailed.

All software/program applications were performed under Microsoft Windows XP.[5]

15.3.1   Software for the continual reassessment method
          and its modifications

The continual reassessment method (CRM) [1] provides a Bayesian estimation of the maximal tolerated dose (MTD) in phase I cancer clinical trials. It estimates the MTD from a fixed set of doses levels, sequentially after each newly included patient, up to a maximal number of 20–25 patients. It is based on parametric modeling of the dose-response relationship and on administrating the dose level closest to the currently estimated MTD after each patient. This method has been largely detailed and discussed in previous chapters, so in this section will only a few of the software be presented to compute and apply this method and its modifications [2–5, 7, 10].

---

[5]Copyright © Microsoft Corporation, Redmond, Washington, USA.

15.3.1.1   CRM and CRM simulator

Method: The CRM software computes the traditional continual reassessment method and the likelihood-based continual reassessment method [1, 4]. Design-based stopping rules can also be computed [2, 3]. The CRM simulator software allows clinical trials conducted with the CRM to be simulated.

Description: These are menu-driven computer programs. A binary source code as well as Win32 and MacOS9 executable are available for download.

Main options: Conduct, analyze and simulate a phase I cancer clinical trial.

Location: M.D. Anderson Cancer Center, Biostatistics Department, University of Texas, Houston, Texas, USA (http://biostatistics.mdanderson.org/ SoftwareDownload/).

Example: Conduction and analysis of a phase I clinical trial with the CRM software. The chosen model was the power model with no restriction in the dose-escalation scheme [4]. Table 15.1 represents the dose level attributed to each patient and the patient's response (1 = toxicity and 0 = no toxicity). The fourth dose level (the dose level associated with the MTD) was assigned for 16 out of 25 patients included in the trial. The output window (Figure 15.2) displays (a) the trial inputs, (b) the number of patients allocated to each dose level, (c) the posterior estimation of the response probabilities associated to each dose level and (d) the posterior estimation of the probability for the dose level estimating the MTD. After the inclusion of 25 patients the estimated MTD is the fourth dose level with the associated response probability of 0.355.

Table 15.1   Dose allocation scheme using CRM.

Patient	Dose	Toxicity	Patient	Dose	Toxicity
1	1	0	14	3	0
2	3	0	15	3	0
3	4	0	16	3	0
4	4	0	17	4	0
5	5	0	18	4	0
6	6	0	19	4	1
7	6	1	20	4	0
8	5	1	21	4	0
9	4	1	22	4	1
10	4	1	23	4	0
11	4	0	24	4	0
12	4	1	25	4	0
13	4	1			

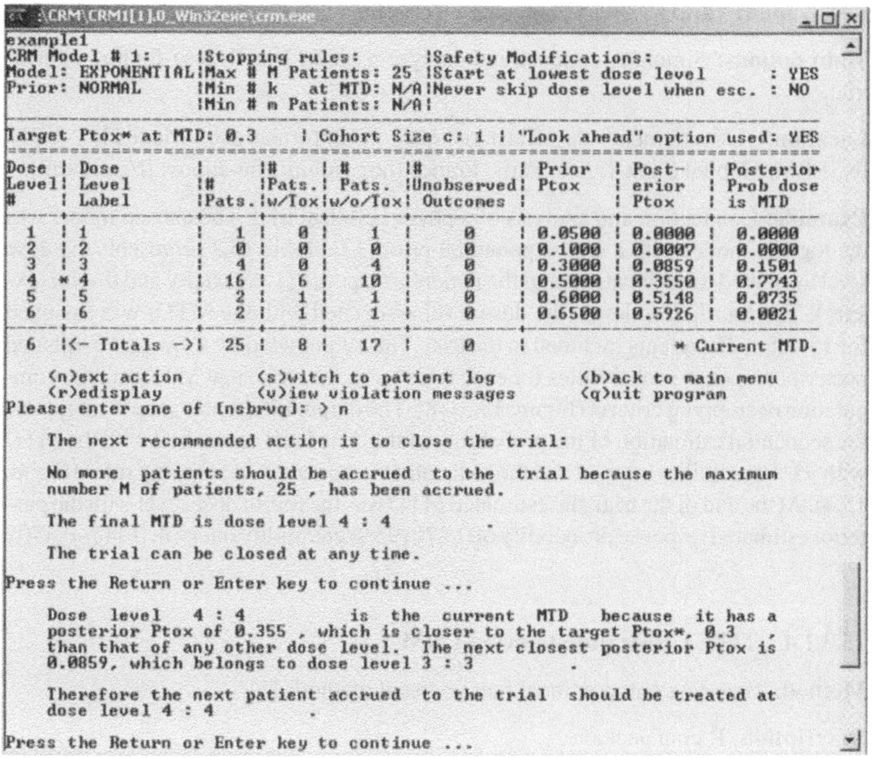

```
CRM\CRM1[1].0_Win32exe\crm.exe                                         _ |□| x|
example1
CRM Model # 1:        |Stopping rules:        |Safety Modifications:
Model: EXPONENTIAL|Max # M Patients: 25 |Start at lowest dose level    : YES
Prior: NORMAL      |Min # k  at MTD: N/A|Never skip dose level when esc. : NO
                   |Min # m Patients: N/A|

Target Ptox* at MTD: 0.3    | Cohort Size c: 1 | "Look ahead" option used: YES
===================================================================================
Dose | Dose     |    |#    | #    |#        | Prior | Post-  | Posterior
Level| Level    |#   |Pats.| Pats.|Unobserved| Ptox  | erior  | Prob dose
#    | Label    |Pats.|w/Tox|w/o/Tox| Outcomes |       | Ptox   | is MTD
-----+----------+----+-----+-----+---------+-------+--------+-----------
  1  | 1        |  1 |  0  |  1  |    0    | 0.0500| 0.0000 |  0.0000
  2  | 2        |  0 |  0  |  0  |    0    | 0.1000| 0.0007 |  0.0000
  3  | 3        |  4 |  0  |  4  |    0    | 0.3000| 0.0859 |  0.1501
  4  * 4        | 16 |  6  | 10  |    0    | 0.5000| 0.3550 |  0.7743
  5  | 5        |  2 |  1  |  1  |    0    | 0.6000| 0.5148 |  0.0735
  6  | 6        |  2 |  1  |  1  |    0    | 0.6500| 0.5926 |  0.0021
-----+----------+----+-----+-----+---------+-------+--------+-----------
  6  |<- Totals ->| 25 |  8  | 17  |    0    |       * Current MTD.

     (n)ext action      (s)witch to patient log      (b)ack to main menu
     (r)edisplay        (v)iew violation messages     (q)uit program
Please enter one of [nsbrvq]: > n

     The next recommended action is to close the trial:

     No more  patients should be accrued  to the  trial because the maximum
     number M of patients, 25 , has been accrued.

     The final MTD is dose level 4 : 4         .

     The trial can be closed at any time.

Press the Return or Enter key to continue ...

     Dose  level   4 : 4      is the  current  MTD   because  it has a
     posterior Ptox of 0.355 , which is closer to the target Ptox*, 0.3 ,
     than that of any other dose level. The next closest posterior Ptox is
     0.0859, which belongs to dose level 3 : 3         .

     Therefore the next patient accrued  to the  trial  should be treated at
     dose level 4 : 4         .

Press the Return or Enter key to continue ...
```

Figure 15.2   Output window for the CRM software where the estimated toxicity probability associated with each dose level, the estimated MTD and the probability for each dose level to be the MTD are represented.

15.3.1.2   CRM using pharmacokinetic measurements

Method: This program computes a modified continual reassessment method where the main modification is a two-parameter logistic curve to model the dose-toxicity relationship [11].

Description: This is a Win32 executable program.

Main options: Conduct and analyze a phase I cancer clinical trial.

Location: Oncology Biostatistics, Johns Hopkins Oncology Center, Johns Hopkins University School of Medicine, Baltimore, Maryland, USA (http://www.cancerbiostats.onc.jhmi.edu/software.cfm).

15.3.1.3   BPCT: Bayesian phase I (or phase II) dose-ranging clinical trials

Method: This software uses the continual reassessment method and allows the computation of statistical-based stopping rules [8, 12].

Description: This is a Win32 executable program.

Main options: Simulate, conduct and analyze a phase I or II dose-finding clinical trial.

Location: Département de Biostatistique et Informatique Médicale, U717 INSERM, Hôpital Saint-Louis, Paris, France (http://dbim.chu-stlouis.fr/soft.html).

Example: Conduction and analysis of a phase I clinical trial. The chosen model was the logistic model with a unit exponential prior [13]. Table 15.2 represents the dose level attributed to each patient and the patient's response (1 = toxicity and 0 = no toxicity). The fourth dose level (the dose level associated with the MTD) was assigned for 15 out of 25 patients included in the trial. The output window shows the estimated posterior response probabilities for each dose level, the estimated MTD and the computation of stopping criteria (Figure 15.3) [8]. The output file contains the main inputs, the sequential estimation of the probability of the dose level associated with the MTD with 95 % credibility interval and the sequential computation of stopping rules (Figure 15.4). At the end of the trial, the estimated MTD was the fourth dose level with the posterior estimated response probability of 0.270 (95 % credibility interval: 0.117–0.470).

15.3.1.4 TITE CRM: time-to-event CRM

Method: Time-to-event continual reassessment methods [5].

Description: R cran package.

Main options: Conduct and analyze a phase I time-to-event phase I clinical trial.

Table 15.2 Dose allocation scheme using BPCT.

Patient	Dose	Toxicity	Patient	Dose	Toxicity
1	1	0	14	3	0
2	5	1	15	4	0
3	2	0	16	4	0
4	3	0	17	4	0
5	4	0	18	4	0
6	4	0	19	4	1
7	5	0	20	4	0
8	5	1	21	4	0
9	4	1	22	4	1
10	4	1	23	4	0
11	3	0	24	4	0
12	3	0	25	4	0
13	3	0			

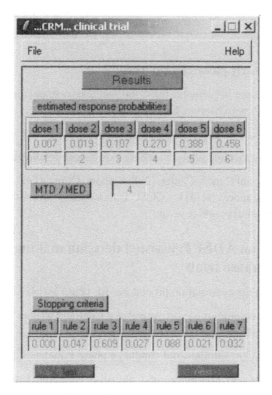

Figure 15.3   Output window, for BPCT software, where the estimated toxicity probability associated with each dose level, the estimated MTD and the stopping rules are represented.

prior probabilities		1.0.050,		2:0.100.		3.0.300.		4:0 500.		5.0.600,		6'0.650.
target . 0 30												
a_zero : 3												
mean prior distribution:		1 00										
subject	rule 1	rule 2	rule 3	rule 4	rule 5	rule 6	rule 7	dose	Pr	inf_CI	sup_CI	
1	0.202	0.319	0.000	0.342	0.561	0.332	0 635	1	0 327	0 000	0 852	
2	0 380	0 050	0.000	0.253	0.591	0.229	0.376	5	0.220	0 147	0.936	
3	0.189	0.076	0.000	0.216	0.474	0.178	0.299	2	0 305	0.001	0 765	
4	0.078	0.119	0.000	0.174	0.354	0.147	0 301	3	0.394	0 006	0.735	
5	0 027	0.192	0.000	0.146	0.364	0.155	0.215	4	0.293	0.024	0.744	
6	0.009	0 271	0.000	0.127	0.310	0.097	0.181	4	0 339	0.016	0 673	
7	0 002	0.373	0.000	0.108	0.297	0.114	0.157	5	0.273	0.030	0.678	
8	0.006	0.156	0.120	0.089	0.270	0.112	0 157	5	0 283	0.102	0 729	
9	0 016	0 043	0 382	0.089	0.225	0.088	0.130	4	0 389	0.109	0.714	
10	0.031	0.011	0.485	0.078	0.282	0.083	0.135	4	0.263	0.172	0.749	
11	0 014	0.015	0.393	0.066	0.222	0.080	0.130	3	0.228	0.046	0 576	
12	0.006	0.019	0 230	0.059	0.208	0.078	0 119	3	0.202	0.042	0.524	
13	0.002	0.024	0.527	0.061	0.172	0.015	0.022	3	0.374	0 038	0 481	
14	0 001	0.029	0.552	0.053	0.169	0.036	0.045	3	0 353	0 035	0 442	
15	0.000	0.041	0.870	0.046	0.149	0.043	0.054	4	0.326	0.115	0.585	
16	0 000	0.056	0 955	0.042	0.126	0.038	0.052	4	0 301	0 105	0.556	
17	0.000	0 073	0.584	0.041	0.125	0.036	0.052	4	0.280	0.095	0.530	
18	0.000	0.093	0.464	0.039	0.123	0.035	0.052	4	0 261	0 088	0.504	
19	0 000	0.035	0 956	0.035	0.106	0.032	0.045	4	0.308	0 123	0 541	
20	0.000	0.046	1.000	0.034	0.105	0.030	0.043	4	0.290	0.115	0.519	
21	0.000	0.058	0 614	0.033	0.103	0.027	0.041	4	0.274	0.108	0 496	
22	0.000	0 022	0.956	0.030	0 092	0.026	0.036	4	0.313	0.136	0.526	
23	0.000	0.029	1.000	0.029	0.091	0.026	0.037	4	0.297	0.130	0.507	
24	0.000	0 037	1 000	0.028	0.089	0.023	0.034	4	0.283	0 123	0 489	
25	0.000	0.047	0.609	0.027	0.088	0.021	0.032	4	0.270	0 117	0 470	

Figure 15.4   Output file, for BPCT software, where the sequential estimation of the toxicity probability associated with the MTD with 95 % credibility intervals and stopping rules are represented.

Location: Department of Biostatistics, Mailman School of Public Health, Columbia University, New York, USA (http://biostat.columbia.edu/~cheung/ftp/).

15.3.1.5   EPCT: early phase clinical trials

Method: This software implements the Continual reassessment method and the standard "3 + 3" design with Storer (2001) changes.

Description: This is a Win32 executable program.

Main options: Conduct and analyze a phase I dose-finding clinical trial.

Location: (1) National Cancer Center, (2) Singapore, Clinical trial and Epidemiology Research Unit, Singapore and (3) UKCCSG Data Center, University of Leicester, UK. To get a copy e-mail ukccsg@le.ac.uk.

15.3.2   Bayesian ADEPT: assisted decision making in early phase trials

Method: Bayesian dose-escalation procedures for phase I trials [14–16].

Description: This commenrcial software uses a front-end written in SAS/AF macro, which uses SAS modules BASE, STAT and GRAPH.

Main options: Design, simulate and conduct a phase I dose-finding clinical trial.

Location: Medical and Pharmaceutical Statistics Research Unit, The University of Reading, Reading, UK (http://www.rdg.ac.uk/mps/mps_home/software/software.htm).

Example: Conduction and analysis of a phase I clinical trial. In this example, the used option was 'design a trial', using a variance gain function with three patients receiving TD30 and TD50 [17]. Table 15.3 represents the dose level attributed to each patient and the patient's response. The fourth dose level (the dose level associated with the MTD) was assigned for 10 out of 25 patients included in the trial. After the inclusion of each new cohort are estimated (a) the posterior dose-response relationship (Figure 15.5), (b) the posterior density of each dose level (Figure 15.6, the fourth dose level) and (c) the dose-response model parameters (Figure 15.7). At the end of the trial the estimated dose level for the MTD was 3.70 (95 % credibility interval: 3.05–4.49).

15.3.3   ATDPH1: accelerated titration designs for phase I clinical trials

Method: Accelerated titration designs for phase I clinical trials [18].

Description: Two programs are available: (a) Microsoft Excel[6] dose allocation macro and (b) S-PLUS script for analysis of the trials.

---

[6]Copyright © Microsoft Corporation, Redmond, Washington, USA.

Table 15.3   Dose allocation scheme using Bayesian ADEPT.

Patient	Dose	Toxicity	Patient	Dose	Toxicity
1	2	0	14	3	0
2	2	0	15	4	0
3	2	0	16	4	0
4	2	0	17	4	0
5	2	0	18	4	0
6	2	0	19	4	1
7	2	0	20	3	0
8	6	1	21	3	0
9	6	1	22	4	1
10	4	1	23	3	0
11	3	0	24	4	0
12	3	0	25	4	0
13	4	1			

Main options: Conduct (under Excel macro) and analyze (under S-PLUS script) a phase I dose-finding clinical trial.

Location: Biometric Research Branch, Cancer Treatment and Diagnosis, National Cancer Institute, Bethesda, Maryland, USA (http://linus.nci.nih.gov/~brb/Methodologic.htm).

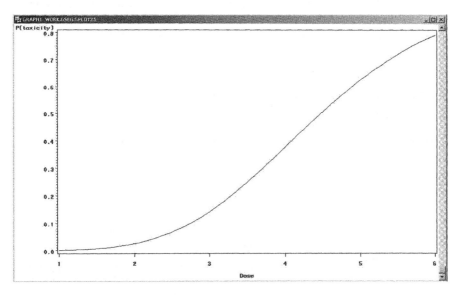

Figure 15.5   Graphic window representing the estimated posterior dose-response relationship after the inclusion of 25 patients using ADEPT software.

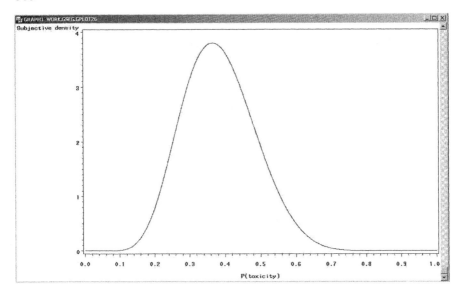

Figure 15.6   Graphic window representing the estimated posterior density of the fourth dose level, i.e. the estimated MTD after the inclusion of 25 patients using ADPT software.

Example: Conduction of a phase I clinical trial (Excel macro). The chosen titration design was $2A$, i.e. no intrapatient dose-escalation. Table 15.4 represents the dose level attributed to each patient and the patient's response ($1 = DLT$ and $0 = no$ toxicity). The trial ended after the inclusion of the 18th patient at dose level 3.

15.3.4   PMTD: traditional algorithm-based designs for phase I

Method: Calculation of the statistical quantities for phase I cancer clinical trials by Lin and Shih [19].

Description: This is an S-PLUS script.

trialno	param	estim	stdev	lower	upper
25	intercept	−6.76582	2.84247	−12.3370	−1.19469
25	slope	4.51993	2.09025	0.4231	8.61675
25	log target dose	1.30943	0.09867	1.1160	1.50282
25	target dose	3.70405	0.36549	3.0527	4.49436

Figure 15.7   Parameter estimation after the last patient using ADPT software.

Table 15.4   Dose allocation scheme using ATDPH1.

Patient	Dose	Toxicity	Patient	Dose	Toxicity
1	1	0	14	3	0
2	2	0	15	3	0
3	3	0	16	3	0
4	4	0	17	3	0
5	5	0	18	3	0
6	6	0	19	End	—
7	6	1	20	—	—
8	6	1	21	—	—
9	5	1	22	—	—
10	5	1	23	—	—
11	4	0	24	—	—
12	4	1	25	—	—
13	4	1			

Main options: Calculation of the statistical quantities of a phase I dose-finding clinical trial.

Location: Division of Biometrics, University of Medicine and Dentistry of New Jersey, School of Public Health, New Brunswick, New Jersey, USA (http://www2. umdnj.edu/~linyo/).

15.3.5   EWOC: escalation with overdose control

Method: Compute the phase I method escalation with overdose control [20, 21].

Description: This is a Win32 executable program.

Main options: Conduct and analyze a phase I dose-finding clinical trial.

Location: Fox Chase Cancer Center, Department of Biostatistics, Cheltenham, Philadelphia, Pennsylvania, USA (http://www.fccc.edu/users/rogatko/ewoc.html).

Example: Conduction and analysis of a phase I clinical trial. The chosen inputs are detailed in Figure 15.8. Table 15.5 represents the dose level attributed to each patient and the patient's response (1 = toxicity and 0 = no toxicity). The fourth dose level (the dose level associated with the MTD) was assigned for 20 out of 25 patients included in the trial. After the inclusion of each cohort is estimated the marginal posterior density for all dose levels (Figure 15.9) and the estimated dose level associated with the MTD are found (Figure 15.10). After the inclusion of 25 patients the estimated MTD is the fourth dose level (95 % credibility interval: 3.42–5.71).

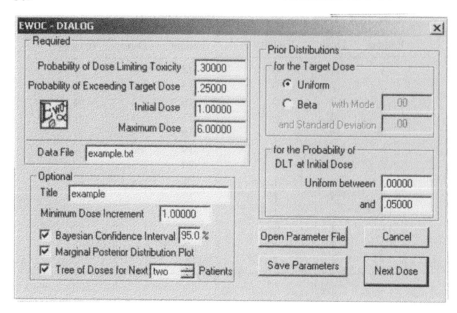

Figure 15.8   Input window using EWOC.

15.4   Phase I/II dose-finding software

15.4.1   EFFTOX2

Method: Phase I/II Bayesian dose-finding satisfying both safety and efficacy requirements [22].

Table 15.5   Dose allocation scheme using EWOC.

Patient	Dose	Toxicity	Patient	Dose	Toxicity
1	1	0	14	4	0
2	2	0	15	4	0
3	3	0	16	4	0
4	3	0	17	4	0
5	4	0	18	4	0
6	4	0	19	4	1
7	4	0	20	4	0
8	4	0	21	4	0
9	5	1	22	4	1
10	4	1	23	4	0
11	4	0	24	4	0
12	4	1	25	4	0
13	4	1			

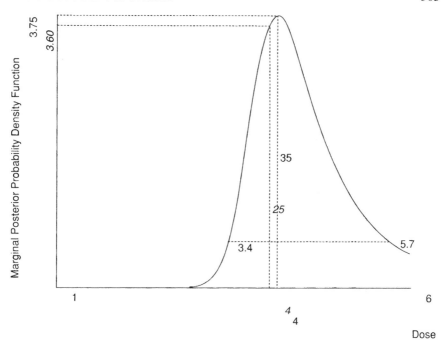

Figure 15.9 Graphic window representing the estimated posterior, the marginal posterior distribution after the inclusion of 25 patients, with EWOC software.

Description: This is a Win32 executable program.

Main options: Simulate and conduct phase I/II dose-finding clinical trials.

Location: M.D. Anderson Cancer Center, Biostatistics Department, University of Texas, Houston, Texas, USA (http://biostatistics.mdanderson.org/SoftwareDownload/).

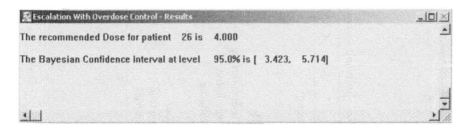

Figure 15.10 Estimated MTD after the inclusion of the last patient, i.e. the dose level recommended for the 'hypothetical' 26th patient using EWOC software.

Table 15.6 Software summary.

	CRM	CRM simulator	CRMp_Pha	BPCT	TITE CRM	ADEPT	ATDPH1	PMTD	EWOC	EFFTOX2
Dose-finding										
Phase I	+	+	+	+	+	+	+	+	+	−
Phase II	−	−	−	+	−	−	−	−	−	−
Phase I/II	−	−	−	−	−	−	−	−	−	+
Graphic user interface	−	+	+	+	−	+	−	−	+	+
Win32 executable	+	+	+	+	−	−	−	+	+	+
Script or macro	−	−	−	−	+	+	+	+	−	−
Options										
Simulations	+	+	+	+	−	+	−	−	+	+
Conduct a trial	+	−	+	+	+	+	+	−	+	−
Analyse a trial	+	−	+	+	+	+	+	−	+	−

15.5 Conclusions

This chapter provided some useful links and material for statisticians and researchers who wish to plan and conduct their own dose-finding trials. This description is not exhaustive but gives an enter point into the subject. However, most well-known and published methods are presented in this software description. The principal characteristics are discussed and summarized in Table 15.6. Finally, if all website addresses were correct at the time this chapter was written, the author does not take the responsibility for any changed in these locations.

References

1. J. O'Quigley, M. Pepe and L. Fisher (1990) Continual reassessment method: a practical design for phase I clinical trials in cancer. *Biometrics*, **46**(1), 33–48.
2. E.L. Korn, D. Midthune, T.T. Chen, L.V. Rubinstein, M.C. Christian and R.M. Simon (1994) A comparison of two phase I trial designs. *Statistics in Medicine*, **13**(18), 1799–806.
3. S.N. Goodman, M.L. Zahurak and S. Piantadosi (1995) Some practical improvements in the continual reassessment method for phase I studies. *Statistics in Medicine*, **14**(11), 1149-61.
4. J. O'Quigley and L.Z. Shen (1996) Continual reassessment method: a likelihood approach. *Biometrics*, **52**(2), 673–84.
5. Y.K. Cheung and R. Chappell (2000) Sequential designs for phase I clinical trials with late-onset toxicities. *Biometrics*, **56**(4), 1177–82.
6. B.E. Storer (2001) An evaluation of phase I clinical trial designs in the continuous dose-response setting, *Stat. Med.*, **20**, 2399–2408.
7. M. Gasparini and J. Eisele (2000) A curve-free method for phase I clinical trials. *Biometrics*, **56**(2), 609–15.
8. S. Zohar and S. Chevret (2001) The continual reassessment method: comparison of Bayesian stopping rules for dose-ranging studies. *Statistics in Medicine*, **20**(19), 2827–43.
9. E. Fabre, S. Chevret, J.F. Piechaud, E. Rey, F. Vauzelle-Kervoedan, P. D'Athis, G. Olive and G. Pons (1998) An approach for dose finding of drugs in infants: sedation by midazolam studied using the continual reassessment method. *Br. J. Clin. Pharmacology*, **46**(4), 395–401.
10. T.B. Dougherty, V.H. Porche and P.F. Thall (2000) Maximum tolerated dose of nalmefene in patients receiving epidural fentanyl and dilute bupivacaine for postoperative analgesia. *Anesthesiology*, **92**(4), 1010–16.
11. S. Piantadosi, J.D. Fisher and S. Grossman (1998) Practical implementation of a modified continual reassessment method for dose-finding trials. *Cancer Chemotherapy and Pharmacology*, **41**(6), 429–36.
12. S. Zohar, A. Latouche, M. Taconnet and S. Chevret (2003) Software to compute and conduct sequential Bayesian phase I or II dose-ranging clinical trials with stopping rules. *Computational Methods, Programs in Biomedicine*, **72**(2), 117–25.
13. S. Chevret (1993) The continual reassessment method in cancer phase I clinical trials: a simulation study. *Statistics in Medicine*, **12**, 1093–8.
14. J. Whitehead and H. Brunier (1995) Bayesian decision procedures for dose determining experiments. *Statistics in Medicine*, **14**(9–10), 885–93; discussion, 895–9.

15. J. Whitehead and D. Williamson (1998) Bayesian decision procedures based on logistic regression models for dose-finding studies. *J. Biopharmaceutical Statistics*, **8**(3), 445–67.
16. Y. Zhou and J. Whitehead (2003) Practical implementation of Bayesian dose-escalation procedures. *Drug Information J.*, **37**(1), 45–59.
17. Y. Zhou and J. Whitehead (2002) *Bayesian ADEPT: Operating Manual*, The University of Reading, Reading.
18. R. Simon, B. Freidlin, L. Rubinstein, S.G. Arbuck, J. Collins and M.C. Christian (1997) Accelerated titration designs for phase I clinical trials in oncology. *J. Natl Cancer Inst.*, **89**(15), 1138–47.
19. Y. Lin and W.J. Shih (2001) Statistical properties of the traditional algorithm-based designs for phase I cancer clinical trials. *Biostatistics*, **2**(2), 203–15.
20. J. Babb, A. Rogatko and S. Zacks (1998) Cancer phase I clinical trials: efficient dose escalation with overdose control. *Statistics in Medicine*, **17**(10), 1103–20.
21. S. Zacks, A. Rogatko and J. Babb (1998) Optimal Bayesian-feasible dose escalation for cancer phase I trials, *Statistics and Probability Letters*, **38**, 215–20.
22. P.F. Thall and D.C. Cook (2005) Dose-finding based on efficacy–toxicity trade-offs. *Biometrics* (to appear).

Appendix: random numbers generation

The random number file was generated with R 2.1:

```
set.seed(33)
runif(25,0,1)
```

Patient number	Random number	Patient number	Random number
1	0.44594048	14	0.34238622
2	0.39465031	15	0.78188794
3	0.48372887	16	0.84324669
4	0.91887596	17	0.77474887
5	0.84388144	18	0.38719298
6	0.51734962	19	0.13576507
7	0.43712500	20	0.90035758
8	0.34319822	21	0.56645266
9	0.01551696	22	0.04273416
10	0.11799116	23	0.48831925
11	0.69098590	24	0.35122322
12	0.26048568	25	0.96966171
13	0.22505121		

If the random number associated with a patient was lower or equal to the true probability of toxicity associated with the given dose level, then the patient observation was a toxicity; otherwise it was not.

Index

Statistical Methods for Dose-Finding Experiments   Edited by S. Chevret
© 2006 John Wiley & Sons, Ltd

STATISTICS IN PRACTICE

Human and Biological Sciences

Berger – Selection Bias and Covariate Imbalances in Randomized Clinical Trials
Brown and Prescott – Applied Mixed Models in Medicine, Second Edition
Chevret (Ed) – Statistical Methods for Dose-Finding Experiments
Ellenberg, Fleming and DeMets – Data Monitoring Committees in Clinical Trials:
    A Practical Perspective
Lawson, Browne and Vidal Rodeiro – Disease Mapping with WinBUGS and
    MLwiN
Lui – Statistical Estimation of Epidemiological Risk
*Marubini and Valsecchi – Analysing Survival Data from Clinical Trials and
    Observation Studies
Parmigiani – Modeling in Medical Decision Making: A Bayesian Approach
Senn – Cross-over Trials in Clinical Research, Second Edition
Senn – Statistical Issues in Drug Development
Spiegelhalter, Abrams and Myles – Bayesian Approaches to Clinical Trials and
    Health-Care Evaluation
Whitehead – Design and Analysis of Sequential Clinical Trials, Revised
    Second Edition
Whitehead – Meta-Analysis of Controlled Clinical Trials

Earth and Environmental Sciences

Buck, Cavanagh and Litton – Bayesian Approach to Interpreting Archaeological
    Data
Glasbey and Horgan – Image Analysis in the Biological Sciences
Helsel – Nondetects and Data Analysis: Statistics for Censored Environmental Data
McBride – Using Statistical Methods for Water Quality Management
Webster and Oliver – Geostatistics for Environmental Scientists

Industry, Commerce and Finance

Aitken and Taroni – Statistics and the Evaluation of Evidence for Forensic Scientists,
    Second Edition
Balding – Weight-of-evidence for Forensic DNA Profiles
Lehtonen and Pahkinen – Practical Methods for Design and Analysis of Complex
    Surveys, Second Edition
Ohser and Mücklich – Statistical Analysis of Microstructures in Materials Science
Taroni, Aitken, Garbolino and Biedermann – Bayesian Networks and Probabilistic
    Inference in Forensic Science

*Now available in paperback

Printed and bound by CPI Group (UK) Ltd, Croydon, CR0 4YY

16/04/2025